Artists of Health

Conversations and Photography
with Practitioners,
Teachers and Innovators of
Natural Health.

Artists of Health

Copyright © 2014 by Tash Mitch

Published by

Chi Evolutionary Publishing

First Printing, 2014

ISBN-10 : 1496107411

Contact: tash@tashmitch.com
Web: www.tashmitch.com

Acknowledgements

To every person who has supported the Artists of Health project, a huge thank you. Your energy and encouragement have been instrumental in creating this book.

To each of the Artists, you have been a huge source of inspiration for me in my work and life, thank you. It is a great pleasure to now extend the inspiration within Artists of Health.

A very special thank you to my partner and best friend, Chris Kain; you have been my sounding board through it all.

To the Artists of Health principle photographer Karyn Schafer Campbell, who has blessed this book with her amazing talent, creativity and vision, I could not have done this without you.

To Artists of Health book designer, Ahad Sheikh, whose patience, diligence and artistic eye has brought my vision to life.

To Wanda Brown and Etty Payne, your help in proofing and editing has been much appreciated.

To my mum, Carol Vasquez, who has been my dearest friend, soul sister and laughing partner.

To Pedro Vasquez, who always brings the salsa and latino vibes.

To Carol Adams and Charade Ibbotson, thanks for being in my life.

To all my Theta Healing Sisters from Intuitive Anatomy, thank you.

For additional free resources to enhance your health
and well being please go to

www.artistsofhealth.com

and sign up with your name and email address.

Body

Massage

Nutrition

Movement Therapy

Osteopathy

Physiotherapy

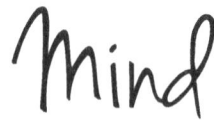

Mind

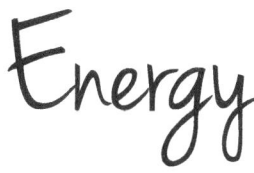

Energy

Yoga

Energy Work

Sound Therapy

Acupuncture

About the Author, Tash Mitch

Tash studied business and finance in university and started her career in media advertising, first for BBC Worldwide magazines and then as a freelancer for Music Week magazine. Her step into the world of complementary therapy took place in 2001 with a Reiki course, which then progressed to a qualification in massage. Seeing how beneficial natural health therapies could be she expanded her knowledge in a broad range of mind, body and energy subjects. Her passion has seen her travelling to Thailand, India and Peru to expand her understanding in the field. She now practises as a well-being coach and teacher with an integrative approach to mind, body and energy work.

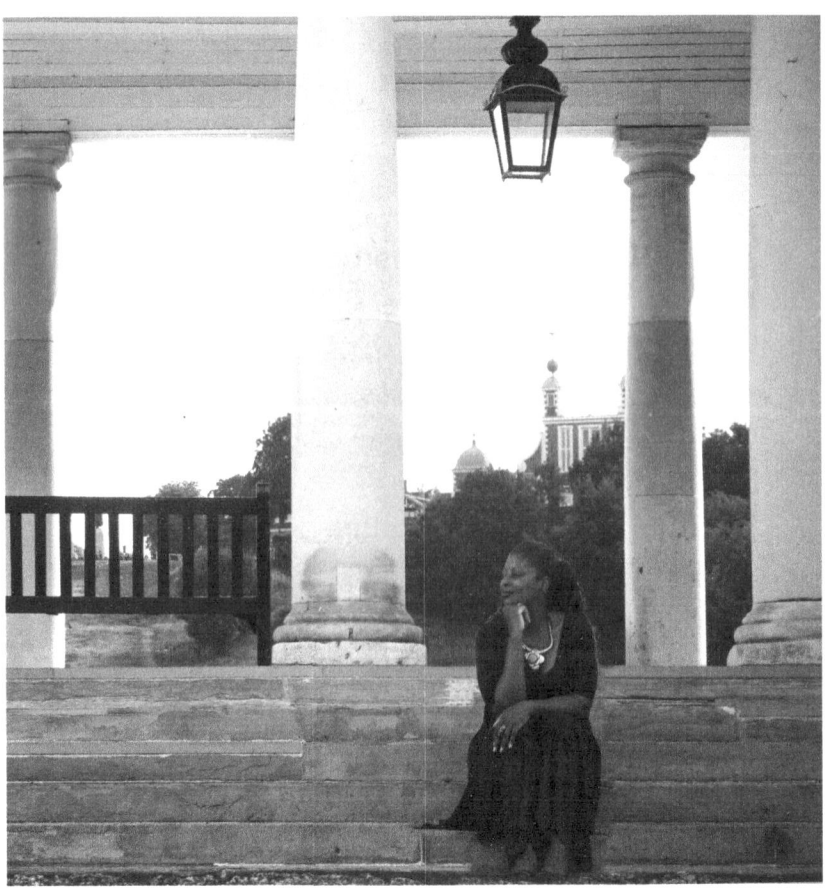

Introduction

When we find the subject of our true passion and we place the energy of our heart and soul into it, the results are always recognisable. We leave a trail in our wake of people, events, happenings and time frames where we have made an impact, a difference, a change and a contribution. This, in my humble opinion, is the stuff of true artistry. By allowing our creativity to flow unhindered we form the tapestries, colours, richness and textures that make up our everyday lives. It leads us to be inspired and is an inspiration.

So, how does health relate to art? I have never really been able to take the mystery and miracle, that is our day-to-day lives, for granted. Because of this, life to me has always been a journey of adventure and discovery. I have found that if we are willing to be opened to the creative flow in our lives, then all our great adventures will eventually lead us to the most amazing journey of all, a journey into ourselves. For me it prompted the question of, 'How do we do this thing called life, with a spring in our step, a smile on our face and the grace of a dancer?' In other words, how do we create health so that we can feel our very best and operate at our optimum? Who better to answer this question than the people who have made the creation of health their art form?

So Artists of Health was born and with it a new journey. This project has led to stimulating, thought-provoking and inspirational conversations with some of the UK's most pioneering and imaginative explorers in the area of complementary therapy. Each person brings a view on how they see their particular area of expertise and what they feel it offers to the healing process and the creation of health.

Along the way I was lucky to meet the lovely Karyn Schafer Campbell, a photographer with a strong vision, who automatically grasped the convergence of Art and Health. She has brought form and amazing visuals to a number of the conversation pieces, bringing each character to life with colour and flair. Additionally, Ahad Sheikh, a very talented graphic designer took the very exact vision I had in my mind for Artists of Health and brought it to life in the form that you will experience in the pages ahead.

Body

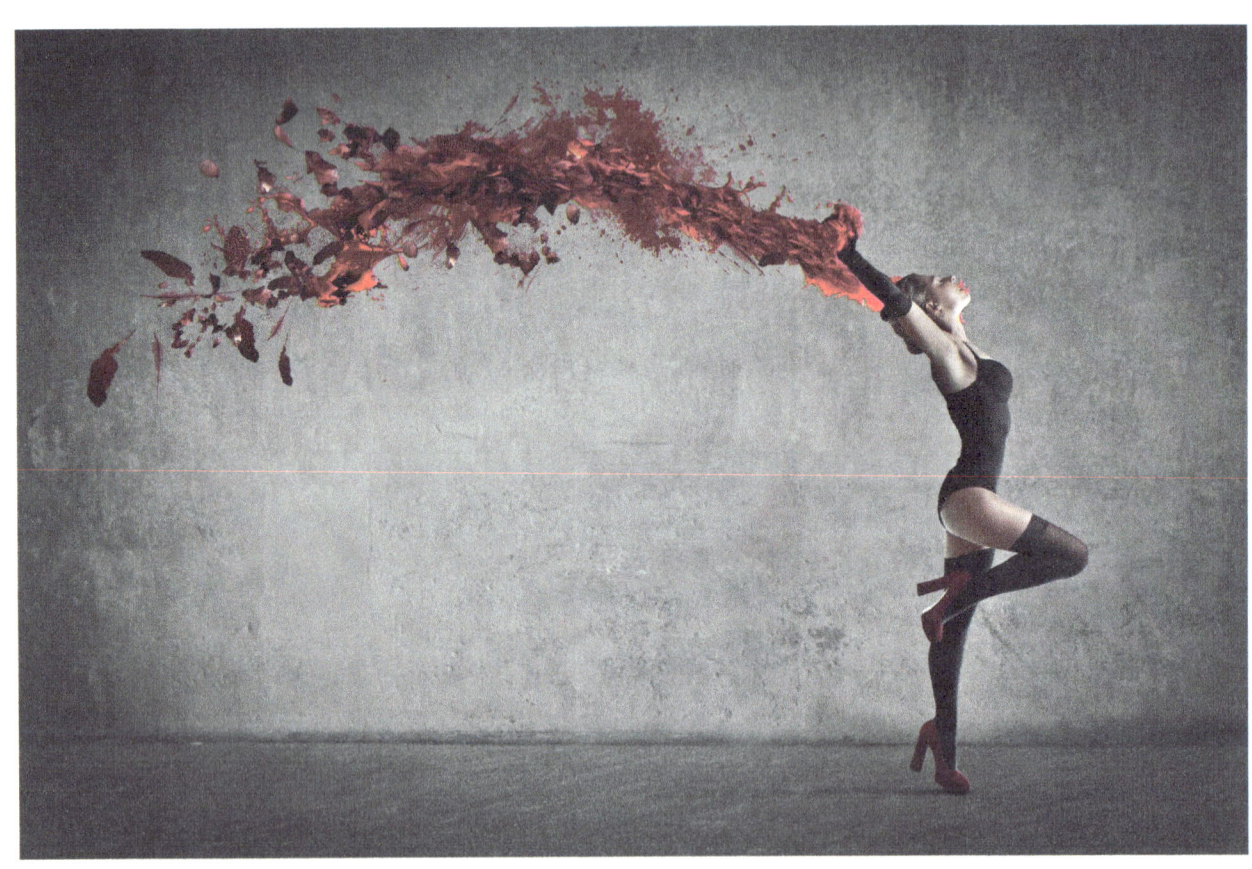

Treatments

Massage

Nutrition

Movement Therapy

Osteopathy

Physiotherapy

"Touch is the most fundamental way of communicating with another human being. It is so powerful that it goes beyond any stories, backgrounds, differences or language barriers."

- Beata Aleksandrowicz

Massage

The benefits of massage as a way to harmonise the body has been understood since the very start of human civilisation. The focus of massage is to work with soft tissue, which includes the muscles, skin, blood, tendons and ligaments. The massage therapist uses a number of techniques, including rubbing, kneading, acupressure and stroking motions to effect change. In our daily use of the body we tend to contract certain muscles to perform specific actions. Likewise, we will hold particular postural positions in walking, running, sitting and standing. Stress and tension is translated by the nervous system as misalignment and it responds with feelings of pain, aches and emotional stress. Massage is very effective at redressing the balance.

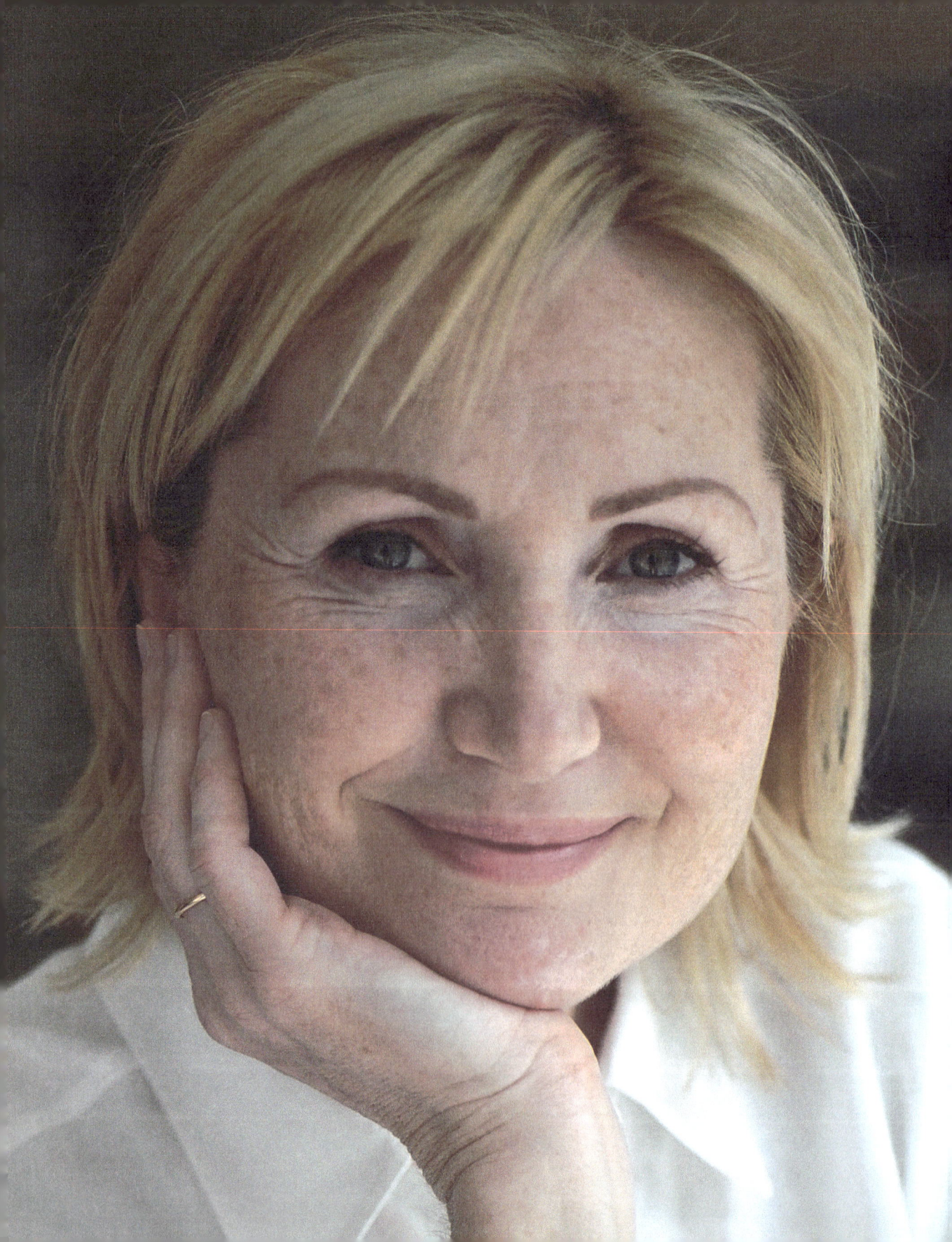

Beata Aleksandrowicz
Director at Pure Massage and Author

Beata Aleksandrowicz is a giant in the field of Massage and Touch Therapy. Her passion for the subject is palpable and infectious. She has a love for the ancient wisdom of the Kalahari Bushmen in Africa and the time she has spent with them has informed every aspect of her expression as a therapist. She has managed to build her practice from being a mobile therapist, to now having Pure Massage operating from three very prominent locations in London. On meeting her you get the sense that when it comes to her work, the sky is the limit.

My company, Pure Massage, is dedicated to massage and human touch. Our mission statement is, 'There is nothing compared to human touch', and this has been present since we opened in 2002. This is because when I had the chance to experience what touch could be, when it is intentionally based on love and gratitude, it made a huge difference in my life. With this understanding came the realisation that when I put my hands on people there was an energy shift within me, as well as the person receiving the treatment.

I did not have the level of understanding when I first started my practice in 1997 to really interpret the depth of my work. I simply knew that people felt better as a result of my treatment, which encouraged me to continue as a massage therapist. When I first started out there was not the same level of acceptance as there is today and people would give you a sceptical look when you said you did massage. I found it a challenge, but I like challenges and I was determined to change people's perceptions about what massage is.

Building my Practice

When I first qualified as a therapist I could not find a place to work that fully allowed me to express my fascination with massage. So I decided to become a mobile massage therapist. I got myself a good table for £700, which was very expensive at the time, but I knew I needed a good table in order to grow as a therapist. The table I found was beautiful, the Rolls Royce of massage tables. It was very stylish, light at seven kg, and made with incredibly strong aluminium. I travelled for years with it on the underground, taking my work to people's homes.

Once I had gained experience I decided to open my own place with my partner Jean-Marc Delacourt, who, among his many talents, has a strong love for designing. We were clear from the beginning that we wanted a place that was solely dedicated to massage. It took two years to find a location, but because of the name 'Pure Massage' no one wanted to work with us. We saw fourteen places in two years and finally we found our first shop in Fulham and opened it successfully. Since then we have developed other places in Bond Street and Surrey.

My Love of This Work

The aspect of massage that really hooked me in was the touch element. Touch is the most fundamental way of communicating with another human being. It is so powerful it goes beyond any stories, backgrounds, differences or language barriers. If, as a therapist, you approach each treatment from the mindset that 'we are all one', then touch gives you the possibility to really experience this paradigm, and the person with whom you are working automatically feels it.

This deeper awareness of touch finally clicked into place when I went to Africa and worked with the Kalahari Bushmen. In my life I have always had enough trust to follow my own intuition. Although at times it has left me feeling lonely and questioning my decisions, it has always worked with providing the best benefits for my clients. Usually my intuition would provide me with valuable information and then lead to a period of experimenting and searching. Each time confirmation and validation would come through intellectually sound resources, letting me know that I was going in the right direction.

Meeting the Bushmen was a real breakthrough in understanding how powerful a connection touch can offer to another person. If massage is only limited to dealing with the physicality of the body, something very precious and unique is missed. Working with this extraordinary tribe, who generously shared with me their very old and powerful traditions, took me to a different level of approaching another person. I got presented with how deep and profound my work could be. It allowed me to see that I can transform a simple back or body massage into an experience that might help my clients to rediscover their essence and themselves.

Professionalism

When you embody the paradigm 'we are all one' in your work with others, you do not need to use words or a narrative to describe this connection. However, you do need to have tools, which can allow you to create the experience. As a therapist your tools are your structure, your knowledge, your professionalism, your awareness, your clarity, your communication and your responsibility. These are all the elements you use to build your work.

In my work it is important to ask questions of myself and constantly look at ways in which I can expand my understanding of what I do. This is important because you never step into the same river twice. To stop asking questions as a practitioner would mean that you know everything. When you start to believe you know everything, it means that you stop listening, you lose your awareness and slowly it all becomes about you, until one day you are not in service anymore.

In any type of service work, with age and experience, there should be a turning point, a moment of maturity and realisation that, if you really want to make a difference, you need to give up the 'me'. You have to have the concept that what you are doing is bigger than yourself. This is such a ceaseless kind of work, especially if you are willing to go deep into the human being.

Influences

Some of my main influences as a therapist have been James Jealous, an osteopath from America, whose CD workshops are an ongoing source of stimulus for me, Alexander Lowen with his concepts surrounding the spirituality of the body, healers from the Kalahari Desert and, of course, life itself! It is important to let life give you experience because all your breakdowns and breakthroughs are a source of knowledge and wisdom, which helps you so much in your connection with your clients.

It is really a pity that generally, when massage therapists reach an understanding of life's greatest wisdoms, they are often burnt out. This is because they were not taught how to develop with synergy. They give everything they have without taking care of themselves both physically and emotionally.

This was the main reason why we opened the school at Pure Massage, to show people that you can work to a late age and avoid being drained. You can have an unlimited source of inspiration from doing this work. It is possible to have a body that is in very good shape, it is possible to not injure yourself and it is possible not to burn out.

Creative inspirations

I sang a lot in the past and then I stopped as other things took over. In 2009 I returned to singing again. I have a huge love of jazz music and love Ástor Piazzolla, an Argentinean composer who specialised in Tango. His music is unbelievably beautiful and I always wanted to sing to it. I performed fourteen of his instrumental tracks and wrote the words myself in Polish and English. This felt very much like it was a completion of my past somehow.

I think I am very lucky to meet some very remarkable and amazing people. They just come into my life and inspire me so very much with their presence. For example, when I worked on my singing, I was coached by an amazing teacher Kevin Leo, who became my dear friend. His love of music and his passion was so powerful that it had an impact on every aspect of my life. Then a pianist, Rick, came along and we spent six months working together and discovered amazing things with Piazzolla. I could feel his enjoyment and dedication for this project. We would play for six or seven hours at a time non-stop on some days, it was beautiful. Over time other musicians joined us, everyone was just happy to be there and be a part of the creative process.

The Future

The future road ahead seems fascinating to me. I am learning every day. I study, I read and I am organising trips to Mongolia as part of my Touch of Trust charity project. I hope to finish my third book at the beginning of next year and I want to develop my school and teach people who want to be massage therapists and those that already are, how to do their work with greatness, so both themselves and their clients can benefit.

All our actions and decisions have an impact on others. Thoughts and words create reality. The good work that you do affects your environment. At Pure Massage we have excellent therapists who work with the highest integrity possible. We provide very good treatments and are recognised for that. Our place emanates with something good, so I want to believe that by doing our work we are creating positive change in the world around us. Somebody once said to me that the work you do is the visible side of your love. This is such a beautiful saying and certainly very true for me.

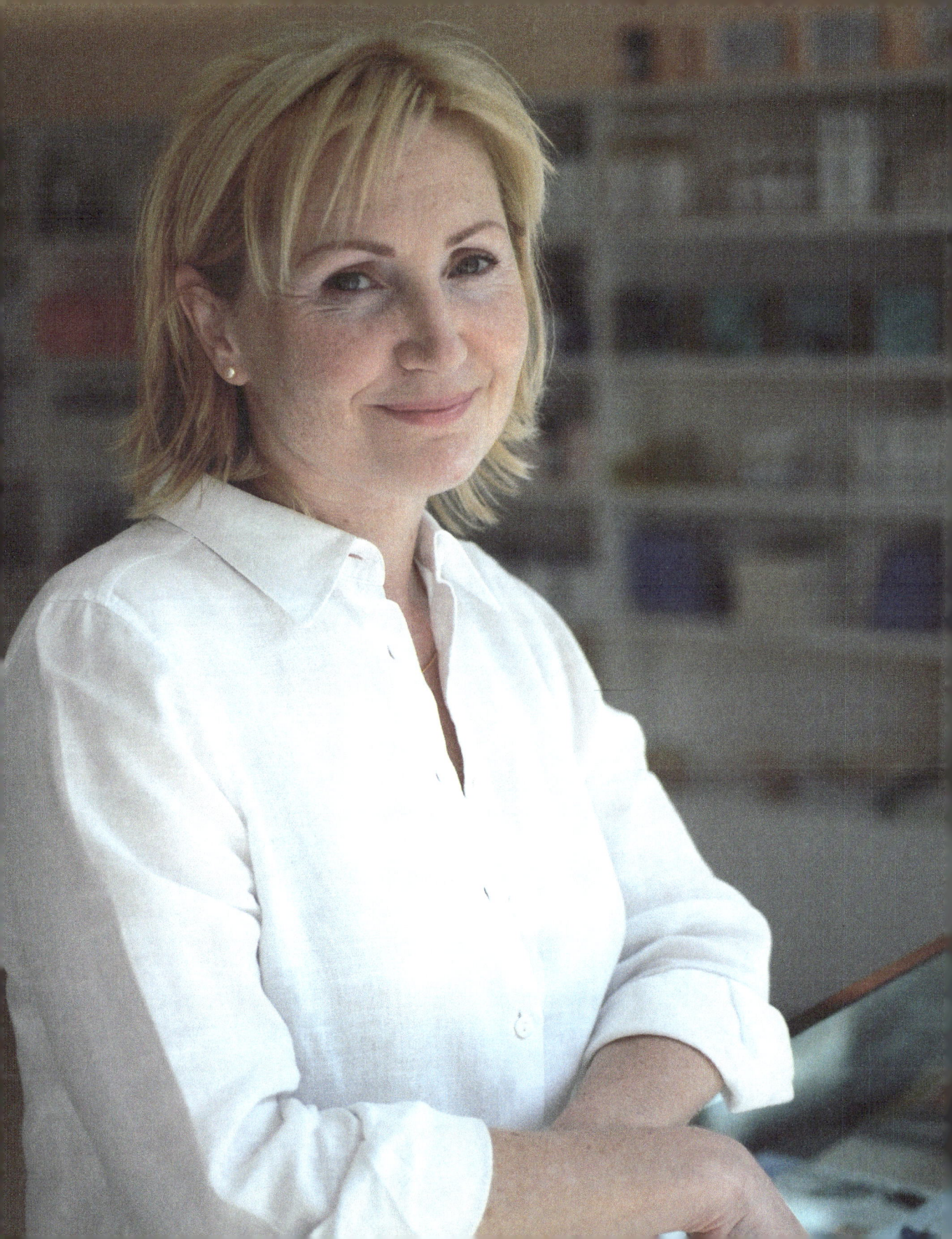

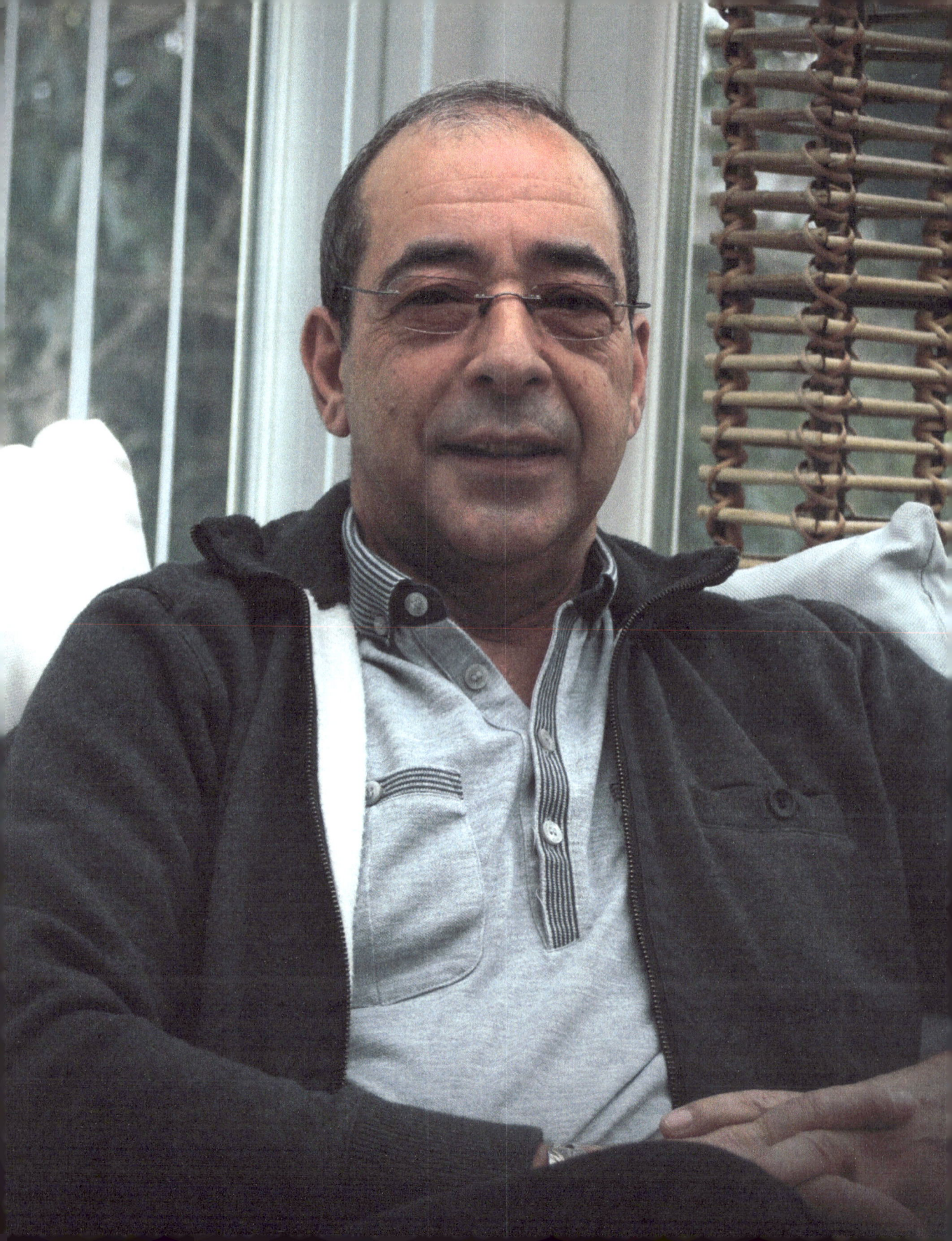

Mel Cash
Author and Director of London School of Sports Massage

For anyone embarking on the journey into remedial therapy and sports massage within the UK, Mel Cash's books on the subject are essential reading. On meeting him you immediately get a sense of why he has made such an impact on the industry. He was an avid sportsman and, with the discovery of massage, he had found a way to enhance his sporting performance and aid his injury recovery time. He was able to do this by working with the muscles and skeletal structure on a deeper level, and has been a massive forerunner in shifting the UK's perceptions surrounding massage.

I was into marathons and triathlons and I was a pretty good club athlete in my 30s. One mid-winter evening I had just finished a fourteen-mile run, I got home and was having something to eat when I began reading a magazine article about massage. It was written by an osteopath who was into sport and at the end there was a snip, about five sentences long, on how to massage your own leg. So I got some salad oil out of the cupboard and massaged my left leg, just using basic strokes. Before doing my right leg, I got up to go to the bathroom and it was walking through the corridor of my flat that changed my life.

I could not believe what a difference that simple massage made. I did the other leg and got in the shower. Up until then I was unhappy with my work and had no idea where I was headed career wise. As I took my shower I thought about all the guys I trained with and how they should have access to massage. I remember thinking about ordinary people with backaches and shoulder aches, I was sure that it would be good for them. So my whole idea of remedial massage came together that night in 1984.

When it came to remedial massage at the start of my journey in 1984, there was nothing at all available. In those days the only place that massage seemed to exist was in the sex industry. I found the only decent massage course I could; by today's standards it was fairly poor, but it got me started.

One of the guys from my athletics club was going out with someone from the Royal

Ballet and through that link I started treating some of the best ballet dancers in the world. The superficial massage strokes that we were taught on my course were a waste of time, so I really had to start teaching myself. I learned from experience using some pretty classy sports people. I had to completely dumb down my practical knowledge in order to do my massage exam, because I had already gone way beyond what I was being taught.

London School Of Sports Massage

After I qualified, the next stage was to get my work out to the public. I decided to write a book and I managed to get a deal with a publisher. We were talking about the title and thought that 'Sports Massage' sounded like a really good name, which I don't think had ever been used before. My dream then was that sports massage would become synonymous with remedial massage. The first book became a rallying point for some other like-minded therapists and this led to the formation of my school.

I wrote my first book because it needed to be written mainly to improve what was available to massage students at the time. Ten years later I could not believe that no one had written anything better, so I wrote another one. Very recently I published my third book, 'Advanced Remedial Massage and Soft Tissue Therapy', which develops a higher level of clinical ability.

The interesting thing is that I am dyslexic so I never thought I would be able to write a book, much less run a school. I wish my English teacher were still alive to see my books, because he once called me 'stupid' as he thought I couldn't write.

Remedial Massage

There are challenges in presenting the remedial aspects of bodywork, because the general public recognises the word massage. A better title for the work I do would be 'Remedial Soft Tissue Therapy'. But the general public may not understand that yet, so we tend to call ourselves Remedial Massage Therapists. Remedial Therapy is far more than just massage and involves the assessment of injury, the treatment within soft tissue context and advice on rehabilitation.

I am very passionate about how working with the fascial system can create positive changes in the body. The reason for success using massage treatment can only be explained if you look at the fascia. When we begin learning about massage we have to study individual muscles because we need bite-size chunks of knowledge.

If we were confronted by the body's complexity all at once, it would just blow us away. But muscles are all, in fact, part of a single fascial system and far more interconnected than we realise.

The thing that gives the fascia its main substance is collagen and elastin. Collagen firms an area up and elastin allows for flexibility. As the body evolves, the arrangement of collagen and elastin begins to structure it. To give an example, my favourite animal is the giraffe. Can you imagine the amount of strength it would take a giraffe to hold its head up? Over the years it has evolved and instead of using the muscle strength it has used collagen. This means that when it puts its head down to take a drink it uses muscles to perform the action, but the neck just springs back up again afterward to normal position. The fascial system forms collagen when we need tension and elastin when we need support.

In essence, the body builds systems of tension areas to support the movements and actions we do every day. On the other hand if you don't move a certain part of your body, over time the fascia starts to stick together. This is why in the morning you need to have a good stretch, which melts the stickiness that forms between the fascia layers. It also explains why some people wake up feeling very inflexible until they begin moving around. If there is a part of your body that you keep in a shortened position, the fascia eventually over time remodels that area and holds it into a position.

The human body is an incredibly versatile machine but it does not like anything for eight plus hours a day, five plus days a week. It does not matter how expensive your office chair is or how many devices you have, if you do something all day every day, your body is going to be upset. We need variety.

How Remedial Massage Works

In order to come up with a remedy for a muscular soft tissue problem it is a three-way split. The therapist needs to work on the fascia to melt the collagen and elastin deposits. The person having the treatment would have to address the positioning that is causing the issue in the first place and functional exercises will have to be given in order to create a lasting change. If one of those is missing then your ability to effect long-term change is going to be reduced. It does not matter how much treatment a person has, if they do not do the remedial exercises and address their postural issues, it is not going to work. In addition, if you just give remedial exercises and postural advice without the soft tissue work, the fascia will pull them back out, so you have to do both. In other words, it is about retraining and remodelling the body, in order to create lasting alignment or balance. This is the area that really excites me!

The Future

My quest in life is to get my students to a point where they are operating as real therapists. I have always had a dream of establishing a recognised form of therapy, which had the same respect as physiotherapy or osteopathy and went way beyond basic massage. Students should be taught how to operate in a clinical context. In training, emphasis should be put on assessment, treatment and rehabilitation. At present the London School of Sports Massage is in the process of establishing a Remedial Massage Therapy course that will have national occupational standards, a core curriculum and a register for Remedial Massage Therapists.

So there is a lot planned for the future. My love of remedial therapy means I am always exploring new ground. In over twenty-seven years of doing this work I am still not bored with it, and this says a lot to me. I know I have found exactly what I am meant to be doing in my life.

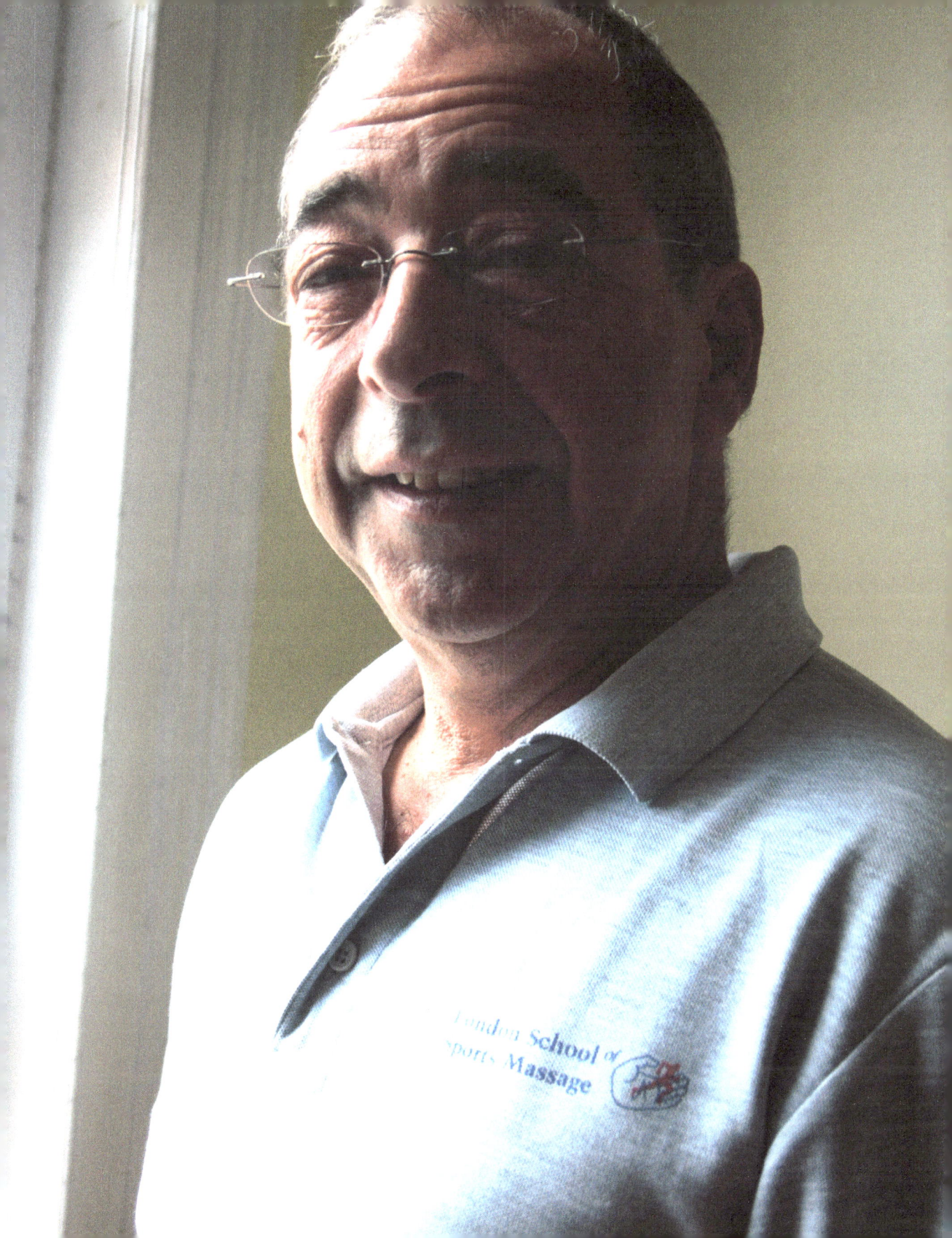

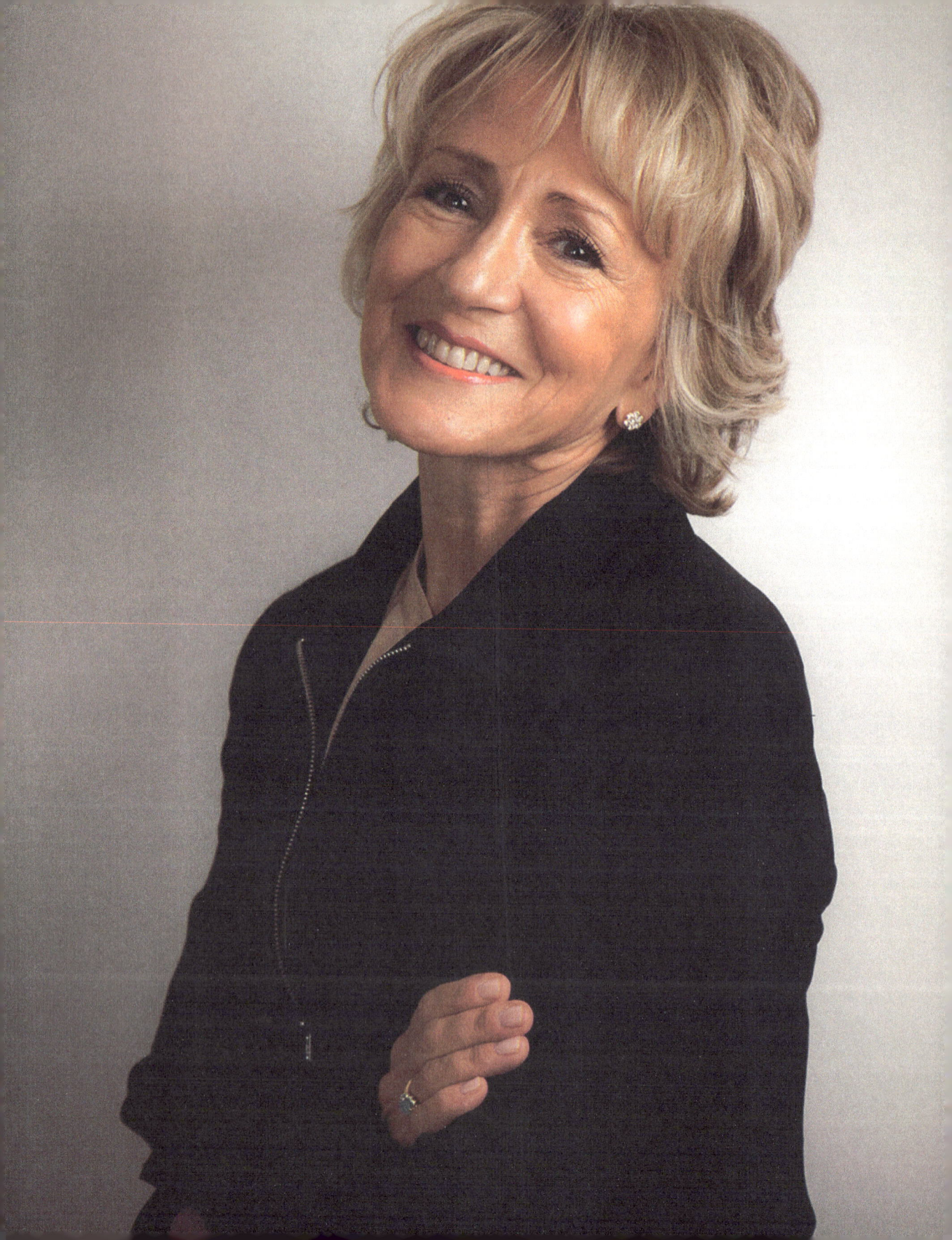

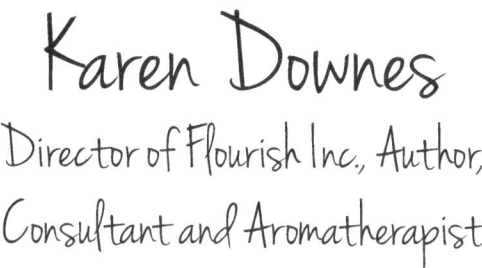

Karen Downes
Director of Flourish Inc., Author,
Consultant and Aromatherapist

Karen has mastered the skill of mixing and blending aromatic essential oils. Her voice, when she speaks of this art, vibrates with both respect and mindfulness. She has a deep awareness of the fact that the oil from a plant represents a gift from the natural world to be cherished and honoured in its use. It is this respect and mindfulness that have been a gift from the natural world to Karen, and the wisdom gained from her work with aromatherapy oils has been used in every aspect of her profession to educate and elevate others.

I was born in a small country town in Australia and grew up on a farm with nature's healing aromas surrounding me. The aromatics of essential oils have always provoked memories and associations with wonderful journeys and adventures, which I found both nurturing and nourishing. From a very young age I would run barefoot in the grass and loved that intimate and immediate connection to nature. Smells have always been evocative and important to the quality of my life.

At the age of twenty-one, I decided to study Beauty Therapy. I had always been very kinaesthetic and loved everything to do with touch, so this seemed the obvious choice, but I soon found that my interests lay in health and well-being. I trained in many mediums including naturopathy and aerobics training as my passion grew.

About six months after qualifying as a beauty therapist, I discovered the Dr Hauschka product range, derived from plants and essential oils. I started to combine these into my treatments with great results and became a devotee of the products, travelling to Germany to train at the Dr Hauschka Institute. That was the start of my journey into aromatherapy. I became aware that the oils worked aesthetically to nourish and rejuvenate the skin and also more deeply to heal us physically and emotionally. During my time in Europe I also studied aromatherapy with Robert Tisserand, which opened a whole new world to me in the effectiveness of essential oils. My clients and my own personal life became the laboratory for testing the applications and effectiveness of essential oils.

In my day-to-day life I discovered I was able to create my own sacred space at any time with the power of the oils. I could use them to create an environment of relaxation, to provoke a connection to my higher self in a spiritual or metaphysical way, or with my daily body rub that would create an aromatic aura around me.

Developing the In Essence Aromatherapy Brand

My sister and I started In Essence together. We had both studied aromatherapy in Europe, along with naturopathy and many other forms of healing. On returning to Australia we saw an opportunity to make aromatherapy available to everyone in all walks of life rather than just through therapeutic practitioners. So, with just $25,000 we put together a concept and product range to go to market. We created the company on a shoestring budget, using our own design and writing skills. We knew that historically women had used herbs within the home for healing and family care. We saw aromatherapy as a pathway for women to be introduced to their inner healer and to actually restore the health of their families and themselves in a very natural way, as essential oils have the potential to be both nurturing and healing.

We created the term 'aromatic dressing' and ran workshops where we encouraged women to be sensual and more connected to themselves and their loved ones. They were taught the therapeutic properties of the oils so they knew how to apply them safely. With a selection of oils we called an 'aromatic wardrobe', we would encourage them to 'dress from the inside out'. We used the wardrobe as a metaphor. Just as they would go to their wardrobe and choose their clothing for the day, they could go to their aromatic wardrobe and choose their essential oils to massage their body with daily. If they were going to a business meeting they could use basil for focus, rosemary for remembrance or lemon to sharpen concentration. By massaging their bodies with those oils they were enveloped by the healing vapour of the oils with which they desired to start their day.

Even though I have now sold the brand and moved into a different arena in my life, I can actually see what In Essence represents and how this is still relevant now, if not more so, because of our demanding lives. I am now working to increasingly raise awareness of how important it is to take care of ourselves first. Nourishing our bodies is so important, the daily massage I do for myself is something I will always benefit from.

Essential oils have a very powerful vibration; they are the final metabolic expression of the plant and a healing gift to us. We are able to take these elements to evoke our emotions, heal our bodies and our minds. When we go out into nature we immediately breathe more deeply and feel healed as a result of our surroundings.. We can actually capture this essence with essential oils and bring it into our city lives to restore and revive us.

Influences

I recently attended a workshop by Sissel Tolass, a German scientist who has made the sense of smell the focus of her work. Her interest lies in what smell actually does to us and how it impacts our lives. She captures the essence of a smell with a little machine that functions almost like a vacuum and picks up aromatic molecules called the headspace of a smell. She then puts the headspace into a jar and analyses its content and impact.

Sissel has taken her work with smells into schools in Mexico and exposed children to the smell of homelessness. Their first reaction was repulsion; however, she kept re-introducing the same aroma over and over again until it was familiar. Once acceptance was gained she was able to reframe the perception of homelessness, from one of repulsion to one of empathy. Through this work the students were able to use their noses as a discerning tool in a way they never could have before.

It is extraordinary what the sense of smell can do; it creates an often unexamined aspect of our world. Our association with aroma influences greatly the things we are either attracted to or repulsed by in the world. By actually training and developing a sense of smell, we become more alert to the world around us. This is one of the most powerful aspects of aromatherapy and, as our ability to smell is one of our main senses, it is a powerful aspect of being human as well.

The Future

Currently, I am creating a consulting business, a series of workshops and eventually a product range called Flourish. This is what I am committed to – people flourishing. Because I have always used my life as a laboratory, the focus for me is women over 45 who are going into menopause and facing dramatic life changes, physically or emotionally. This is the time when children typically leave home and the mothering role changes, or they may have lost a partner or a parent. It is a time to flourish not flounder. To truly flourish, I see there are five essential well-being components – physical, financial, spiritual, relationship and career.

My aim is to support people to be inspired by life, their own life, life around them in their communities, and the natural world, so they can truly reach their full potential and flourish.

I love the fact that the title of this book refers to us as artists. I think all of us have a palette to work with. Life is all about what colours we put onto our palette and what we choose to paint with those colours. My palette has been aromatherapy, I started with a blank canvas, so to speak, and then just asked myself where to begin. From that passion, I found a vehicle to express. I formulated both a company and college that created the richest experiences of my life. For many months I would work seven days a week, but it didn't matter because I was doing what I loved. Malcolm Gladwell wrote the book *Outliers* and in it he studied what it took to be a master of something. He examined people like Bill Gates and the Beatles and discovered that, although it looked like they were an overnight success, it actually took 10,000 hours to be masterful. The time you put in is what creates the quality of the work. I have met and worked with some phenomenal leaders who are passionate about their art. As I listened to their stories the common element in all of them is curiosity. Without curiosity and wonder an explorer won't take the next step. Start with passion and always be curious.

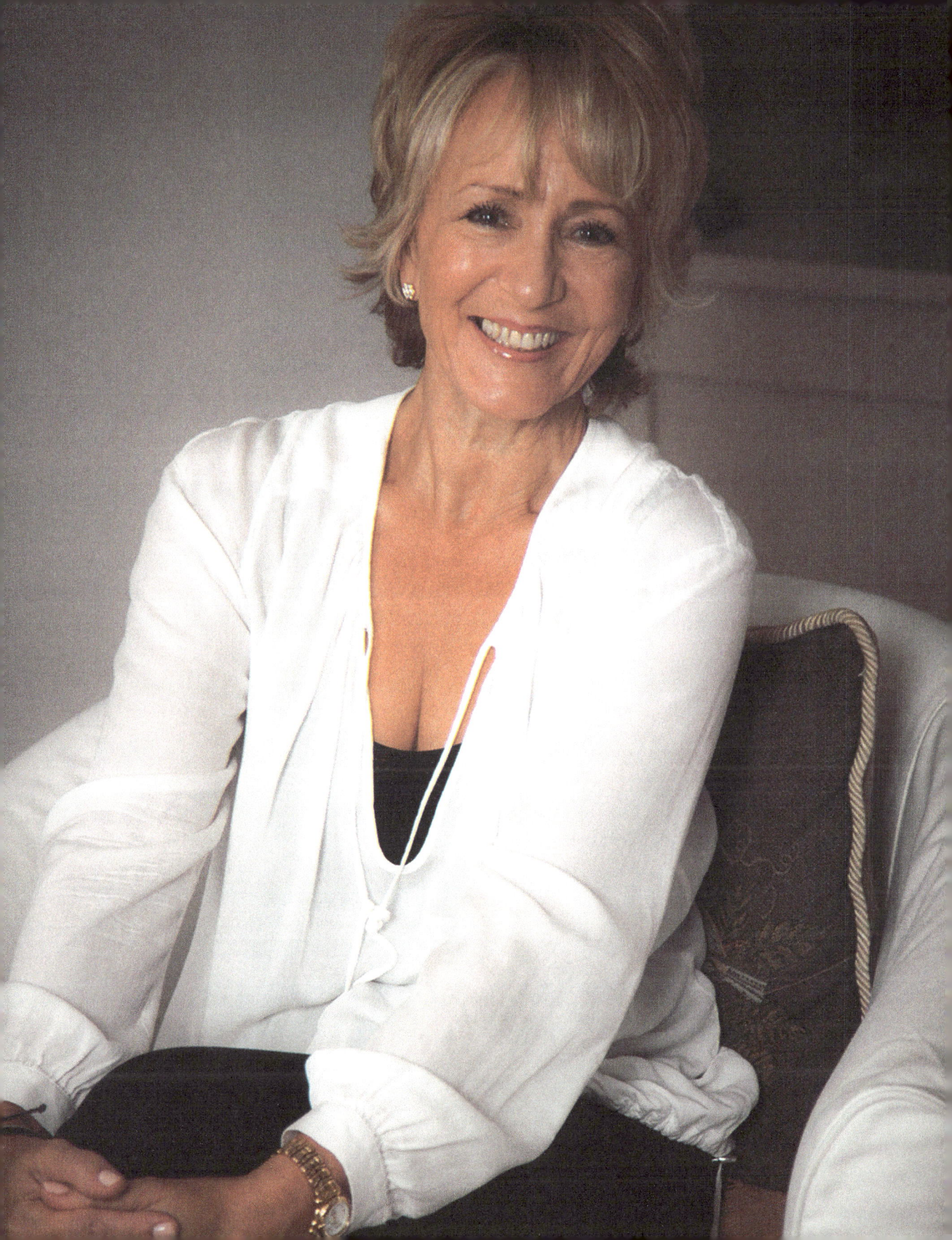

"One thing I did learn quite early on is that in order to make a difference you have to be appealing to people, you have to present information in a way that they can identify with, understand and use."

- Ian Marber

Nutrition

Nutritionists seek to avoid health issues by adopting a healthy and balanced diet. Attention is placed on putting structure to the eating habits, ensuring that the contents of the diet are supportive of health. In some cases nutrition is used on an even deeper level as medicine, designed to restructure the biochemistry of the body. It is clear that a poor diet makes a huge contribution to a number of modern day diseases, such as heart issues, diabetes, osteoporosis and digestive problems. Nutrition is considered a very important part of the equation when it comes to restoring and maintaining health.

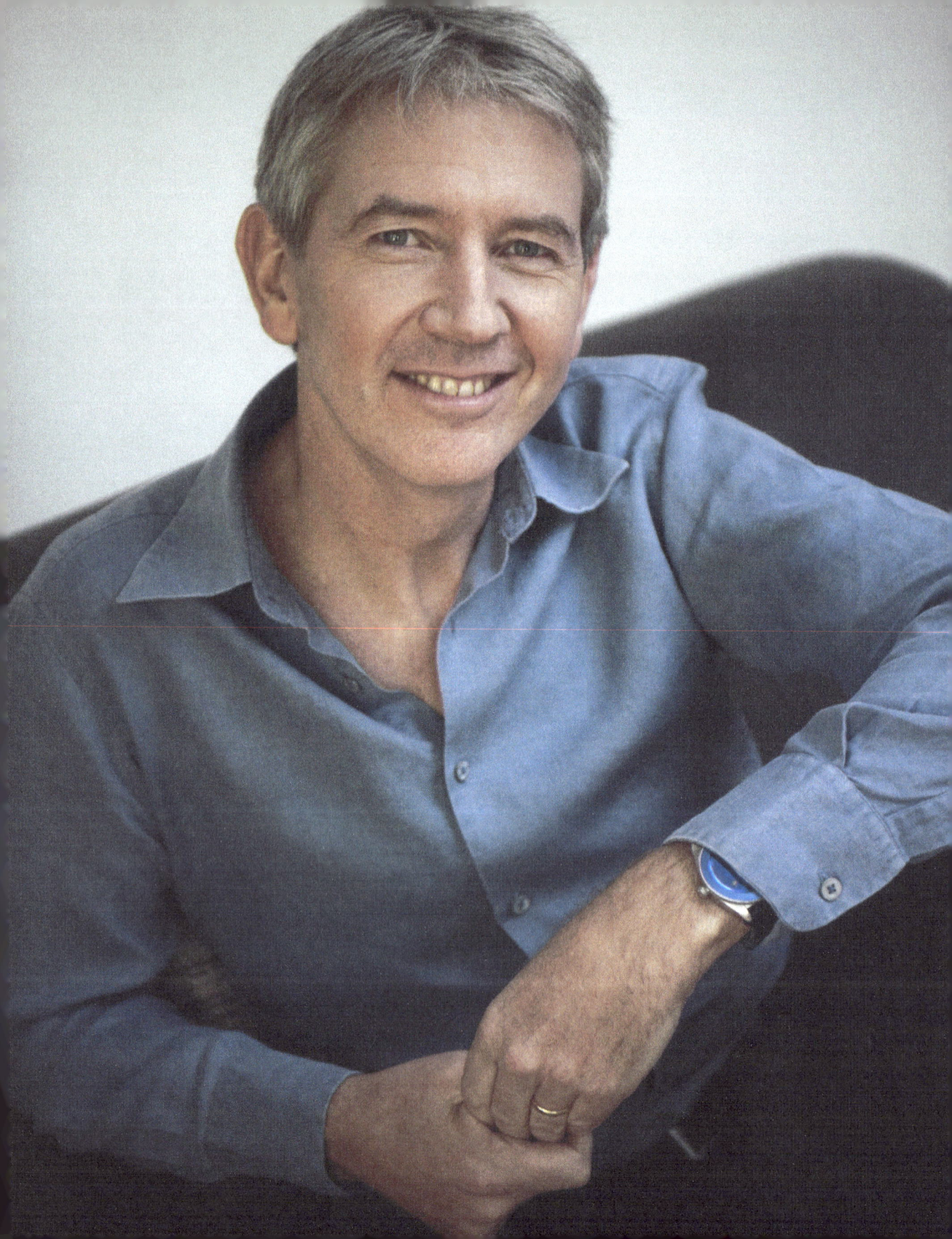

Patrick Holford
Founder of The Institute for Optimum Nutrition, Author and Teacher

Patrick Holford started his career in the field of psychology but came to the realisation that nutrition was a key link in the chain of mental health and well-being. He has become a global pioneer in the nutritional world, studying and presenting cutting edge developments in the use of nutrition to reverse and prevent modern illnesses, such as heart disease, Alzheimer's, obesity and schizophrenia. His goal is to present the scientific facts that nutrients and nutrition are undeniable factors in both our prevention and cure of numerous physical ailments.

I started my career as a psychotherapist and I was very interested in the treatment of schizophrenia. I believed that psychotherapy was the way forward for mental illness at the time, but it wasn't proving to be very effective for schizophrenia. I was not a fan of the medication that was being used because in my opinion it was basically a chemical straitjacket. It may stop people harming themselves, but does not actually cure anything.

Then I came across very good research by a man called Dr Abram Hoffer, who did the first double-blind placebo controlled experiments in psychiatry. He discovered that large doses of vitamins B3, folic acid and vitamin C can help psychosis and restore normal brain function in schizophrenia. I met Dr Hoffer in Canada a few years later and learnt about his approach. I asked him how many people he had treated and he said over 5,000, and his success rate was 85% cure. I asked him what he meant by cure and he said free of symptoms, able to socialise with family and friends and pay income tax. I became his student and started to get really interested in what nutrition actually was, and what the role of vitamins, minerals and essential fats were. My study in this area convinced me that one of the major driving factors behind the patterns of modern western diseases, from cancer to diabetes to heart disease, was nutrition on some level. In 1984, I founded the Institute for Optimum Nutrition in the UK to study the subject.

Nutrition

I spend most of my time talking about nutrition because that's my speciality. But I think that we get sick because we're not living in accordance with our natural design and that includes nutrition, exercise and our state of mind. The fundamental thing to get across is the discovery that quite a large amount of nutrients can restore natural function. What Hoffer and other key people in science discovered is that when you're sick and your biochemistry is out of balance, you need substantially larger amounts of specific nutrients than you could ever eat to bring you back into balance.

I think that, as much as stress can create problems in our physical health, exercise is important. Obviously things like smoking and alcohol can also play a big role. The single biggest driving factor of modern day diseases has been a fundamental shift in our nutrition. But this has not just been caused by a lack of the appropriate nutrients, there is also an excess of anti-nutrients, meaning that we consume a lot of substances that actually destroy nutrients, including refined foods like sugar, alcohol, drugs and medications. So there are two objectives, one is to get optimum nutrition and the right nutrients. The other is to minimise anti-nutrients. They are two sides of the same coin.

We are learning so much. Recently, I've been very involved in promoting a low glycaemic load diet, or a low GL diet. This is all about how to eat to stabilise your blood sugar. Loss of blood sugar control is something that's absolutely rampant in the 21st century because we have much more availability of carbohydrates, sugar, sugar drinks, refined foods, and much less need to exercise. In fact, we can go a year without any exercise and still function. There was a time when this was unheard of because you had to exercise to get food.

You can't just say we should all eat like Stone Age people because we don't live in a Stone Age world. We have to process a lot more information, so there has been a huge increase in psychological stress in the 21st century, compared to the 16th century, and the brain works much harder. The role of essential nutrients for brain function is really important and I think that it is the brain stress of modern living that has led to a very big increase in mental illness from depression and schizophrenia.

Educating the Public on the Importance of Nutrition

Most of my work now is actually teaching the public in whatever way I can through books, seminars, websites and so on. I set up the Institute for Optimum Nutrition in the 80s, which is one of the largest and longest running training centres for nutritional care. I left there in the late 90s because I felt my job was done, but it continues to train people. My focus has been on writing books to get this work out there and I've just finished my 36th. So I've spent the last 14 years really focusing on making this information available to millions of people.

We are badly in need of a revolution in healthcare. The question is, will it come through the medical system or will it be driven by people? I think it has to be driven by people. I think people have to want a different way of treating diseases, so most of my work now is focusing on reaching as many people as possible.

Yes, I think there is a growing awareness among people of the importance of nutrition. But as new people are born and new generations arrive, there's still an incredibly large amount of ignorance. While there is a subset of society who aren't necessarily toeing the line in terms of conventional medicine, there are an awful lot of people who really know very little about nutrition. We're expecting to have over half a billion people in the world with diabetes by 2030 and this is a totally preventable and reversible disease. Incidences of Alzheimer's are set to go through the roof and, again, it's a preventable disease. Corporate food companies are pouring money into India, Africa and China, so we can expect a massive increase in these places of 21st century western diseases, such as diabetes, heart disease and obesity.

So while there is more awareness, health issues globally are getting worse. The World Health Organization has said that people being overweight has become a bigger health issue in the world than undernourishment. For every one million people starving, there are three million people who are obese. This was not so in the 1970s. My work over the last 20-30 years has been about finding solutions, but you can't reverse a disease until you understand it. Diseases are not cured by a life of drugs. If you're not really dealing with underlying causes then you're not going to stop diseases.

A 360 view of Nutrition

All the various elements of our health feed into each other. For example, if someone is feeling stressed or depressed, they might choose to eat sugar or drink alcohol in order to deal with the problem. If this becomes a habit, it depresses the mood even more. So there's a strong link between obesity and depression, for example. The worse you feel, the more sugar or alcohol you consume and your energy gets lower and lower. You have no desire to exercise and the more overweight you are, the harder it is to exercise anyway. So you get really big vicious cycles. But similarly, if you radically improve your nutrition, after only five days your energy will start to go up. If you've got more energy, then you're more inclined to exercise. If you exercise, it it actually helps to improve your mood. You look better and feel happier, so all of these factors, psychological, physical or chemical, all feed into each other.

The Future

Modern diseases are driven not solely, but largely, by sub-optimal nutrition and the science is really streaming in to support that view. So I'm delighted at the way this whole new paradigm has been unravelling. There have been so many incredible discoveries made in relation to nutrients and part of my role has been to highlight the areas of nutrition where science shows there are effective cures. There's a lovely quote by Marcel Proust, who said that 'the real act of discovery consists not in finding new lands, but in seeing with new eyes'.

Nutrients and vitamins have only been discovered in the last 100 years. In this period we have begun to understand the essential nutrients and have made huge leaps in our learnings. But the idea that we can reverse disease processes with large amounts of specific nutrients is a paradigm shift. I am very happy to help in bringing the knowledge of this shift to the public in any way I can.

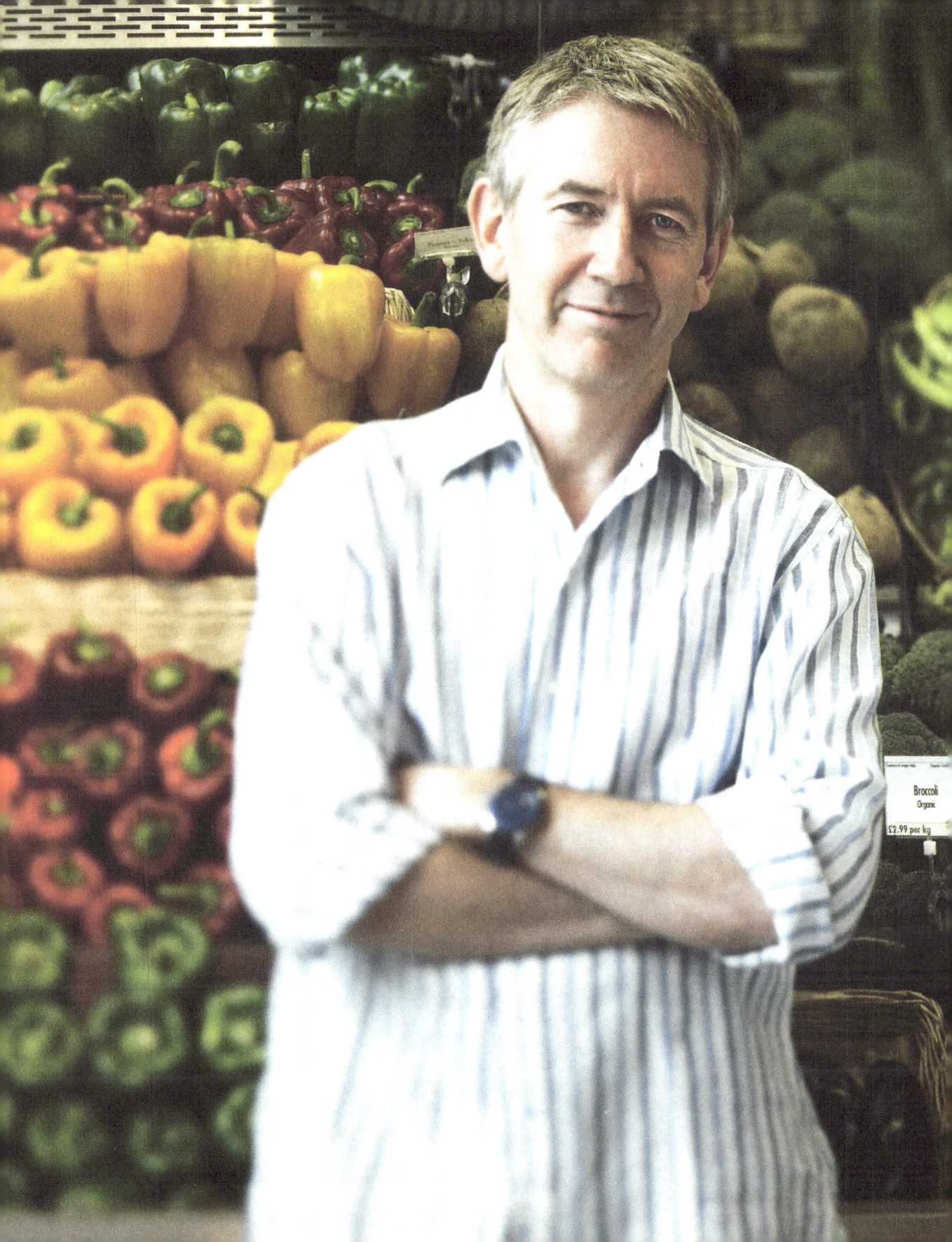

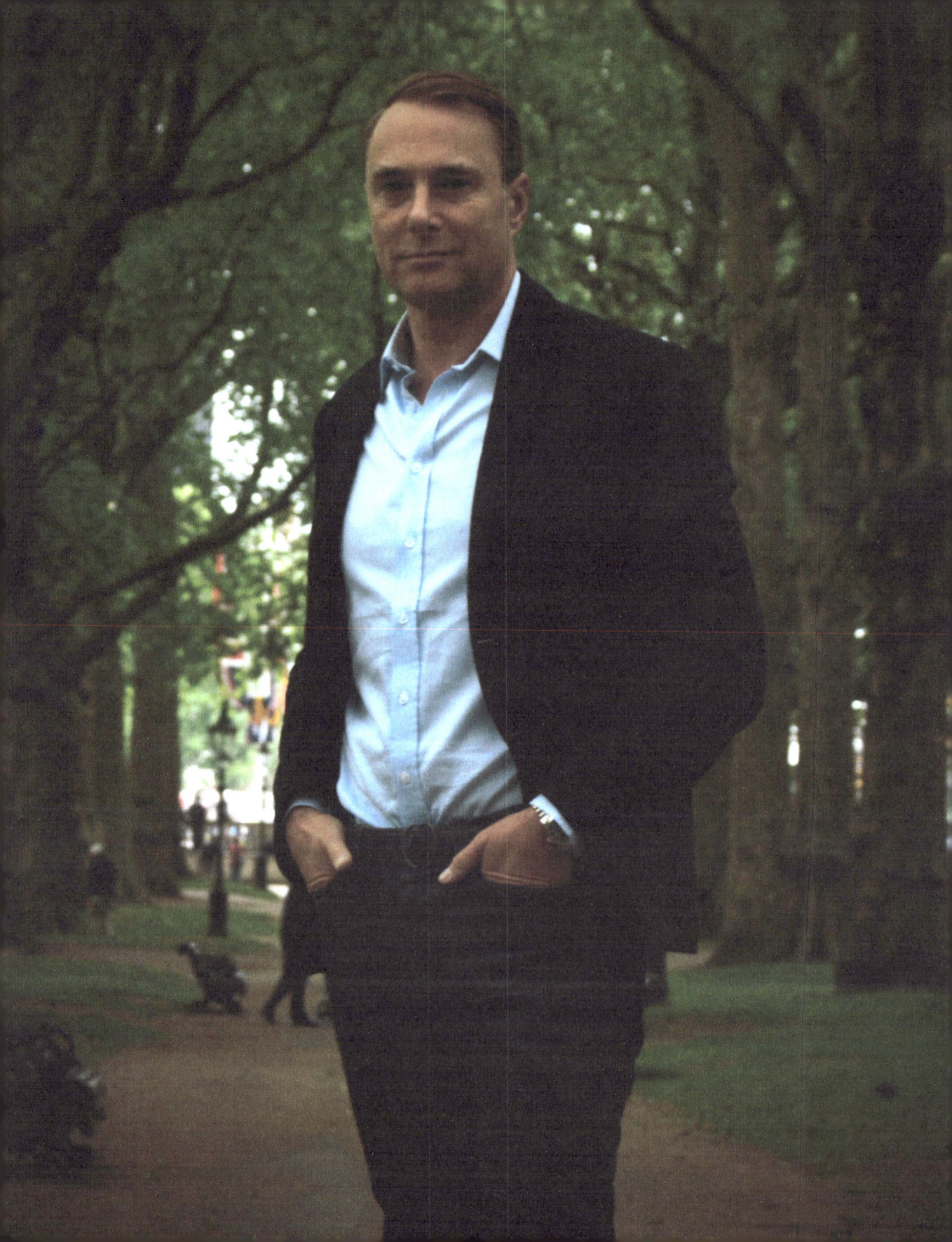

Ian Marber

Founder of the Food Doctor brand,
Author and Nutritionist

Ian Marber has been incredibly influential within the field of nutrition. He came to the industry at a time when the subject of healthy food was being presented as alternative, New Age and very niche. His success as a television presenter and author has seen him championing nutrition and making it a much more accessible area for the general public. The clarity in his communication has ensured that people could apply his nutritional advice to their real life, everyday situations in a simple way. It was fascinating to speak with Ian about the journey he undertook to become a nutritionist.

I grew up in a middle class Jewish family in London with a comfortable life. When I got to my mid-twenties I became aware of how privileged my lifestyle was, as well as how hedonistic it could be. It was all very pleasurable but I was yearning to experience more depth, so I volunteered as a buddy for the Terrence Higgins Trust in 1991. In those days the vast majority of people diagnosed with HIV went on to develop AIDS and ended up dying. There was a huge stigma involved, so the Terrence Higgins Trust set up a system where a buddy would work with AIDS and HIV victims in the capacity of an unbiased friend, and that's what I did. Eventually I become a coordinator for the Council of Chelsea buddy group for two years and then went back to being a buddy again.

This was a very powerful introduction to the value of health and I became much more aware of my own personal health. I was in my twenties when I started working with the Terrence Higgins Trust, which is an age when we usually see ourselves as invincible. I was diagnosed with coeliac disease at this time, which is a gluten intolerance, and I went to see a dietician whose advice was to avoid gluten. It seemed such a simple solution that I began to wonder why all other people were not seeing nutritionists. My thoughts started to snowball on how better nutrition could affect our health. Cooking and eating always interested me and it seemed an obvious way of combining nutrition with something I enjoyed.

At the time I was quite unsettled and not particularly happy in what I was doing career wise, so I was looking for a way out. This for me was a big factor in the whole thing. If you are not looking to make a change, it is quite possible that you will ignore all the signs pointing to a different path.

Nutrition

On a personal level there were two parts to my experience with nutrition that piqued my interest. One was cutting out gluten, which was very easy and greatly improved my health. The other was the fact that I started to get better nutrition.

The changes I made really increased my energy levels, which caught my attention, as I had not realised that I was in a low-level malaise the whole time. If low energy is generally the way you feel in life, it becomes normal to you. I did not have a major transformation, because I was not unwell, but I felt better. My energy levels, concentration and mood all improved. The effects were so positive I ended up leaving my job, selling my flat and enrolling on a nutrition course, which I studied at the Institute of Optimum Nutrition for three years.

While I was there I kept asking why there were no great books on nutrition. There were either textbooks or what were described as Californian New Age nutritional books. But there was nothing that the mainstream public could relate to. My first book was published at the same time that I graduated, which is pretty pushy, but it was very much about being in the right place at the right time.

My Work

I never knew that the work I did would make such an impact. I always thought that I would be working one to one with people, but I was not hugely confident that so many people would buy and remember the book. A couple of weeks before the book was published, the publishers faxed through the schedule and I was shocked there were interviews, radio and all sorts of things. I had never anticipated this amount of media coverage and its reach. In some ways it was terrifying, but a lot of fun.

At the time I would talk to intelligent people about nutrition and they would have no clue about it. This was before the internet, so if you wanted to know something you had to look it up in a library or buy a book. My first book contained basic us-er-friendly information in order to make nutrition more accessible, more day-to-day and, in a way, more pedestrian. I learnt quite early on that, in order to make a difference, you have to appeal to people and present information in a way that they can identify with, understand and use. So it was more about pointing out different options that were available to them in real life situations.

Once the first book was released, we started a consultancy in Notting Hill. It all happened very quickly. In a matter of weeks we had people asking us to set up a business with them, which gave birth to the Food Doctor products. At the time nutrition was viewed as being really alternative and New Age. The only books out there for the public seemed to be about vegan or raw food diets. What we were doing was more understandable because we were asking people to make small adaptations and changes to their lifestyle, as opposed to a complete turnaround.

Passion

My passion in nutrition fluctuates but, even at its weakest, it's still pretty passionate. I think the difficulty has always been that you can have a passion, but you've also got to pay the mortgage. You may be passionate about writing, for example, but you can't always write what you want to because you may have an editor who has commissioned you. So it's finding a balance between what you want to say and how the person that's editing the piece wants it to be presented. When it comes to being passionate creatively, there is always going to be a level of compromise if you work commercially. This causes your passion to get channelled in different ways to how you may first have imagined. For example, clients are incredibly enthused about doing weight loss programmes in January, when the gyms are full, the supermarkets sell more of their low-fat ranges and fewer people are drinking in restaurants; at that point everyone is really serious about nutrition. But by February, people are talking about Valentine's Day and eating chocolate again. The gyms are less full and the level of gusto is declining. So when I take away all the commercial aspects of my work and get right back to the nutritional part, I become inspired all over again.

The Future

I view my time as the Food Doctor as something I did in the past. Things are very different now to how they were a decade ago. I think the Food Doctor helped to make nutrition more mainstream in the UK. Some people say that when your identity is wrapped up with a brand, you've got to be quite careful not to draw that identity into your personal boundaries. Letting go of the brand definitely took adjustment at the time, but now it just seems like a chapter of my life.

I am now a consultant to several food brands and have just completed a project for a multinational company. But mainly I am writing and have eight regular feature columns. Additionally, I have a new book out in 2014 and an online weight management plan due to be launched. I also do seminars and conferences and enjoy the public speaking aspects of my work.

Apart from nutrition, I am a patron of the Mulberry Bush charity in Witney, just outside of Oxford, which works with children who have been completely excluded from mainstream education. It looks after thirty children a year who've been failed by the system. They may have grown up in homes that contained violence, domestic abuse, drug abuse and/or prostitution. Often they are angry and troubled and the charity works to make them feel safe and secure within themselves and to integrate them into society. So in the future I anticipate that my time will continue to be both busy and varied.

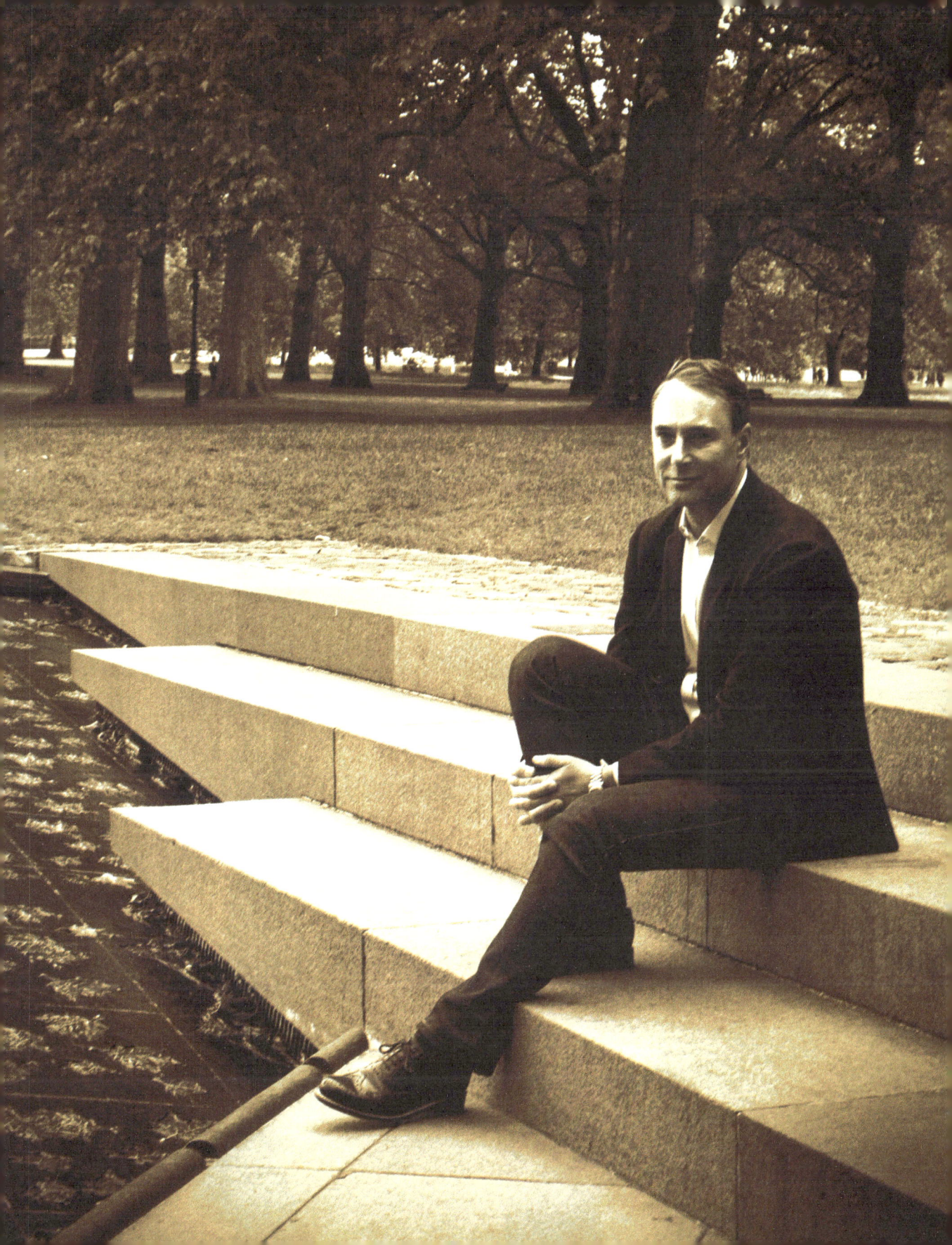

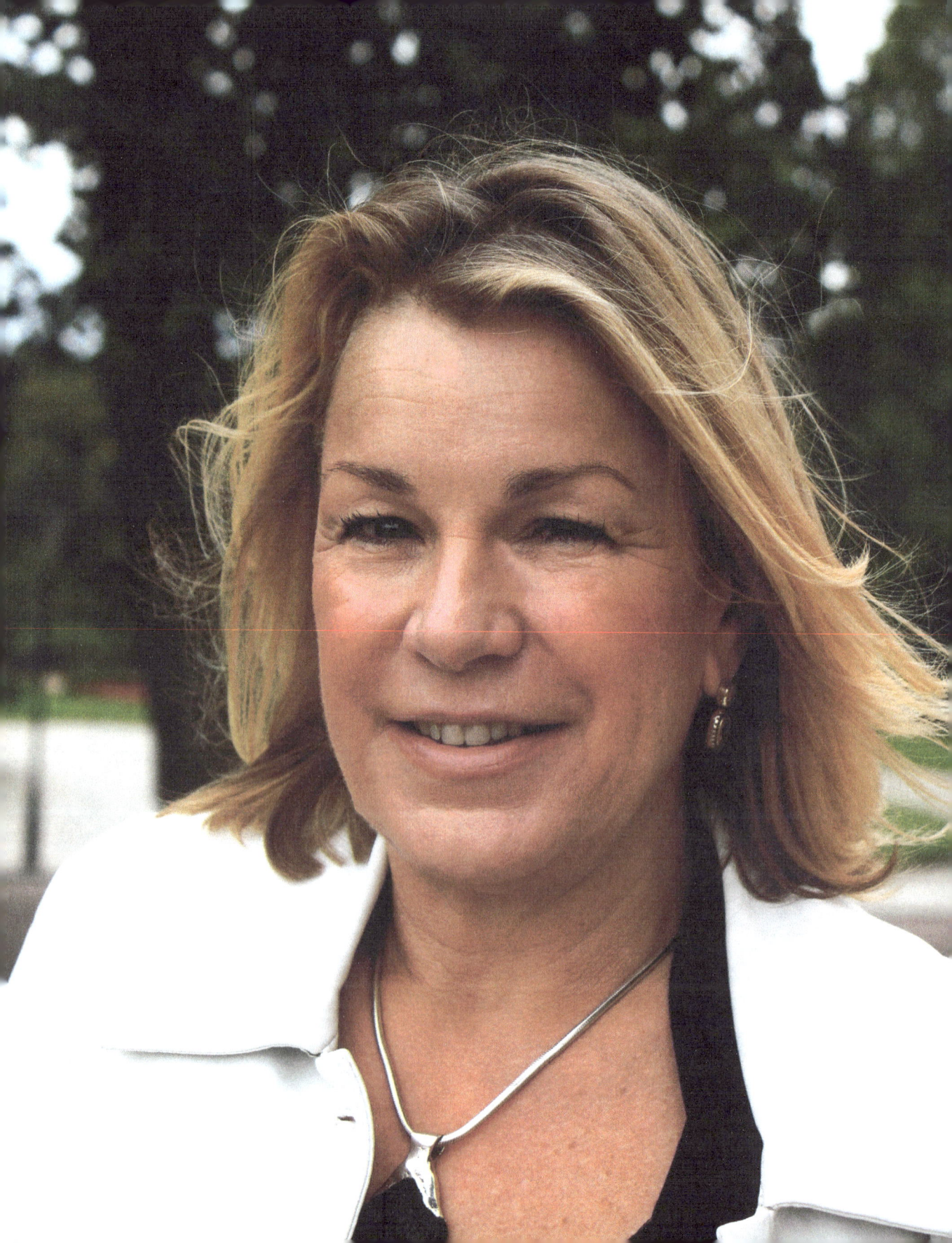

Gloria Parfitt
Founder of GP Natural Weight Management Ltd, Director of Metabolic Balance UK and Nutritionist

When it comes to nutrition there is so much information out there. It can be hard to know what our best course of action is or what our perfect food match is. This is what makes Metabolic Balance stand out so much. It is an individualised health plan based on balancing the chemical composition in the body, using only natural foods. Gloria Parfitt, the UK Director, is an interesting mix of creative adventurer and health academic. Her career path has led from nursing to aviation to nutrition, a journey which reflects how open she is to exploration. It was great to get her perspective on food as therapy.

I got into nutrition through personal experience. I did not have a great time during my midlife changes because hormonal issues led to me piling on weight. As a nutritionist, I knew about the importance of blood sugar control. I had used nutrition to sort out both my Irritable Bowel Syndrome and blood sugar issues, but I could not seem to shift my weight and this began to depress me.

While on a retreat in Mauritius I met a lady in her late sixties who was absolutely stunning. She was also wearing a swimming costume that I had my eye on here in the UK, but could not get into because of my size. She told me that Metabolic Balance was responsible for how well she looked. She was German and the programme had been created by a German doctor called Wolf Funfack. At that time it was saturated in the German market, but had no presence in the UK. I got in contact with Dr Funfack and he put me in touch with his son who was working in America. I flew over to meet him, got trained in the methodology, and was offered the UK licence.

I discovered Metabolic Balance two years after qualifying as a nutritionist. At the time I had a few clients but I found it hard to break into the industry without a niche or specialty. After I completed the programme I felt amazing and people who knew me were really shocked at the transformation. Through this experience I realised that the general model nutritionists follow – of three meals and two snacks a day – was heightening our blood sugar rather than controlling it. A high blood sugar level in the body leads to an overproduction of insulin and this becomes a problem because once insulin has done its job, it then turns into a fat storing hormone.

How Metabolic Balance Works

Metabolic Balance is very straightforward. The programme is based on your blood result, which offers a snapshot of where you are in terms of the biochemical composition within your body. Its main aim is to address digestion and give the digestive system the opportunity to rest and heal itself. It allows a person to learn about the impact and therapeutics of natural food on the body.

A review is done on 34 different elements within a person's blood sample and the data is entered into a computerised programme generating a result. This gives a view on what the body needs chemically to balance its hormonal and metabolic functions. Foods are selected in order to create this balance. The influence of the nutritionist or practitioner is in their understanding of the various processes that take place. There are dramatic changes to the body composition of each individual who does the programme. At the start some people experience inch loss as opposed to weight loss because they are in the fat burning mode. So they may have lost three kilos of fat while increasing their muscle mass. Increased muscle mass vastly improves the efficiency of the metabolism.

Metabolic Balance is a process that eventually becomes a lifestyle with rules and boundaries. By doing the programme, a person begins to realise that snacking is not necessary to control blood sugar and can lead to exacerbated stress levels if there is imbalance. I have put over one hundred nutritionists and health practitioners through the training weekend, so that they can practice this modality in their own clinics. Metabolic Balance has become really well sought after because it is such an easy and successful tool to work with. It forces you to have a greater variety of vegetables and balances protein intake. There is also some fruit involved, but at the beginning it is very limited.

The programme encourages people to be creative with healthy food and many people say that they did not think they would enjoy a particular vegetable, because they had never had it before. Becoming a therapist of the programme is most popular with nutritionists because it focuses on the nutritional aspects of wellness. But it is attractive to a variety of individuals because it causes weight loss. Depending on the desired result, food can also be chosen for weight gain and weight maintenance. Once certain parameters are put in place, the body responds quite positively.

My Work Previous to Nutrition

I was a private jet pilot before I became a nutritionist and enjoyed every aspect of flying. From my very first flight I loved the amazing and unrivalled peace that I experienced while being in the air, but I felt as though I was on borrowed time. When I started out I was really sought after as there were only a few people and private jets offering the same service within the industry. But, with time, the industry began to boom and things started to change.

Nutrition seemed like a natural course for my next choice of career because I was a nurse before working in aviation. Healthcare had always held an attraction for me and I also understood that nutrition was one of the main keys to optimum health. So it ticked all the boxes.

Building Metabolic Balance in the UK

I have had a huge amount of support from some very special people, such as Petronella Ravenshear from Chelsea Nutrition and two amazing instructors who deliver the weekend programme to Metabolic Balance Coaches. These are Anthony Haynes, a very well respected nutritionist and author, and Gerry Gajadharsingh, an osteopath with a very integrative approach. I have found that if someone works on a therapeutic basis with others and has an understanding of the implications associated with nutritional issues, then Metabolic Balance serves what they are doing very well. The way that it is structured makes it easy to implement within their work. Anthony and Gerry are a perfect combination in their presentation and teaching of the programme.

There is a great support system within Metabolic Balance, so the coach does not have to make the choices in terms of the dietary plan. This is formulated automatically in response to the blood test results. Their role is simply to provide support and guidance to the client through the process.

As a coach there needs to be an awareness about the effects of the programme, especially if the person undertaking it is on medication. Obviously medication is determined through the client's relationship with their doctor. For example, if the client is on high blood pressure pills and during the programme they start feeling dizzy, then they would be advised to go to their doctor and check whether the dosage of their medication needs to be lowered or stopped. High blood pressure and high cholesterol are two examples of what is being addressed within Metabolic Balance.

So far the programme has had some amazing success stories, including Boy George, who has had a lot of media coverage surrounding his successful weight loss on Metabolic Balance. There has also been a lot of publicity about Jemma Kidd. Her results were so positive that she has now begun to champion the system, which has gained more and more popularity as people have begun to experience the positive effects of Metabolic Balance.

The Future

Metabolic Balance and nutrition as a whole are very important pieces of the puzzle. But when you look at the holistic picture of the body, it is necessary to look at things from other angles as well. I am currently doing the most amazing course in Clinical Psycho Neuro Immunology or cPNI. It is a study of how our psychological, nervous and immune systems all interrelate and evolve. The science is very cutting edge and a lot of what we have learnt is yet to be made public, I find this very exciting.

One thing I have discovered over the years is that my strength lies in my creativity as opposed to my ability to be an academic. This being the case, it will always be important for me to explore new grounds and to diversify into new areas in the future.

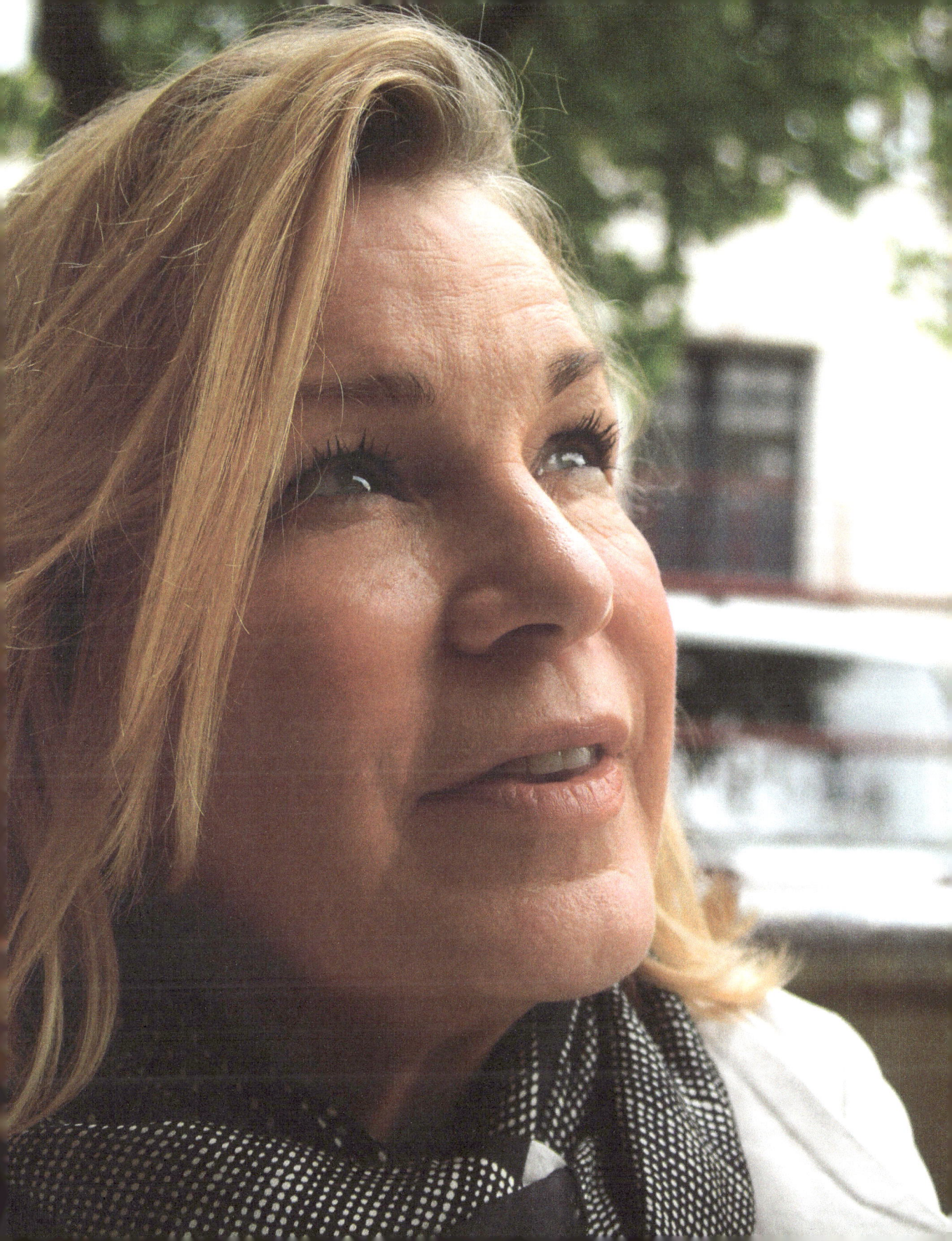

"Culture, family, life experience, our gender, our race, all of these incorporate the programming that we use to create our body. We live in a space of habits where we do what we have always done. To find our true potential we have to be willing to be in a place where we have no idea what it is we want to plug into, which takes us past the limits of what we know."

- Emma Roberts

Movement Therapy

This section was created to spotlight the areas of physical care that focus on movement in order to enhance function and create structural changes. The three examples used here are Pilates, Feldenkrais Method and Dance Therapy. Pilates was developed by Joseph Pilates with the specific goal of strengthening the mind/body connection. The Feldenkrais Method, developed by Moshe Feldenkrais, aims to increase awareness of movement as a way to promote smooth and unhindered function. Dance Therapy gives the body an expressive way to channel and release emotions through movement.

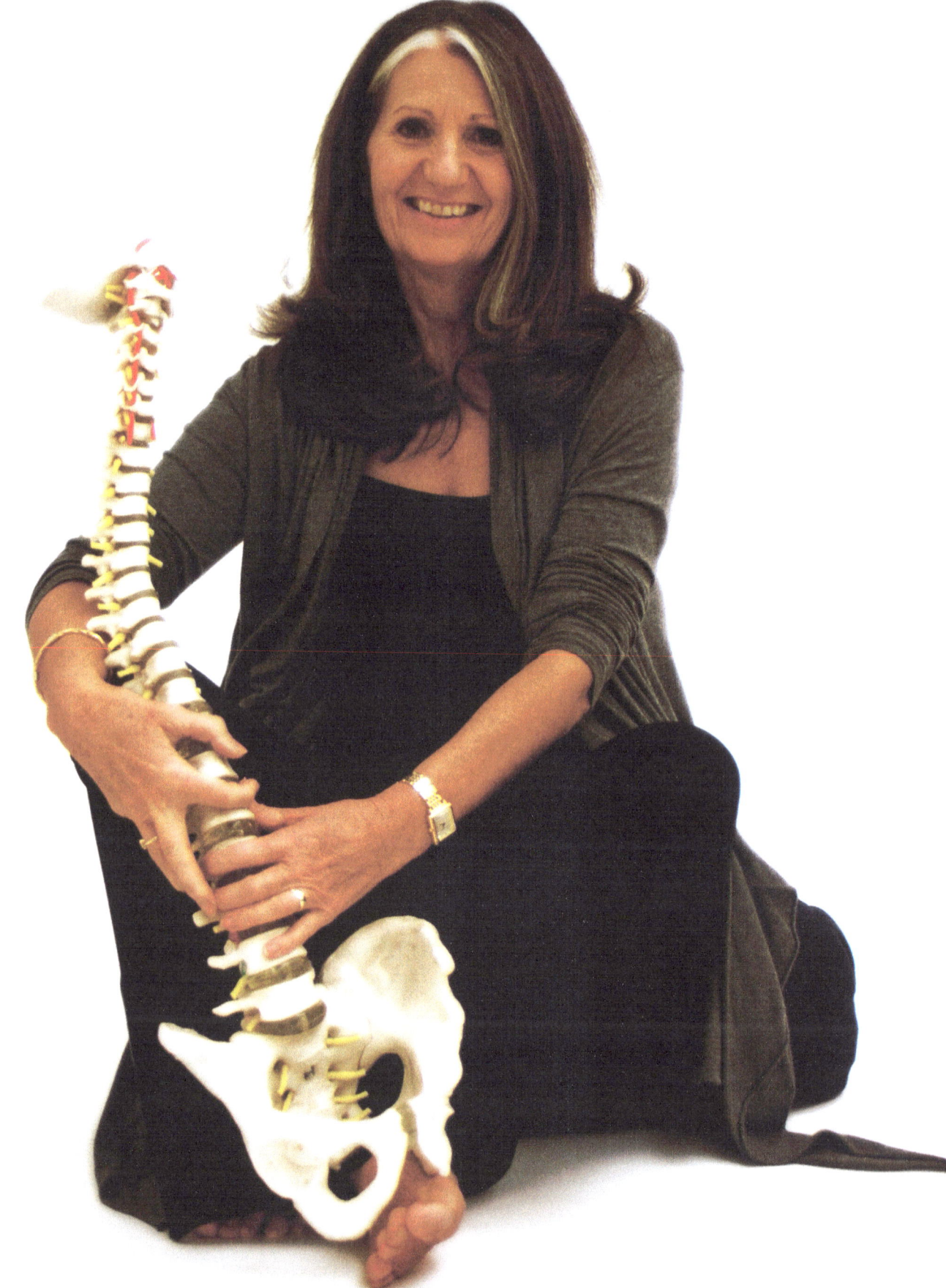

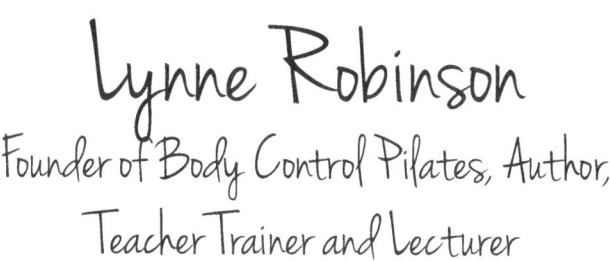

Lynne Robinson
Founder of Body Control Pilates, Author, Teacher Trainer and Lecturer

Lynne Robinson's journey into Pilates has been very personal. It was responsible for helping her to manoeuvre through life with a herniated disc in her back and still maintain a full and challenging schedule that sees her flying all over the world teaching her art. Because of the part it has played in her own life, Lynne has picked the most direct and influential route to get Pilates out to the general public, by teaching people who themselves want to teach with excellence, integrity and solid knowledge. It was a pleasure to meet this very warm and very humble lady.

I found Pilates by fate when I turned up for a yoga class at the wrong time. The truth is that I am your least likely fitness guru because I used to avoid any form of exercise. I inherited quite a slouchy posture from my parents, had a tendency to be overweight and was a real academic. Added to this I am really uncoordinated; if you ask me to raise my right arm I will most likely raise my left leg. Career wise I studied history at university and trained to be a secondary school teacher.

My physical issues started after I gave birth to two large babies and didn't do any of the exercises that you are supposed to do afterwards. Over time this began to have a negative impact on my back. Then I decided to start playing golf and that was when what was just a bad back became herniated. At the time we were living an ex-pat life, I did not have much information on exercises that could help me so I began doing regular yoga. I am quite hyper mobile and without core stability and awareness of what I was doing, yoga was not effective. My body was moving where it could move and not where it should move.

We emigrated to Sydney, Australia, and I thought I would try doing a yoga class there, but I got the timing wrong on the schedule and a 'pilots' class was on, which I was told I could come in and join. I couldn't do it very well and we had to adapt the exercises to suit me, but I ended up doing it five times a week, I loved it that much. Because my husband's job meant we moved from one country to the next, I was worried we might get sent to a place where Pilates would not be available, so I trained to become a teacher. Being quite an academic and given the challenges I had with my back, I tended to dissect and analyse each movement and write everything down, so my first book developed naturally from this.

Pilates

Pilates is mind and body conditioning. Basically it teaches you how to use your body well. It is a system that will improve your posture, it will help you breath more efficiently and it will increase your core stability. Its ultimate goal is to help you to move within your body in an aligned way. Pilates is a traditional exercise performed by doing repetitions and as a result it also helps in toning the muscles in a more general sense.

My success with Pilates in the UK is really down to timing, we were very lucky. Whilst Pilates was quite big in Australia and America, when I started as a Pilates teacher, it hadn't really hit the public market in the UK. There were a few select private studios in Central London, which was obviously not accessible to everyone. As a teacher I could see that in order for the exercises to be taught safely in groups, they had to be modified. The traditional work is best taught one to one unless you know what you are doing.

I started teaching Pilates classes in Sevenoaks; nobody had heard of it there. But as luck would have it, a local osteopath liked what I did and started supporting me by sending his patients to me. Things just grew from there. Suddenly, I went from two classes to so many I could hardly cope. I was teaching in church halls, village halls and community centres all around the area.

Because of my passion for Pilates, I put a lot of work into getting it to as many people as I could. The DVDs and the books are the very glamorous side of what I do. I have also done television and radio as well and it all has been great. But once the first book was written we turned our attention to creating a training programme. My focus was on training teachers well, so they could teach a maximum of 12 people in small groups really effectively. This is where my true passion lies and now we are training teachers all over the world.

My Personal Journey with Pilates

Once I started doing Pilates regularly I felt so good after every class. It doesn't cure your back problems overnight; you have to be committed to work at it. The fact is that I still have a herniated disk in my back, which has not disappeared, but neither have I had to have a back operation. Through Pilates I have both managed and controlled the problem and it has connected me consciously to my body and the ways in which I use it. Before finding Pilates, I was getting to the point where I couldn't sit and do yoga. Each flight I took was agony. I was waking up every morning with terrible sciatica, whereas now I am flying all over the place teaching. Because of my own experience, I have a particular interest in Pilates for pregnancy and postnatal, as this was where my problems started.

A healthy spine and core are really influential factors in how we manoeuvre ourselves within the world. Although we technically do not talk about Pilates from an energetic or spiritual viewpoint, there is an understanding that, because we are working with the mind and the body through the musculoskeletal system, the effects go much deeper. You can't work on the mind and body and not work on the soul as well. Once I had been doing Pilates for a while, I was able to breathe better, I was more confident and felt centred within myself.

The Success of the Body Control Brand

We are in a great position with Body Control, in that we do not go out looking for business, it tends to come to us. For example, I have worked with the Chelsea football team. We do British Airways in-flight exercises. In terms of our worldwide teachers, we train people from other countries at our London studio. They eventually go home and contact us, when and if they feel they are ready to progress to training other teachers themselves. When they contact us, we send them a teacher and all the course materials that they need to take this step. So it all happens organically, we are really not aggressive with our marketing. Everything is done on request.

Because of my passion and the groundwork I did through books, DVDs and media, it has built trust. I think people know that if they come to Body Control, they can trust us to deliver. It is a system that has been tried, tested and we know that it works. There are several areas of teacher training that I am working on developing at the moment, one of them is Pilates for children, which I am setting up with a paediatric physiotherapist. My aim is to get government backing so that our teachers can teach in schools. We are also working on a new course in Pilates for older people. We already have a version of this, but I want to sharpen and hone it.

Pilates as my Life's Purpose

I can definitely say I am fulfilling my life's purpose through Pilates. When I take a step back and look at the schedule that I have at times, with all the travelling and training

I do, I know I couldn't successfully get so much done if it wasn't what I am meant to be doing. I have to pinch myself sometimes in order to make sure it is real, because I love my work. I love all the people I meet through it. I love that this has become a family business, with both my husband and daughter helping me run it. There have been some scary challenges, like going on live television, or doing a conference for 300 orthopaedic surgeons from the British Institute of Muscular Skeletal Medicine. Every time I teach a new group for the first time I get nervous. But I recognise that with each great challenge, there is on offer a great opportunity, which gives me a surge of energy and adrenaline that carries me along with it.

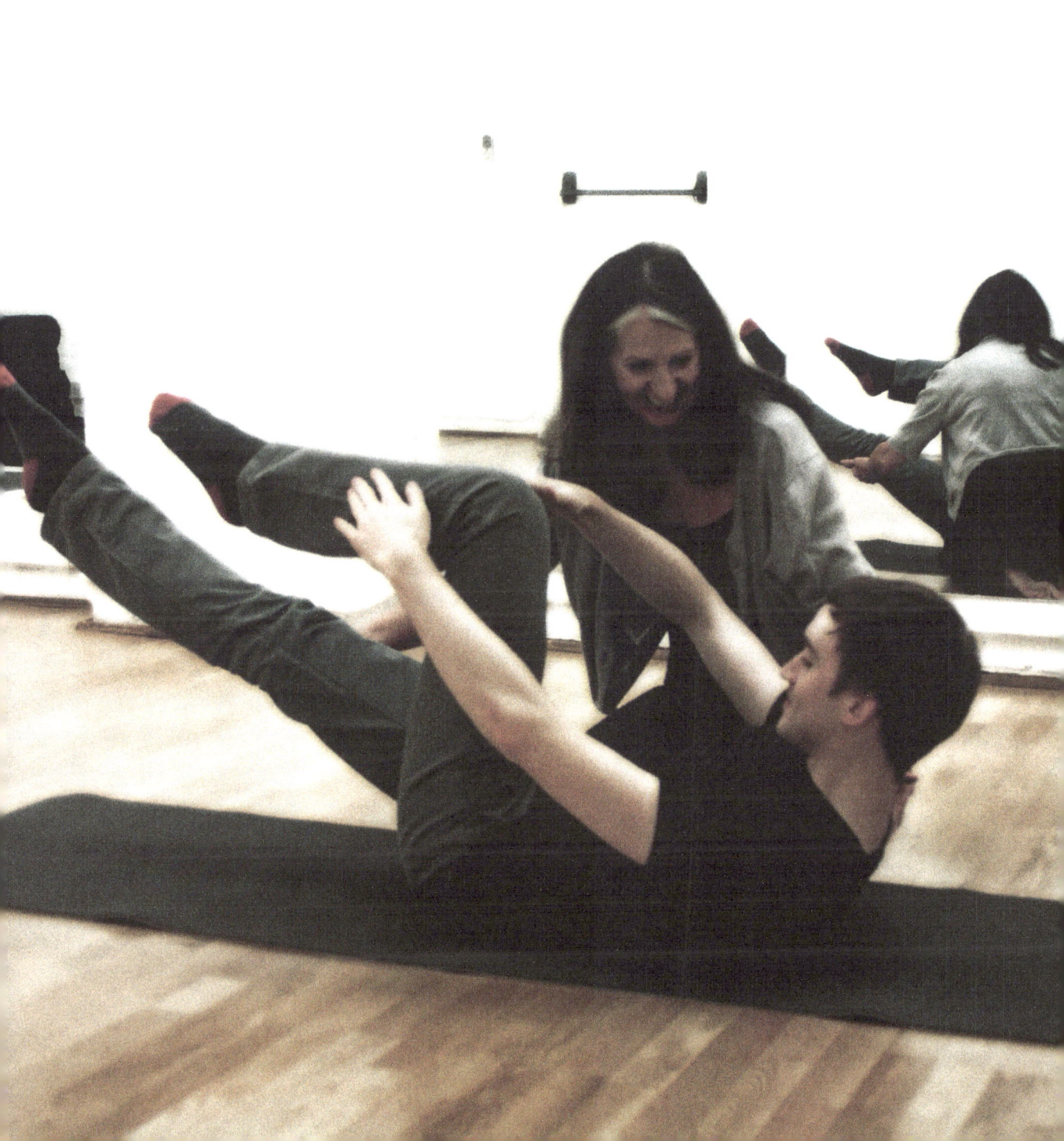

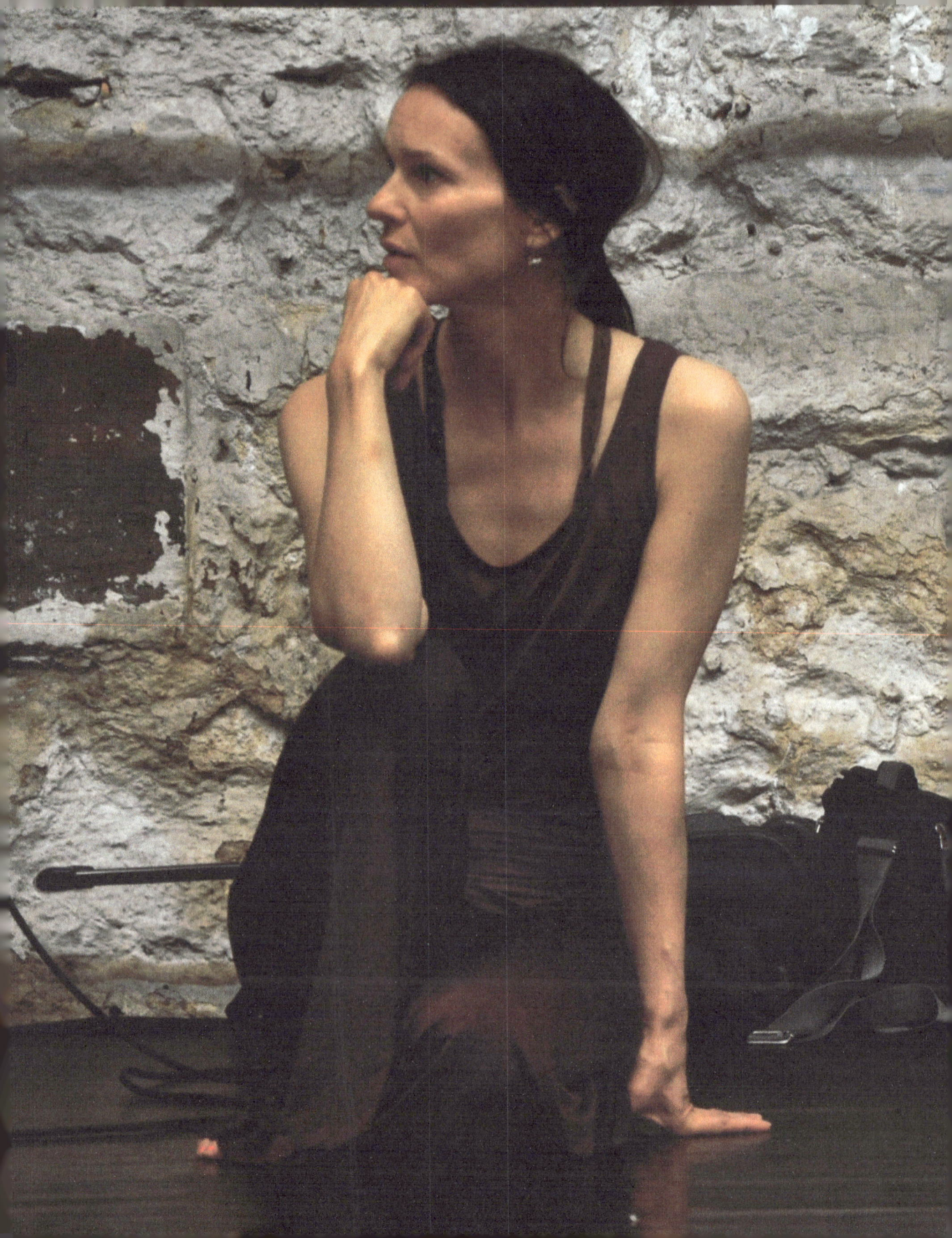

Emma Roberts
Director of Shaping the Invisible,
Choreographer and Five Rhythms Teacher

Through dance, Emma Roberts takes self-development to a whole different dimension. Using the body, the context of a group dynamic and the imagination, her students are enfolded in a space where they can explore their edges and boundaries, as well as their infinite and unknown. They get to play with what it means to be a human being, what it means to be in community with others and what it means to allow the body's intelligence the free rein to truly communicate.

My lineage is originally dance, and then I went into theatre, into therapy, into improvisation, back into theatre and now I have started a company called Shaping the Invisible, which feels like an umbrella name for all the aspects I have been pulling on. It is about accessing what is in the unseen world and giving it a physical outlet through exploration, expression and engagement.

I was an actress for a number of years, but was a reluctant performer at that time. This was mainly because, as I got older, I became less and less layered and so felt too transparent. I moved away from the acting world when I was twenty-eight even though I was pretty successful with it. This decision was made because I thought that doing well would make me feel well, but it didn't. It just brought up more and more questions. All my creativity was waking up and I did not feel like I was being used to my capacity, which I found quite limiting. My next move was to be a director and so I did my MA in directing at Middlesex University, but things were still not fitting. I then decided to do drama with movement therapy when I was twenty-eight and in 2010 I embarked on Gabrielle Roth's 5 Rhythms Teacher Training, which brought all the pieces of the puzzle together.

I was attracted to the therapy side of things because I was interested in the enquiry it presented. I think some of my own demons meant that I was quite plugged into the darker side of the world, which prompted the question, 'How do we work with darkness?' Ultimately this led to the greater question of what it means to be a human being.

My Work

I would say my work is about self-development. I am interested in the intelligence of the body and I feel like its humble student. Even though I have been working with movement since childhood, I am only now beginning to understand the size of the intelligence the body contains. The work that I do with others is about holding the space for each individual to discover this intelligence inside their own body; not just in relation to themselves, but also within the relationship of the group. It offers the person a way to experience the play between the micro and macro detail.

There are times when I work as a movement director in theatre; this means that we are aiming to create something specific. Dance is used as a transmission to an audience and we work with clear ideas that will look at things philosophically and psychologically. The focus is on how people are receiving the information in their bodies, minds and questioning. There is a conscious creation of a beginning, middle and end. When I am working creatively with a group I try to keep things in the context of the enquiry.

Other times I work within a workshop or class setting and in this context we have a clear theme from the very beginning. So, for example, we may make an enquiry about the use of imagination through the body. We look at what we are able to feel within the body by tapping into the imaginative space. We look at the concept of how far our mind can expand our feelings. We explore ourselves physically through the fact that, although we can't see our spine, our bones or any other part of our internal body, we have the ability to imagine them and keep expanding this vision. Dance in this way allows us to see that our imagination can become a big ally in helping us to experience life.

Feeling, rather than thinking, the body

When I take this work into theatre we use a live musician and an exploration is made on how, from empty space where you can't see anything, there is the living potential of anything being created, and that all creation is based on a relationship experience. My material is formed on exercises that wake up the intelligence inside the body. I try to do very little theory because it brings people too much into their heads. In contrast, when I am working in the space, my approach is about getting people's bodies to a receptive point, so that it can access the intelligence of the material. From this place I can use words and language, which will facilitate it even more powerfully into their experience. I have to work from a deeply intuitive tract in order to follow what I am seeing and to allow the potential, that I sense is there, to emerge.

Dance for me personally is a language. Out of all the languages that you could possibly have, dance is universal. Every culture has created some kind of origins of dance as a way to unify and express itself within groups or within the individual. It is a three-dimensional language, which involves your cells, your blood, your spirit and your soul. Everything becomes engaged when you dance and when you witness it or are part of a dance, the energy is tangible and pure. You feel everything in the language of movement, it does not lie and it has a much greater intelligence. We can be very articulate and yet be very separated from who we really are. In other words, we can talk a very beautiful life but not actually live a very beautiful life.

Something about dance and movement embodies all the different landscapes of who we are, from the very lightest to the very darkest, and from the most acceptable to the most unacceptable. When we put this into movement it transforms into art and beauty. It is the most healing contribution to life. When someone who is suffering finds a beautiful dance that really expresses their pain, every cell is transported and it becomes an alchemical experience. The real aspect of creativity and evolution is that it has an expansive nature, which embraces everything and does not judge it.

Dance has been the purest holding space for me to be able to express who I am as a human being. I think most people are quite complex, but the question is whether they are engaged enough to experience all levels of their complexity. It is beautiful for me on a witnessing level, during a class or workshop, to see people at their most utterly naked and beautiful. I have the most profound conversations of my life on the dance floor. I might know nothing about the person's job, where they come from, how old they are, but on the dance floor I meet something really essential and direct in who they are.

The creative process

I think I am quite the perpetual student, it is just the way my brain is plugged in. I am restlessly curious all the time. I love that Martha Graham quote where she says that the artist is always in a place of divine dissatisfaction. There is never a sense of fully arriving.

Through my study of improvisation we played with the idea that there is this empty space. Culture, family, life experiences, our gender, our race, all of these incorporate the programming that we use to create our body. We live in a space of habits where we do what we have always done. To find our true potential we have to be willing to be in a place where we have no idea what it is we want to plug into, which takes us past the limits of what we know.

The same applies to me as a dancer and performer, the question is always, 'How can I plug into a place where I can truly be with the unknown?' Within the unknown lies an infinity of creativity.

The Future

I am really interested in microbiology, cell consciousness, a study on how the body has evolved through time and how this intelligence lives within us and connects to the rest of life. Additionally, I am becoming more interested in quantum theories. I feel that the world works on a fractal basis, meaning the whole is contained in the smallest particle and the smallest particle is an integral part of the whole. From this level the more I can understand the universe within myself the more I can be a proactive and positive contributor to life. Part of my being here is to be in service to life in the greatest sense; there is a deep-seated need to create a meaningful life and to understand how all experience is connected.

I don't feel like I am necessarily looking for answers; it is about creating the possibility and potential for brilliance and addressing all the things which inhibit that.

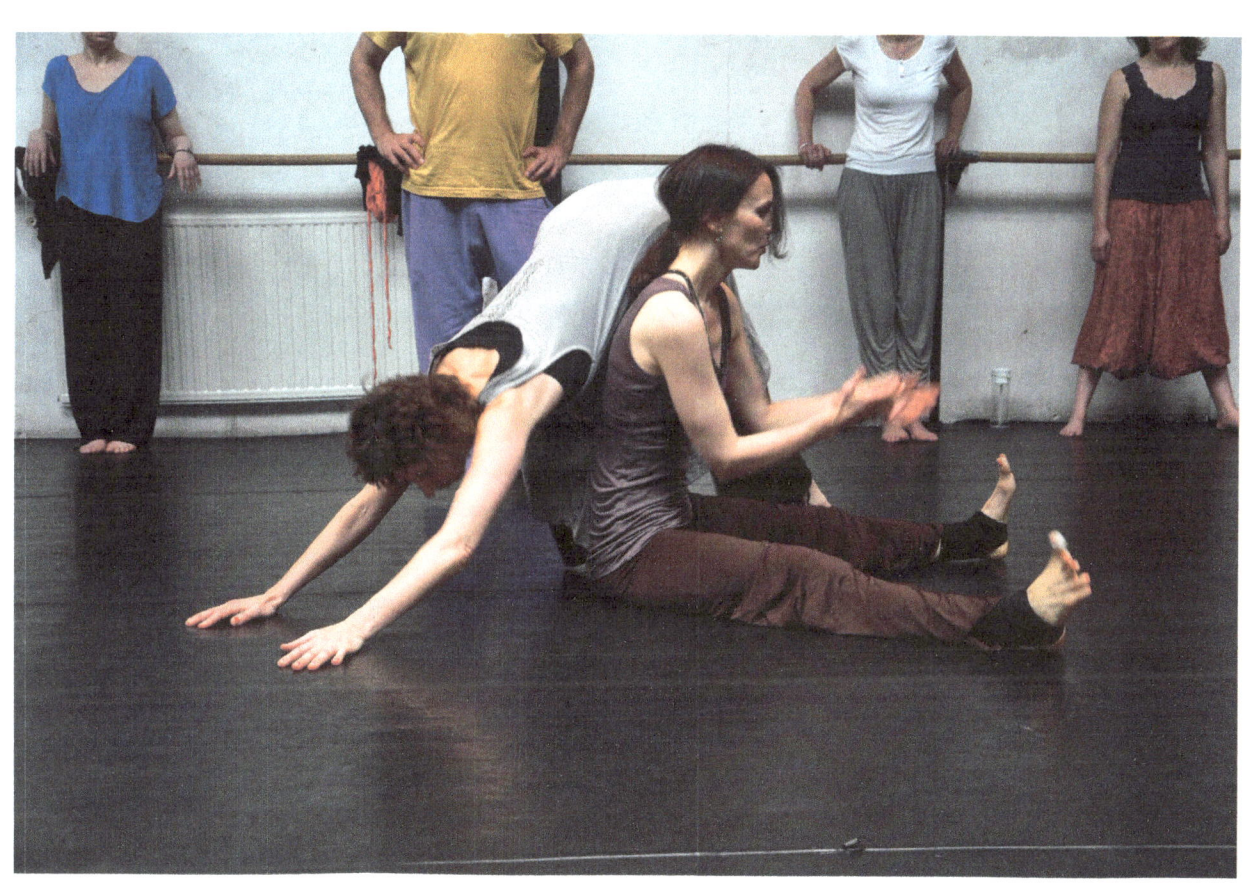

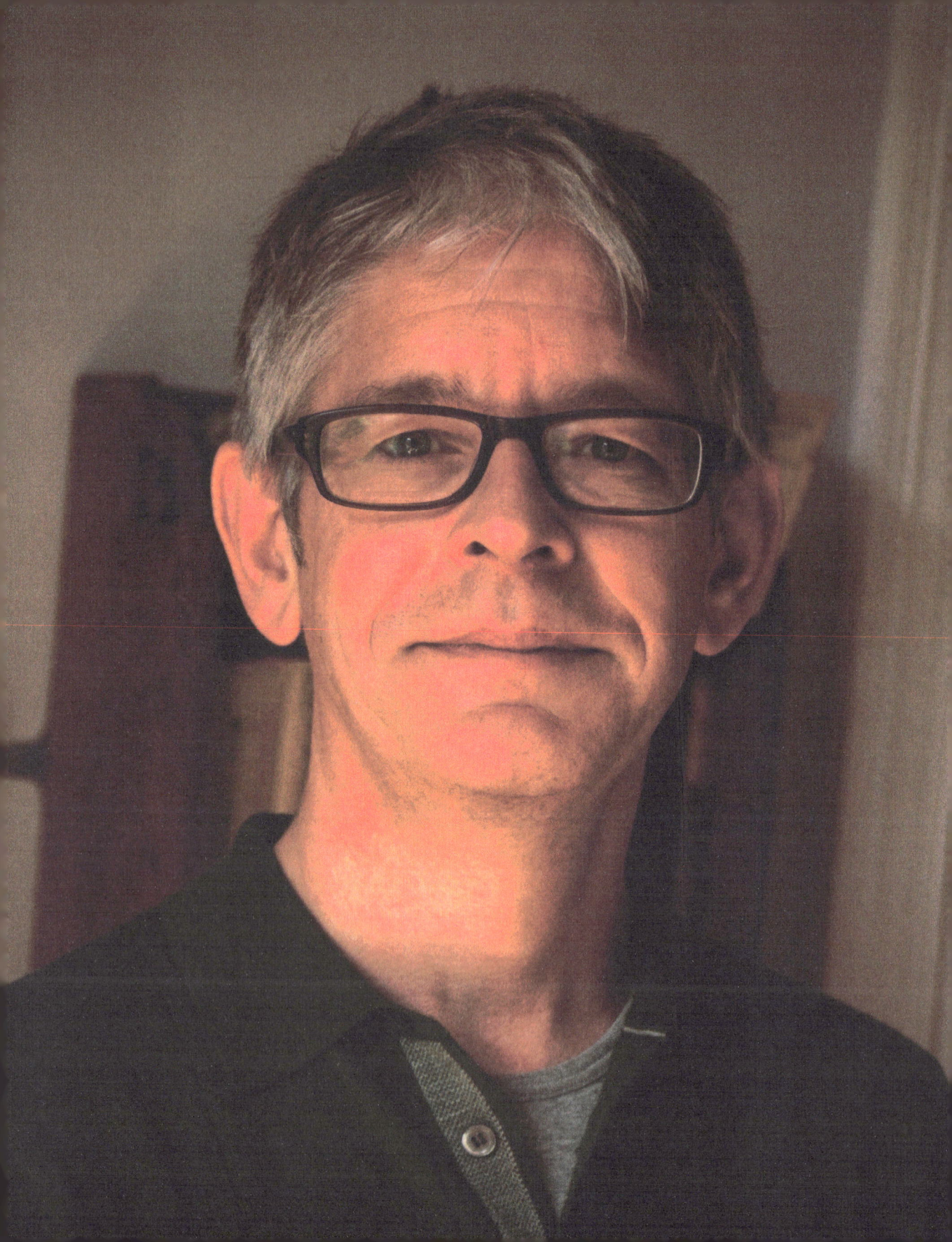

Andrew Dawson
Performer, Choreographer and Feldenkrais Method Teacher

Andrew Dawson has been gifted with a curiosity about how movement shapes, creates, animates and informs us. This curiosity has taken him into illusion, mime, acting, dance and has led him to the Feldenkrais Method. He is a global performer who seeks to engage his audience with their own perception of space, their bodies and the textures, sensations, emotions and artistry that movement can invoke. It was great to take a look at the Feldenkrais Method from his own expert view of the world.

I started off doing mime, which got me into dance and then developed into a fascination with movement. I was interested in theatre and performance, but discovered quite early on that acting did not come naturally to me, which opened me up to exploring. In one of the workshops I went to, the teacher taught me some old-fashioned illusions and I found that I was good at it. Mime stemmed from there. At the time movement and illusion were so exciting to me, I was like a kid with a new toy. I could make things that did not exist appear and disappear. Also this sort of theatre was a world that felt possible for me, while mainstream acting didn't. Mime is all about creative movement, so dance seemed a logical extension from this. I joined a local youth dance theatre at nineteen, which is quite a late stage to start getting into dancing.

Through it all, movement was what held the main attraction for me. Although I loved dance, I was never going to be the kind of dancer that would be in a company. I came to the realisation that I wanted to tell quite definitive stories through movement, rather than being involved in abstract dance performances. At the heart of my fascination was the way in which we can play with the textures of movement, in order to create something that is unique. This is where my interest in theatre developed, as I started to focus on how to create a narrative using movement as the central point. I am always looking for new ways to explore, perceive and interact with movement, so all my work has been based on my own relationships and life.

Bodywork

If you think about it, the whole essence of bodywork is based on movement and the body's relationship with space. So it is either about moving in space, moving the space, or moving the awareness within the body to create internal space. Whichever way we focus, it represents a conscious choice that we make for the body. Where performance illustrates the external interaction between the body and space, bodywork illustrates the internal interaction.

I studied acting with Monica Pagneux, a renowned teacher in Paris. She would conduct the movement element of the course in the morning and another tutor, Phillipe Gaulier, taught the acting element in the afternoon and, in order to demonstrate the directing element, they brought the two together. It was through Monica that I made the connection with how valuable our internal awareness of movement was. By engaging our awareness with our movement, the focus of the audience is taken off their relationship with the actor and put onto their relationship with themselves. This is what eventually sparked my interest in the Feldenkrais Method.

Movement

I am interested in authentic movement, which is something that can be missed when working with choreographed dance. I am also interested in the movement of the everyday and using this to create with. For example, you can make a simple gesture. Then you can start to repeat it, which gives it a different layer. Then you can teach it to someone else, which breathes a new life into it. From there you can both start doing it together, which now creates a framework. Add music to it and you give it a rhythm. This is the sort of awareness I like to bring to the attention of others through my workshops. If a movement is authentic it does not look imposed or weird or strange, it just seems really natural. There are no gaps between the mind and the body, they move as one. The question here is can we get out of our own way, to allow this process to happen.

When you invite others to explore who they are, they then reveal a truth about themselves. This can be both amazing and reflective and in a nutshell it is really what my work is about. It invites others to find their own truth and to really feel it. As a facilitator, it resonates with me when a person in my workshop has managed to do this. There are some movements that can be so descriptive, they are almost like a painting

The Feldenkrais Method

The Feldenkrais Method brings the connectedness and awareness that a dancer develops in the process of embodying the dance to everyday life and everyday people, which is why the work of its founder, Moshe Feldenkrais, was so brilliant. The movements he formulated relate to our day-to-day use of our body. He called his one-to-one work Functional Integration. This may seem a boring phrase to use but it describes exactly what it does, which is integrate seamless functional movement through your body and into your own life. It brings your awareness to how you sit, how you shift, how you use your back. There are unlimited choices available to us in how we move our bodies and our attention is brought to the fact that we do not have to move the same way all of the time.

The bones are constantly regenerating and if we keep moving the same way, it begins to create a different template within the body. You do not have the same skeleton you had seven years ago. The bones are malleable and can be pulled and sculptured by the muscles. The only reason they have the shapes they do is because of the muscles and the tendons that pull on them. If in our day-to-day life we use them in a way that continuously pulls them in one direction, then we need to balance this by creating a pull in the other direction. By keeping our whole body moving, we reduce injuries and degeneration of the bones as we grow older, so there is less of a need to engage with health professionals to help us with our physical pain and imbalances.

The nice thing about facilitating the Feldenkrais Method in a group dynamic, is that people get on the floor and their awareness is completely on the movements they are doing. In this way we work on an individual basis. So I may be teaching everyone the same move, but they all do it in their own individual way; everyone has to find their own place. For example, we may explore lifting the arm. With just that simple movement there are so many choices and it is up to the person which way works best for them.

If you take the act of sitting, for example, people often find that just changing their position will make a whole host of changes to their internal dynamic. I really enjoy exploring that. So if sitting in one way is difficult, we then need to look at why it is difficult. Where does it feel difficult and why does another posture feel easier?

People can use their bodies in quite habitual ways and then the work becomes about breaking the habit. Habitual patterns can end up carving a groove in our body that begins to fix us in certain ways. With posture you can do so many things, depending on what is appropriate in any given moment. There are movements that you travel through and are never static because they are part of a journey to the next movement. It is about awareness and getting into the internal energy of a movement so that you become less externally based.

My Personal View of Feldenkrais

It does not work so well for me to be overly academic about things. I have to be in the fabric of life. That is why I love doing workshops, because everything happens right there and then, so you have to be really present in the moment. I would love to go back to the time before I discovered Feldenkrais to see what the difference was. That would be a profound thing to do. On a practical level, I am a runner and it has kept me injury free. It is something amazing to grow old with. Some of the greatest teachers I know are in their 80s and they can sit on the floor and get back up with no issues whatsoever. It has shown me that it really does work to keep your functions healthy. With each workshop I do, people go away feeling better and I also leave feeling much better, so it creates a circle.

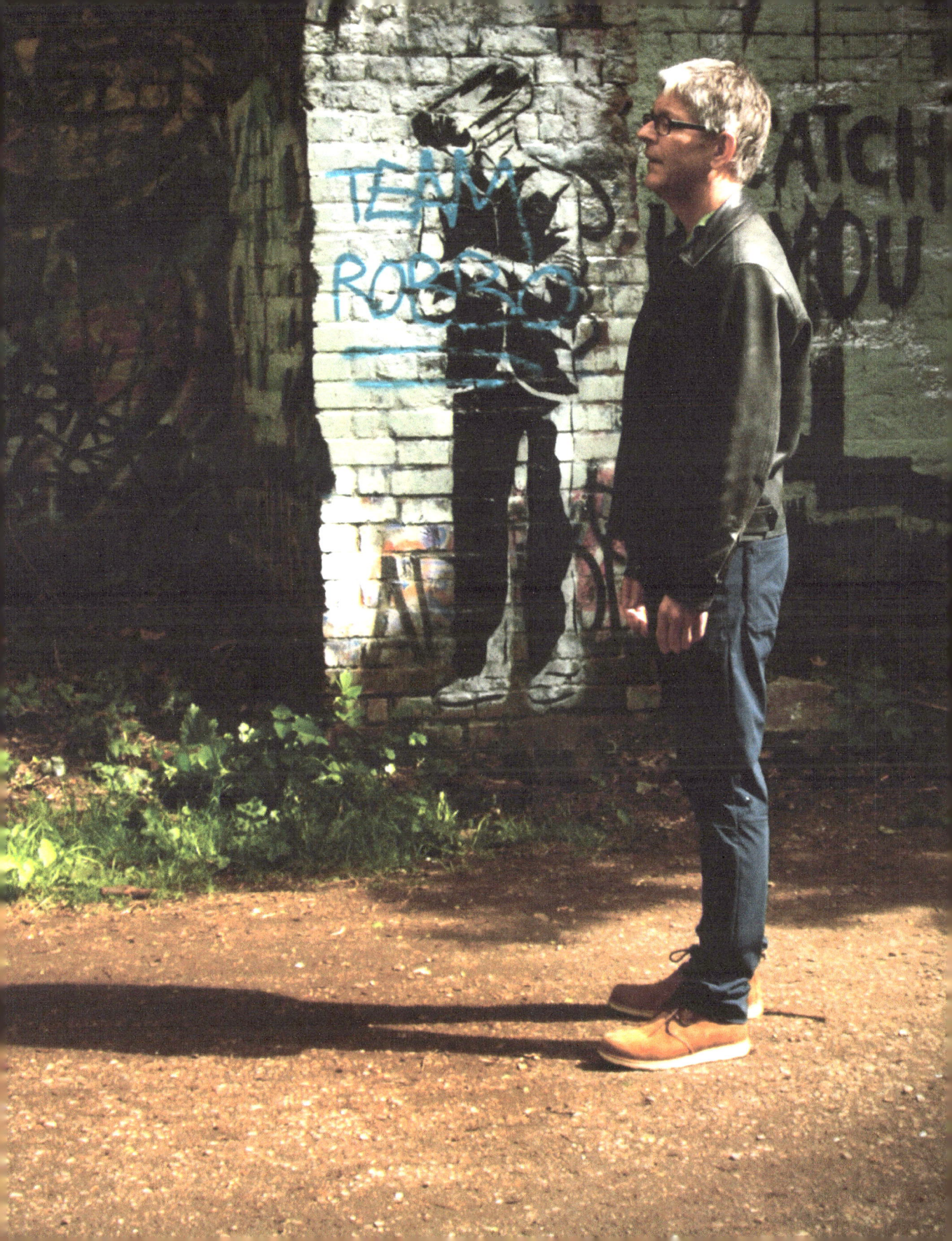

"As an osteopath I know we are all built exactly the same way, we may be varying sizes or we may be older or younger, but what really makes us different is our story."

- Indera Ajimal

Osteopathy

A physician and surgeon called Andrew Taylor Still developed osteopathy in 1874. It is mainly concerned with how the structure of the body relates to its function. The osteopath will focus primarily on the skeletal building blocks of the body together with the person's history, range of movement, ease of movement and how the soft tissue of the body looks, feels and responds to motion, in order to track where misalignments exist. The founding surmise of osteopathy is that the body has an inherent intelligence to heal itself. Various manual manipulations are applied to remind the body of where its equilibrium and balance is.

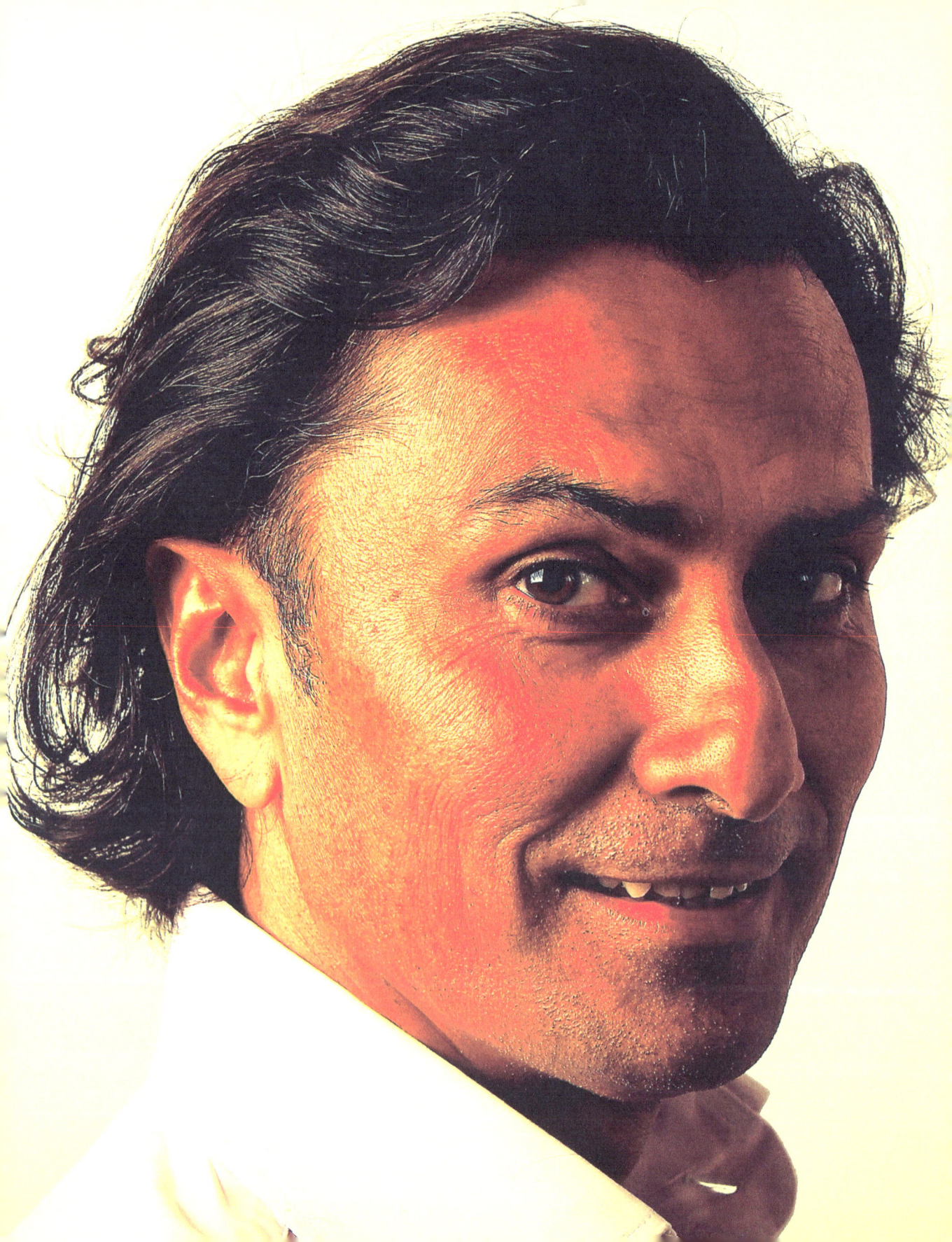

Gerry Gajadharsingh DO
Founder of The Health Equation, Osteopath, Diagnostic Consultant and Lecturer

Gerry Gajadharsingh is what one could call a modern medicine man. He is an osteopath who is highly versed in nutrition, biochemistry and psychology. He lectures globally and uses the teaching element of his work, to hone and craft his knowledge and understanding in his chosen subjects. To Gerry the most important element in achieving wellness is diagnosis. This means as his patient you are given an accurate and thorough assessment of where your imbalances are and empowered with the tools to make permanent change. Through him I got a glimpse of what integrative medicine can truly offer.

When I was at school fencing was my passion. During a fencing competition I lunged and unintentionally did the splits, sustaining a really bad groin injury. At the time neither orthopaedics nor physiotherapy could help. I saw an osteopath and because it was a straightforward muscular skeletal injury, I had full exposure to the medicine of osteopathy and it cured me. I was truly fascinated and this became my career path. Before I began my training in osteopathy, I was always under the impression that it was a holistic form of medicine. However, although I did a year each of clinical psychology and clinical nutrition as an undergraduate, my knowledge was inadequate when applied to the real life scenarios of my patients. In the years after I qualified as an osteopath, I have been lucky to work with some amazing people who have cemented me and encouraged me to holistically develop my speciality.

Another influential factor in my career was that I became very ill around fifteen years ago with a rheumatological condition. I then realised that general medicine was very limited in its understanding of the causes of diseases and its strategy for treatment was exclusively limited to drugs. While I needed drugs in the beginning, it was never really going to cure my problem. So that set me on the pathway of exploring what illness actually was. The reason I set up The Health Equation was because I thought that there had to be a more expansive viewpoint on illness and the creation of wellness.

I qualified twenty-six years ago as an osteopath and, whilst palpation and Osteopathic Manual Techniques (structural, soft tissue, fascial, cranial and visceral) are still a large part of my job, diagnostic medicine is also a major component.

In order to do a treatment, you first really have to understand what the patient's issue is. For the majority of my new patients, our first appointment is spent giving light to why they may be ill. It is then a case of deciding which clinician is best suited to get them better. That may mean referring them to a psychological team, an exercise team, nutritional medicine or osteopathic manual treatment. To me this initial stage is critical. Patients have a habit of exploring treatments, so they would say for example that one modality was not good because it didn't help them and another was brilliant because it did. However, treatments are only really helpful if the patient is directed to the right one, so the first step is always diagnostic.

The Importance of Diagnosis

Making an accurate diagnosis requires good listening skills. I personally believe that the focus of the history is to listen to what the patient has to say. So you are using your intelligence, clinical background and knowledge to try to make sense of them and gently explore what might be relevant on a deeper level. During a consultation I usually start with a blank sheet of paper and invite the patient to tell me their story. We have a saying that everything is always about something else. So the patient may come in with a problem, but that problem normally has nothing to do with what is actually going on. Sometimes you have to manage their symptoms in the short term, but often there is an underlying story and you need to find out what that story happens to be.

I truly believe in individualised medicine, meaning that every single history is completely different. The only questionnaire I give patients to complete is an online psychological profile because I am very interested in where their mind is. With someone who is psychologically and emotionally aware we may be able to take a more expansive view. Whereas with the person who isn't we would, for example, concentrate on the strained muscles in their shoulder, until we were able to build a rapport with them and help them understand a bit more about what their overriding issue may be.

Ultimately, what I do is help people to change their belief systems. Part of the process of being an osteopath is using my hands as diagnostic tools, so I can feel what is happening within the body structure. I am then able to gauge the relationship between the body structure and function and the person's emotional patterns. Generally in day-to-day interactions we use 5% of our brains consciously. The other 95% is the subconscious nervous system, which drives every single thing within the body. So if a person's issue is musculoskeletal, I then need to see if there is an underlying subconscious pattern that is not allowing good muscle function.

For most new patients there will be a comprehensive report that would most likely include a number of health tests. I believe in keeping extensive notes, partly from a research perspective and also because I think patients need to understand what is actually wrong. Sometimes when a patient receives a treatment it appears to be magical. They lie down, someone does something and then they are better. They do not necessarily engage with the process. However, I believe that the aim of the treatment is to empower the patient so that ongoing treatment is minimal. This is done firstly with accurate information on why their system has gone wrong. Then by giving them the educational tools, including awareness on eating, breathing, psychology and mechanical and muscular function, once they have this knowledge most people can do without having any treatment whatsoever.

Making a Diagnosis

A patient may come in to see me with a shoulder pain and musculoskeletal examination may show that they have pulled a muscle. The next level is, why has that muscle been pulled? So I would look at what is going on with their life at the moment. Are they an upper ribcage breather? If they are it may make those muscles even more tense, which could have led to the injury. Do they carry the weight of the world on their shoulders? Are there disagreements going on with their spouse? Is there something that they are stressing about psychologically that may be relevant? Are they a big drinker? The liver may be connected to the right shoulder. So there are many ways to approach the subject, it just depends on what the patient is able to take and how willing they are to explore.

Patients never get better until they understand what is wrong with them. The understanding can come in a flashing lightbulb moment or they may need therapy. If a patient has struggled in the past, often they may have had many different treatments with no positive outcomes. 99% of the time it is not because they didn't have successful therapy, instead the diagnosis is usually incorrect and the patient does not understand why they are ill. Until their belief surrounding why they are ill is brought to their awareness, there is no therapist in the world that can truly get them better.

The Future

The challenge is that there are not many people who like to think outside the box, because it requires an enormous amount of work. So nutritionists will probably remain nutritionists, osteopaths remain as osteopaths and General Practitioners probably stay as GPs. My own view is that if we were able to educate enough people in truly integrative medicine, we would actually save the NHS billions of pounds.

For my 50th birthday I was given a book called *The Doctor, His Patient and The Illness*. It was a story of fourteen GPs in London and their selected patients, who were followed over a period of five years. The questions were: What did the GPs think was wrong with the patients? How did they treat them? Who did they refer them to? What did they think the x-rays showed? The whole exercise was supported by a psychiatrist and a team of psychotherapists at the world famous Tavistock Clinic. The conclusions were that at least half of the patients' illnesses were psychologically linked. What the GPs thought they were doing for the patient they weren't, and what the patients thought the GPs were doing they weren't. The fascinating thing about this book is that it was published in 1952 but it is still very relevant now.

My workload is taken up by so many people who have had extensive medical investigations and they are still no better off. You have a massive waste of resources in the NHS, and in the private sector, either the insurance or the patient pays. But, a lot of the time, they are not really discovering what is wrong with them. Taking the route of accurately diagnosing the issue may require some time to reach a conclusion because it is about identifying the belief system that is causing the malfunction. However, once you manage to get people on the right belief system, things change radically and they get better.

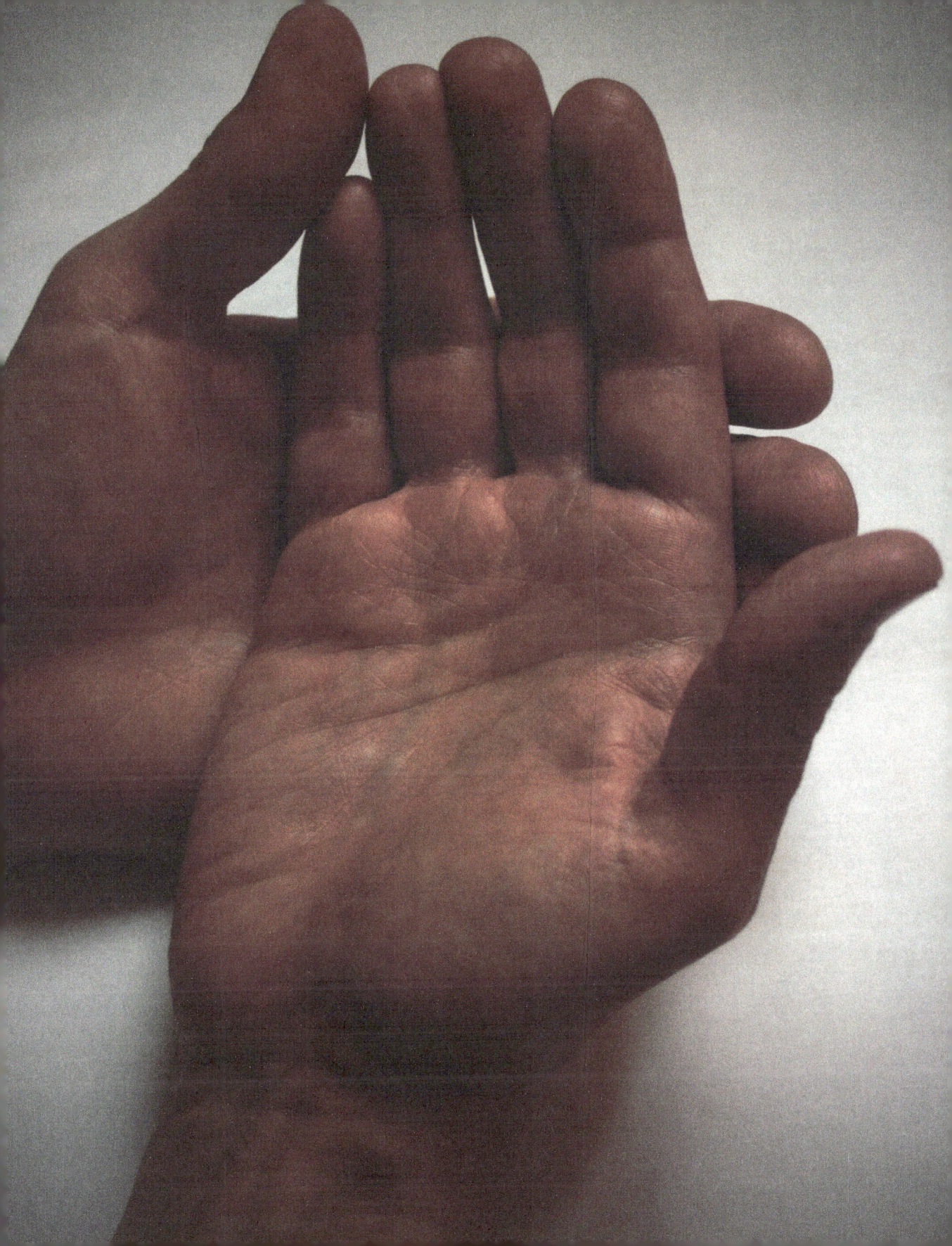

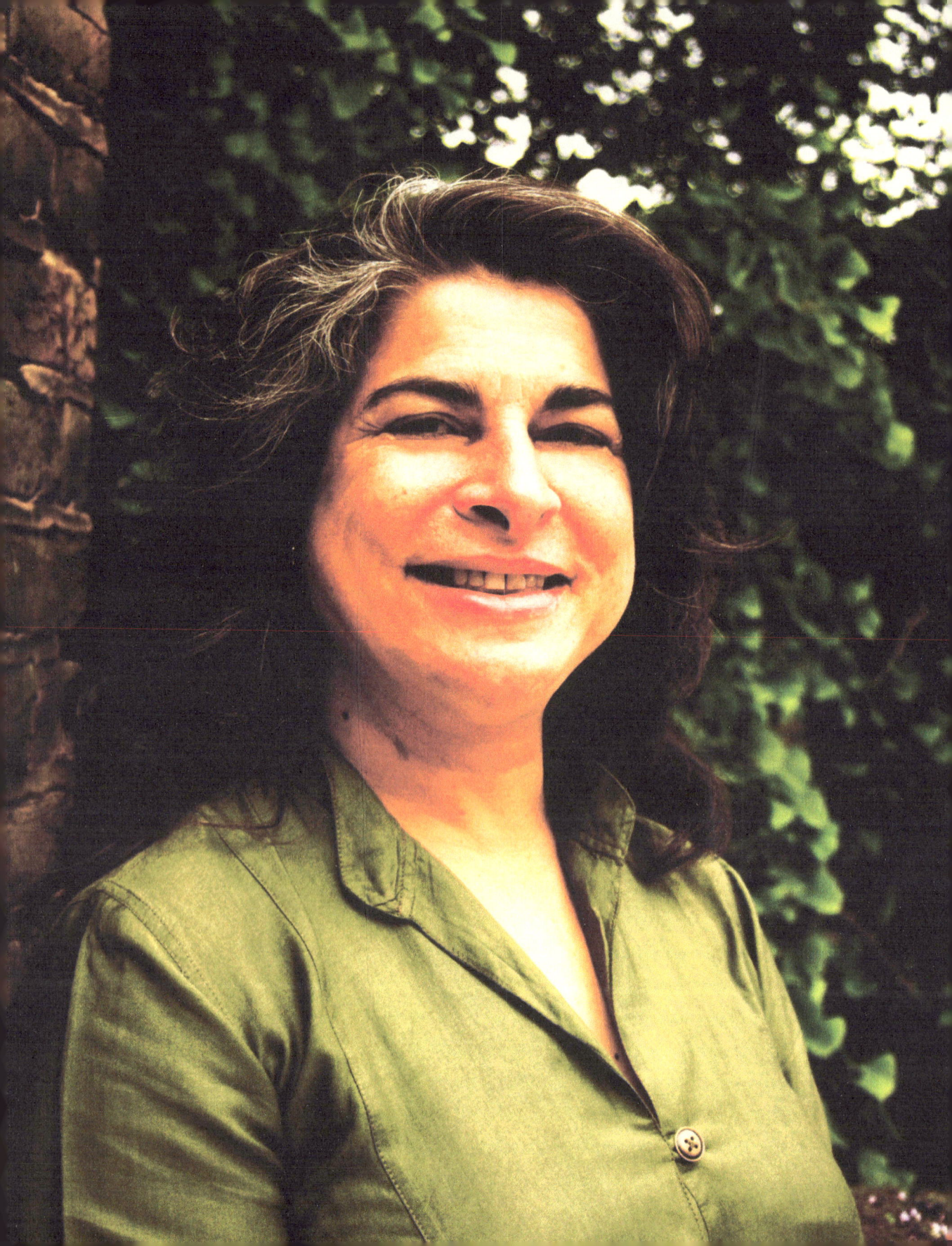

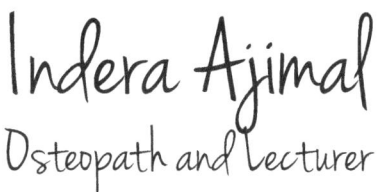

Indera Ajimal
Osteopath and Lecturer

Indera Ajimal, or Indi as she is known informally, exudes a warmth and genuineness that makes you feel immediately at ease with her. As an osteopath it is clear that she is passionate and really cares for her patients, over and above what would be considered standard. Although she would describe herself as a general health practitioner, treating from the cradle to the grave, as she calls it, the area closest to her heart is women's health. She offers a solid support system and knowledgeable voice of wisdom to both mothers and parents pre and post pregnancy. She is truly a rare gem in her field and it was an honour speaking to her about her work.

I started my career in nursing and it was the best decision I made because I loved meeting such a wide variety of people through my work. I started off on a Medical Ward and after some time moved to a Children's Ward. Part of my role in the children's department was to act as a support system for both the parents and particularly the mothers. Once I discovered how much I enjoyed this aspect of the job, I trained to become a midwife. People think that midwifery is all about babies, when it is really about being a voice of knowledge for the parents, and this role encouraged me to train as a health visitor in London.

I developed an urge to go travelling, which I did for two years and ended up working as a midwife teacher at a mission hospital in Uganda, where my dad was born. When I returned to the UK, I knew I wanted to expand my studies, so I applied for a traditional birthing teaching course in Kerala, India, but, before a firm commitment was made, a friend of mine introduced me to the idea of osteopathy. She said that she thought I would be really good at it and outlined the reasons why. I loved the idea, so I changed my study to a four-year full-time degree. Having worked in midwifery, I had learnt anatomy, physiology and the birthing ways of the baby. Osteopathy deepened my level of understanding of the body and its structures. It allowed me to put the pieces of my previous roles together under one umbrella.

Supporting Mothers

After the birthing process has taken place, everyone focuses on the baby postnatally, but forgets about all the pushing and shoving of the mother's internal tissues as it made its way into the world. One of my greatest passions is postnatal care and support for mothers. Even women between the ages of 50 and 70 come to see me about a current issue, where the dysfunction has its root in their pregnancy or birthing experience. It presents itself through things like incontinence, back pain or abdominal separation. Most of these are preventable, given the right action and information.

As women, we are generally very body aware. The cyclical aspect of our body functions through periods and fertility brings that awareness to us. Women often talk freely about their issues and have immense wisdom surrounding their bodies, but need access to a sound source of knowledge. In my ten years of doing osteopathy and thirty years of working within women's health, I have had a lengthy period of time to evaluate the results of my own care. This has brought me a lot of confidence because I know osteopathy works.

I also do a birth home visit at one or two weeks post pregnancy. Left alone, the woman will usually wait around four to six weeks before she comes to the clinic. By that time feeding problems have kicked in, maybe because the baby can't turn its head or the woman is not eating enough, or she is in pain. When I see the mother at her home, one or two weeks post pregnancy, I am able to treat her and the baby straight away. I do another visit between two and four weeks and then I will ask them to come to the clinic. This works well for them and they love it.

In some of the situations where there is a traumatic delivery and emergency caesarean, women end up with post traumatic stress syndrome. I had a lady who came to get treatment for her six-year-old child. I began asking her about her pregnancy history and she started crying, six years after the event. She came for her child, but she was the one who needed the support the most. In many cases young mothers are homesick because their support systems are not around them, or may be in a different country or city. Often their husbands are working long hours, which means that the woman ends up being very lonely. At times like this, my role is to be the mother who isn't there.

I really disagree with this thing called postnatal depression. Everyone is quite happy to label the woman as having postnatal depression, but if anyone has to stay in a house 24/7 with a screaming baby, I think it is possible that they would go slightly bonkers. It is important to allow the woman to express what she is feeling, because what she really needs during this time is support. It does not matter if it comes from her family, her husband or the woman next door, as long as there is help available. There are times when she needs an hour off to wash her hair or walk around the Park, or to go shopping for a dress. One woman told me that everyone thought she was had postnatal depression, but she did not feel that way.

What she was actually feeling was homesick. She was missing having her friends and family around her. She was from Australia and had only been in the UK for six months. They relocated because of her husband's job and once she realised what the cause of her unhappiness was, she was able to move past it. But sometimes the labelling that goes on is horrendous. I strongly feel that it is necessary for women to be given a combination of time and support before they go down the route of antidepressant medication.

Treating Children

I treat a number of issues in children. For example, one of my patients is a four-and-a-half-year-old who has the reading ability of a child of eight, but can't write. It was a really traumatic birth and somewhere along the line their neurological connections are not working. Neurological testing and MRIs have been done through the medical system, but to no avail. I am providing regular osteopathic treatments and monitoring the response. Another patient is a 22-month-old baby who is not walking or talking and has a squint. Once again, in this case, there was a very traumatic delivery. It is my belief that with every traumatic delivery the baby should automatically go to see a cranial osteopath.

One of my patients was a seventeen-year-old boy. He was physically big and played as a forward in rugby. He got into a pile-up during a game, where everyone landed on top of him causing him to have a prolapsed disc. We had to treat him in rehab so he could grow properly. Another rugby player was headbutted by accident as he was going for the ball, and experienced a personality change at the age of seventeen. He was refusing to study for his 'A' level exams and had become terribly rude to his parents, which was very unusual for him. His mother was trying every possible treatment she thought may be of help and I mentioned cranial osteopathy, because it was possible that he may have had whiplash in his neck and suffered damage to the frontal lobe of his brain, where the personality lives. With cranial sacral osteopathy he completely changed. It is in cases like these where I truly get to evaluate the results of my care.

Teaching

As well as being an osteopathic practitioner, I am a clinical tutor for the London School of Osteopathy. We have a student clinic where the students bring the patients in, take their history and present it to us. We then examine the history in order to determine if there is enough detail to provide a diagnosis. We watch them do the examinations, clinical tests, make a decision on the diagnosis and perform the treatment. I have been doing that for three years and love it. I also teach women's health, contraception and fertility at an academic level, including anatomy and physiology of the female reproductive system and the pathologies that affect this area, particularly the cancers.

My Work

I am a primary health care practitioner and I love to treat people from the cradle to the grave, it is not about being a specialist in one area for me. As an osteopath, I know we are all built exactly the same way. We may be different sizes or be older or younger, but the design is the same and we all have changing tissues and changing histories. I always tell my students that we are designed and built in exactly the same way, what makes us different is our story. This is why I place a great importance on the taking of a person's history.

With regards to my own work, I made the decision a long time ago that my ultimate life's choice was to be a teacher, on a community level, and provide support to women in a vulnerable stage of their lives and as a student teacher. I definitely feel that I am living my purpose.

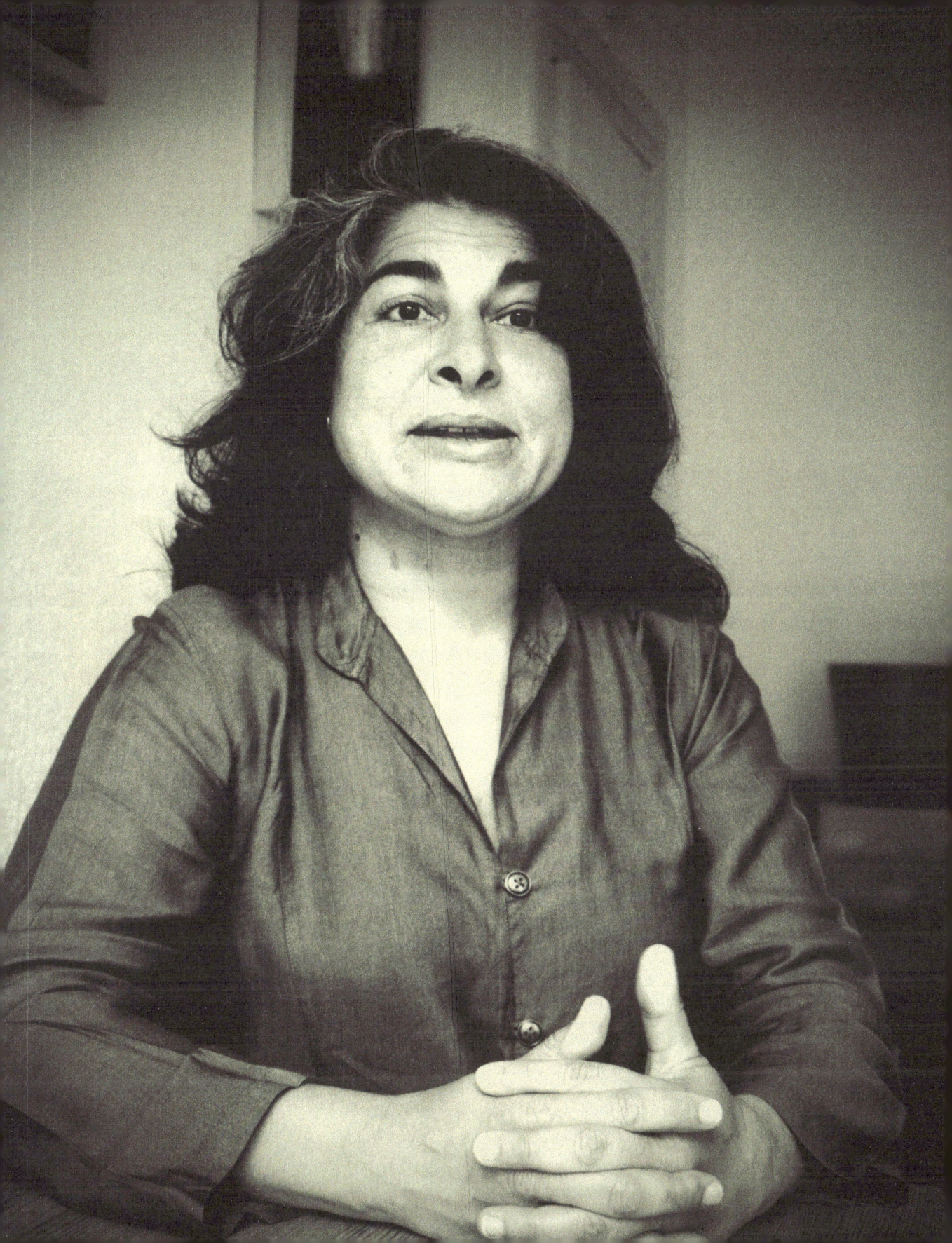

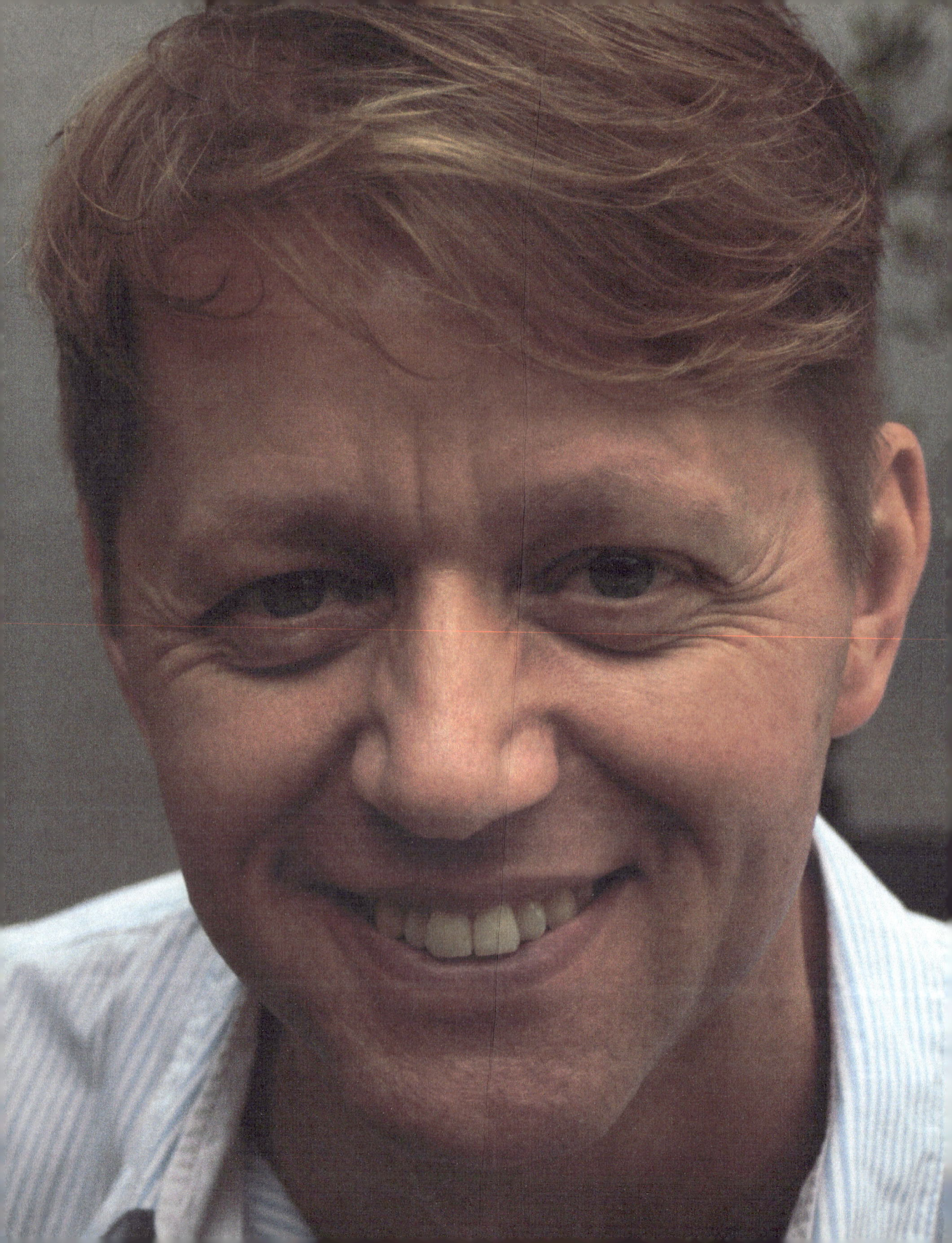

David Sheriff
Director of Vital Osteopathy and Lecturer

David came to osteopathy as a result of a willingness to redesign and recreate his career path. Ten years after qualifying he has built a hugely successful practice, lectured at The British College of Osteopathic Medicine and not looked back. He has a deep curiosity about the body and what it means to be performing at an optimum level, as well as a drive to continuously expand his knowledge and understanding of his field of work.

Before coming to osteopathy I worked in Cornwall for the National Rivers Authority. I loved it and worked very long hours and most weekends, but I got to the point where I knew I could not go on unless I studied as a scientist. There was no way I could study and work because I was working all the hours I could, so I decided to take three years out to do a degree.

It then occurred to me that if I had to stop working to study I could do anything I wanted to, which opened up a world of possibilities. I began to figure out what I truly wanted from my career. I knew I wanted to do something that was professionally respected, helped others and would enable me to work with my hands. It was also important for me to have a medical link, but I did not want to work in an environment where I did not see the body and health in a deeper setting. I did not want health to be impersonal and to be sending patients away with pills and instructions. Instead, I wanted to have a wider and more holistic approach and so osteopathy fulfilled everything on my list.

My attraction to natural health stems from my mother, who was a spiritualist, a healer and was quite well known in our area of Cornwall. She got involved in environmental groups, ran the vegetarian society, did vegetarian open days and ran a meditation and spiritual group. Both my parents embraced the whole new age thing in a big way, although my father was also in the oil industry, until they sold up and moved to Cornwall to enjoy life and get away from the pressures of modern living. My mother was always in touch with her own healing abilities, which came as a result of her upbringing. Her parents ran a spiritualist church in Wales and this had a huge impact on her.

My Work

When it came to my own work, I wanted a scientific and recognised way of looking at the body, as well as a sound knowledge base. I chose The British College of Osteopathic Medicine above the others because I thought it had the right mix. It did not just focus on osteopathy, we were also taught naturopathy, which involved studying nutrition, psychology and counselling. We were taught about the triangular link between the emotional, the physical and the nutritional, and so it offered a very good basis.

I do not go into people's diet and nutrition. This is not because I am not interested, but because it is very in depth and you need to keep up-to-date. I'm here to do the physical stuff, but when I am treating someone I am very conscious of the link with their emotions. So I am as likely to ask them about how life has been, as I am to ask what they have been doing physically. It is interesting when you can get people to make the link between how they are feeling and why they are expressing pain. I am usually the person during the healing process who is there to help my client through a difficult patch in life. I not only give them the physical help that they need, but I give them a little bit of comfort and understanding. I am someone they can let off steam to.

My Clients

In my work I see a huge variety of people, my youngest patient is four and my oldest ninety-two. The reasons why people come to me really varies and depends on the individual. Some people are in touch with their instincts and are in tune when their body is out of kilter, others who come in are physical wrecks but have absolutely no knowledge of this. Their bodies could be tumbling down but as long as the pain is gone, they are ok. These people are more likely to be taking painkillers in order to rid themselves of the pain, so that they can keep going. When people are more in tune with their bodies they are more likely to come in and say, I am not in pain, but I just don't feel right, I feel out. I fully understand what they mean by that.

There is a huge lifestyle aspect to osteopathy and, after being here all this time, there are a number of people who just drop in and use me as they would an aspirin. I have a lot of clients that I see three to five times a year and they come because they recognise that their aches and pains are not something they have to put up with; they know they can get them treated. There are also a lot of people with whom I have quite a close bond and it is a social thing now, which is great, and others come in just to offload as they have a lot going on in their lives.

Fulfilment

There are a number of things I find gratifying about my work. There is the physical healing element that people receive and the immense job satisfaction, as 99.9% of the time people you treat experience some form of improvement, which is very rewarding. I am also fulfilling my need to learn a lot more about the human body, the way it works and how it is interconnected, and there is also a drive to learn what the physical optimum performance of the body is.

I have no desire to study Pilates or yoga at this point, but I am beginning to understand the contribution they make in creating a balanced physical structure, and how this equates very much spiritually with the concept of being completely aware of what is going on, and living in the now. Living in the now is about centring yourself both mentally and physically and, in doing so, there seems to be a kind of unifying factor.

Osteopathy

The physical and energetic bodies are completely interlinked. But many people are often either deeply reflective of the past or so wound up in the future they continually think about what they have to achieve, where they are going and what they need to do to get there. They have 101 things on their mind - the kids, the lists and all the things that have to be done to keep juggling the balls in the air. As they are walking along they are bent forward, hunched over as all their energy is in front of them. You need to withdraw back from that, in order to return back to yourself.

The great thing about osteopathy is that when people come in for treatment you can start reading them. You are able to read where they are in their lives and what they are doing by their body shape and structure. So half the time my role is about holding a mirror up to people and reflecting themselves back to them. I give people gentle nudges. You have to be realistic about what they can and can't do, but there is nothing wrong with gently nudging them towards positive changes.

On the other side, though, it is really funny when I come across people who come in and want to know everything, right now. They want to know all their exercises and instructions on what they have to do because they want to change their life, right now, in this instant. With the impatience and frustration they are expressing, you know it is just not going to happen. It is then important to bring their attention to the fact that the body responds best to kindness and patience.

The Future

As an osteopath, through my interaction with a huge cross section of people, there have been opportunities for personal growth, as well as a lot of professional knowledge that has been gained. Here I am 12 years after graduating, really hungry to learn a lot more and I know that I will never get to a place where I will stop learning, which is really nice. I am embodying what I am here to do, and I can say this without a doubt and with a smile on my face.

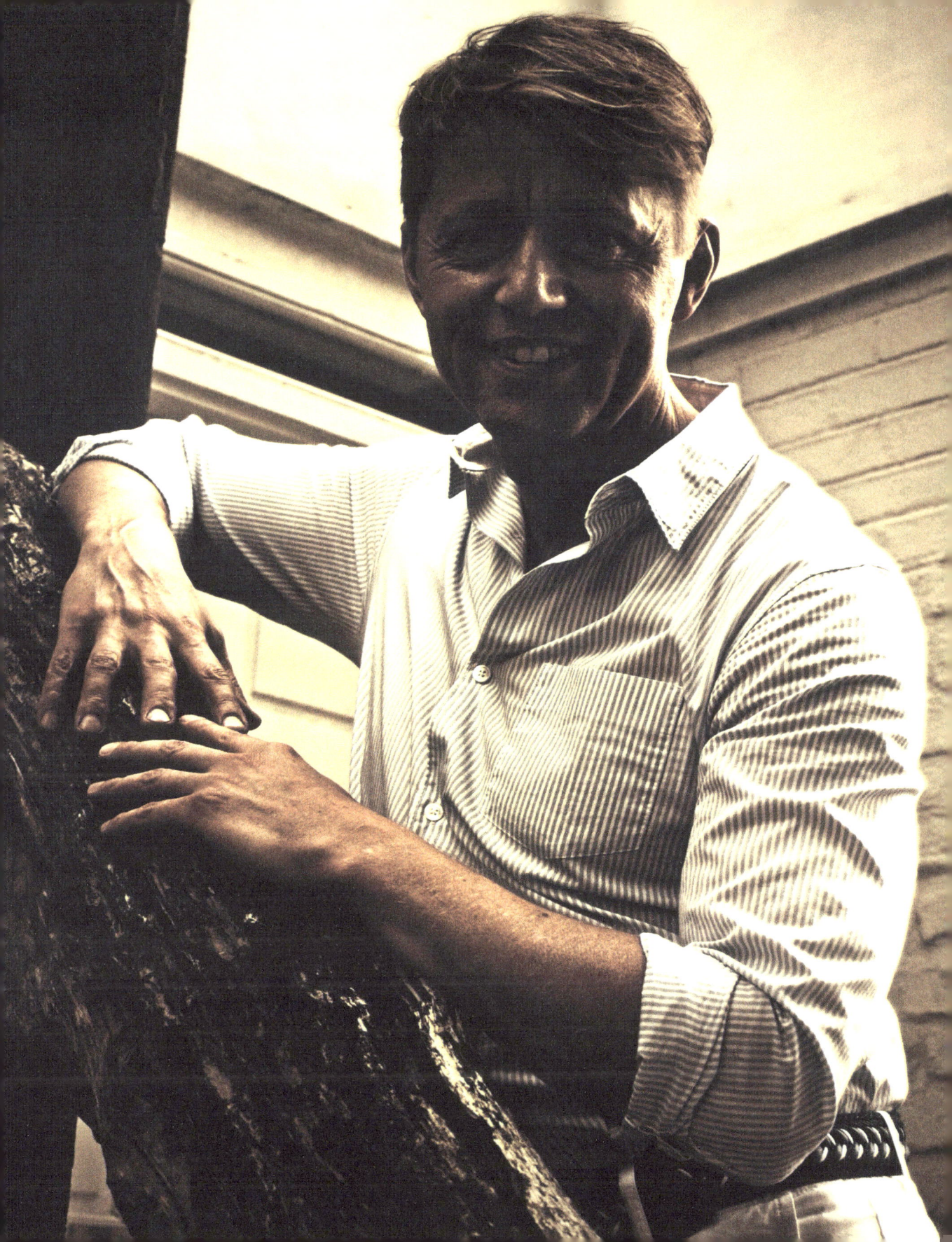

"While I was doing my A Levels, we were sent to do some community work, which took us to a centre with people who had learning difficulties. There was a physio there working with a little boy who had cerebral palsy. I watched as she turned this tight, angst-ridden child, into a fluid movable being and I was completely blown away."

- Anna Barnsley

Physiotherapy

Physiotherapy was designed to treat individuals who are being rehabilitated because of physical dysfunction, which could be due to injury, illness or structural misalignments within the body. After a diagnosis has been made the Physiotherapist would use manual manipulation, prescribed exercises and stretches and lifestyle advice in order to create change. The educational element is seen as vastly important because the assumption is made that knowledge is power, so the more supportive, positive information the patient has at their disposal the greater their ability to heal and return to optimal function.

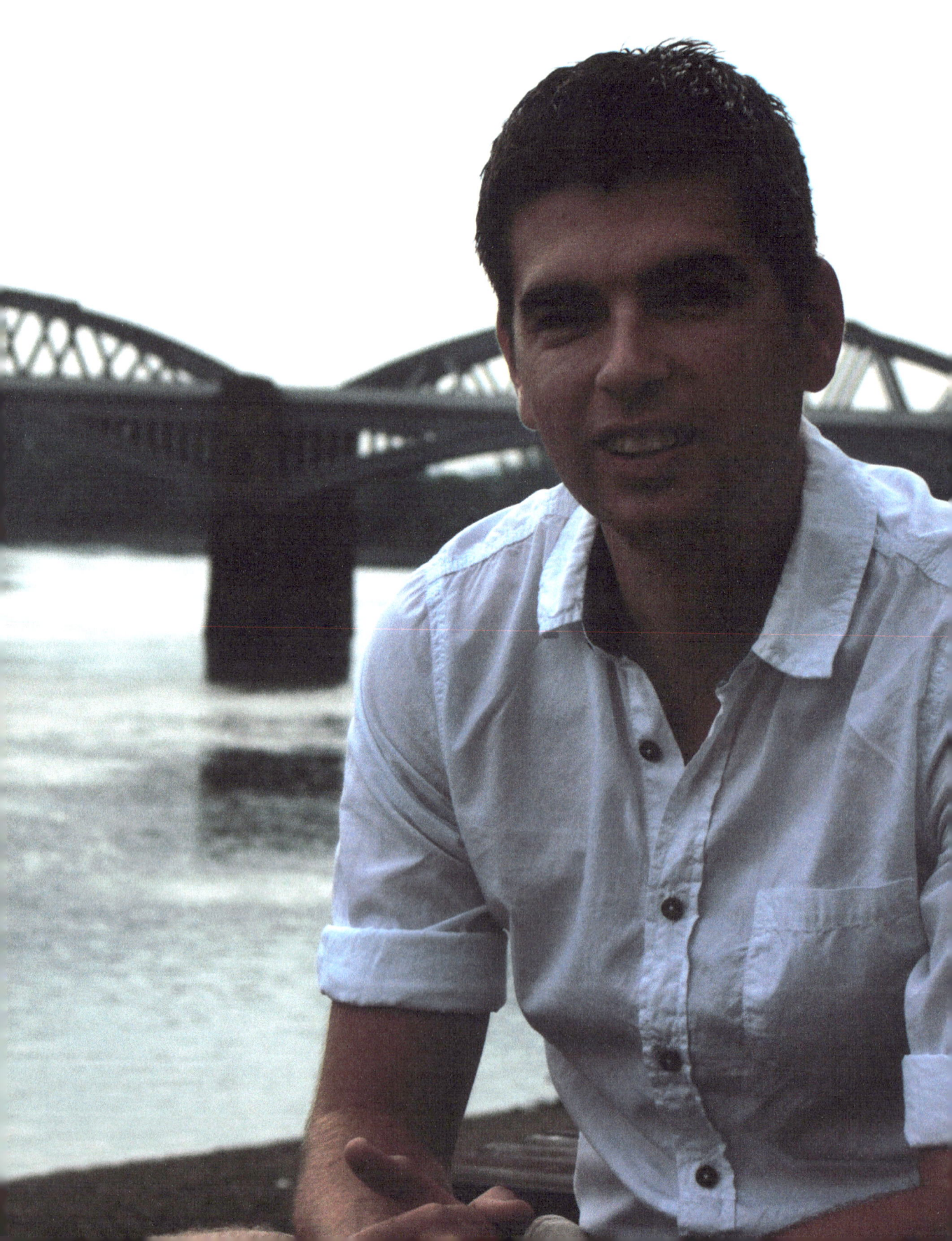

Martin Baker
Chelsea Football Club Physiotherapist

Martin Baker worked as a physiotherapist on a part-time basis for Chelsea Football Club and built a very successful private practice. He now works for Chelsea full time and at the age of twenty-nine he exudes an air of assurance and confidence in his abilities. But this aura is not by chance, he has built up his experience by working gruelling hours in intense situations within an NHS hospital. This has allowed him to craft, hone and meld his discipline in physiotherapy, getting him on a fast track to a place of wealth in understanding, knowledge and wisdom.

I got into physiotherapy purely by accident. When I picked my 'A' levels, I chose the subjects I liked studying the most, which were sports, physical education and biology. Following on from that I did sports science, which included injury prevention work and anatomy at a very basic level, both of which I liked. When I came to choosing a career path I looked for something that utilised my education and physiotherapy was a natural progression.

I always had a clear idea of what I loved doing but I think my parents had quite an influence in this, because they always made it understood that I should do what I enjoyed. They warned me to avoid choosing a career in something I did not like because I would not want to complete it or do it to the best of my ability. They also identified the fact that I had the temperament to be a good teacher. I knew I did not want to be deskbound in my job, so physiotherapy seemed to tick all the boxes. This was mainly because I would work to help, teach and inform people, and I would still be using the elements of sports science and biology, which I loved.

Working within the NHS

I found the work I did within the NHS to be really stressful and I wasn't happy, but I knew I was learning a lot. I wanted to pick up and absorb as much of the information as I could, but in order to do that within physiotherapy at that time, I had to be in an environment that didn't suit me, so it was always a tricky trade-off.

I found working within a hospital environment to be quite draining. A lot of people I dealt with were in the outpatients unit; however, they didn't really want to get better and didn't listen to my advice. Although this was great for me in terms of developing my communication skills, I found the work a massive challenge. Everyday the people I treated were coming back and saying that there was no improvement in their condition, but when I questioned them I would realise that they were not doing any of the exercises or taking on any of the aftercare advice given to them. It was like banging my head against a brick wall and that was just very frustrating. Additionally, the work required long hours and at one point I had gone for sixty-seven days without a day off.

On the other hand, I loved being on the wards and doing post-op care, because in that environment physiotherapy made a massive difference really quickly. People in the position of recovering after an operation were always appreciative and they had a great desire to get better. I also loved working in intensive care, but I found aspects of it quite depressing, as I was not able to emotionally separate the patient from the work. I was quite miserable when end of life decisions were made for patients on whom I had done physiotherapy. Having said all that though, when I look back on this period, the lessons I learnt were amazing. I am thankful for the experience, because it got me where I am today and has given me a strong knowledge base.

Physiotherapy for the Chelsea Football Club

One of my lecturers who I became good friends with knew my capabilities and, through a contact, found out that Chelsea FC were looking for a physiotherapist. She recommended me and I started with the club straight from university, working part-time and later on a full-time basis. Part of my job is to do game cover, so that means dealing with injuries, assessments, emergency aid and physiotherapy during match times. When the team is training, I am in the physiotherapy room or the gym doing rehabilitation and injury treatments.

Defining Physiotherapy

In defining physiotherapy, I would say that when a person has a physical impairment or is in pain due to injury, having physio enables them to achieve their goal of getting better in the shortest possible time. It creates an environment, where they can get back to performing the same actions they did before the physical impairment. The practice involves problem solving and finding a cure.

I think physiotherapists are very good at picking up on different pain states and how pain is being conceptualised. Pain is only an interpretation of the mind; it is a feeling rather than a physical symptom.

When people have had chronic pain for a while, they tend to see it as being a physical manifestation rather than a mental interpretation. Additionally, there is a lot of research into physiotherapy, which shows that stress massively feeds into pain interpretation. So, whether pain is a perception or an actuality really just depends on the experience of the person and their interpretation. As a physiotherapist, to get to the root of the issue, you sometimes have to dig really deeply while at the same time not being intrusive. The aim is not only to get rid of the pain, but also to keep it away.

So, for example, one of my patients was told that their back was unstable. There are words in physiotherapy that research has shown should never be used within a consultation. From the viewpoint of medical diagnosis, an unstable area of the body means simply that the area cannot be fully controlled by the person. But if a patient is told that their back is unstable it triggers fear, they immediately hold it in a locked position and minimise their movements. Over time, an injury may have healed, but because of overcompensation, the back becomes locked into place and the range of movement completely inhibited.

This can also happen when someone is told that there is degeneration of the spine. In medical terms degeneration describes an aging or a wear and tear process. However, when you tell a patient who hasn't got that background that they are degenerated, they see it as something that is going to progressively worsen. They begin to hold themselves in quite a rigid way, which leads to pain. The pain acts as confirmation to them that damage in the back is occurring, when in fact there are three distinct areas that flow into creating an interpretation of the pain. These are emotional, physical and neurological, and all of these factors need to be addressed.

In terms of neuromuscular control, the muscles switch on and off to move a body part or to keep a body part in position, by neural pathways. The brain has to tell the muscles and the joints what to do. Equally, if you touch the skin the nerve sends a message to the brain to interpret the sensation. There is a condition called allodynia where normal touch gets interpreted as excruciatingly painful because the nerve sends a message to the brain that touch is dangerous. Since there is no damage to the area, if you get the person to rub their skin for extended periods the pain will dampen over time and eventually normal sensation will return.

To be successful with physiotherapy, which means curing rather than just treating a problem, you have to take into account that people will go back into their home en-vironment. Meaning that they may be stressed at work, they may have bad working postures – which they maintain throughout the day – or they may have kids, worries postures – which they maintain throughout the day – or they may have kids, worries and illness to contend with. It all relates.

Being a physiotherapist

I always wanted to enjoy my work by making a difference, being a good physiotherapist and not getting complacent as time goes on. But I think it is also important to have time to go away for the weekend or to see my family and friends.

A lot was put into perspective when my best friend, who had studied physiotherapy with me, passed away four years ago. This experience massively shifted my emphasis on life. It may sound a bit clichéd, but he was my age and was aiming for exactly the same things, when he had a cardiac arrest while running a race and that was it, game over. It is easy to say, but you have got to just enjoy life while you are here and I suppose that is what I am doing with my job. I am aiming to work in a way that makes me happy. In the meantime, through physiotherapy, I not only help people to be pain free, I am actually making a difference to them and assisting them to a position where they can use their bodies efficiently, for which they are really thankful. For me this is a great place to be.

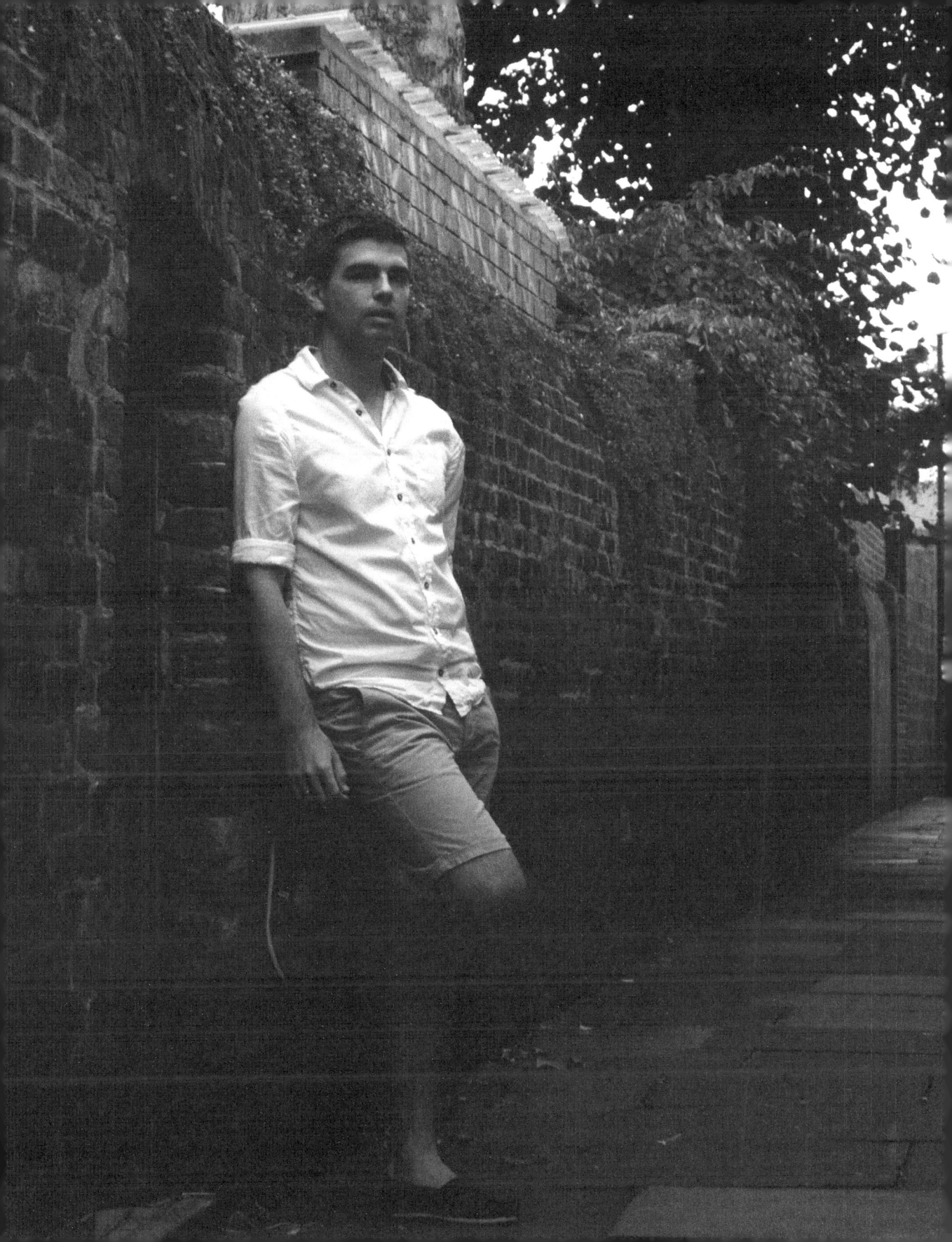

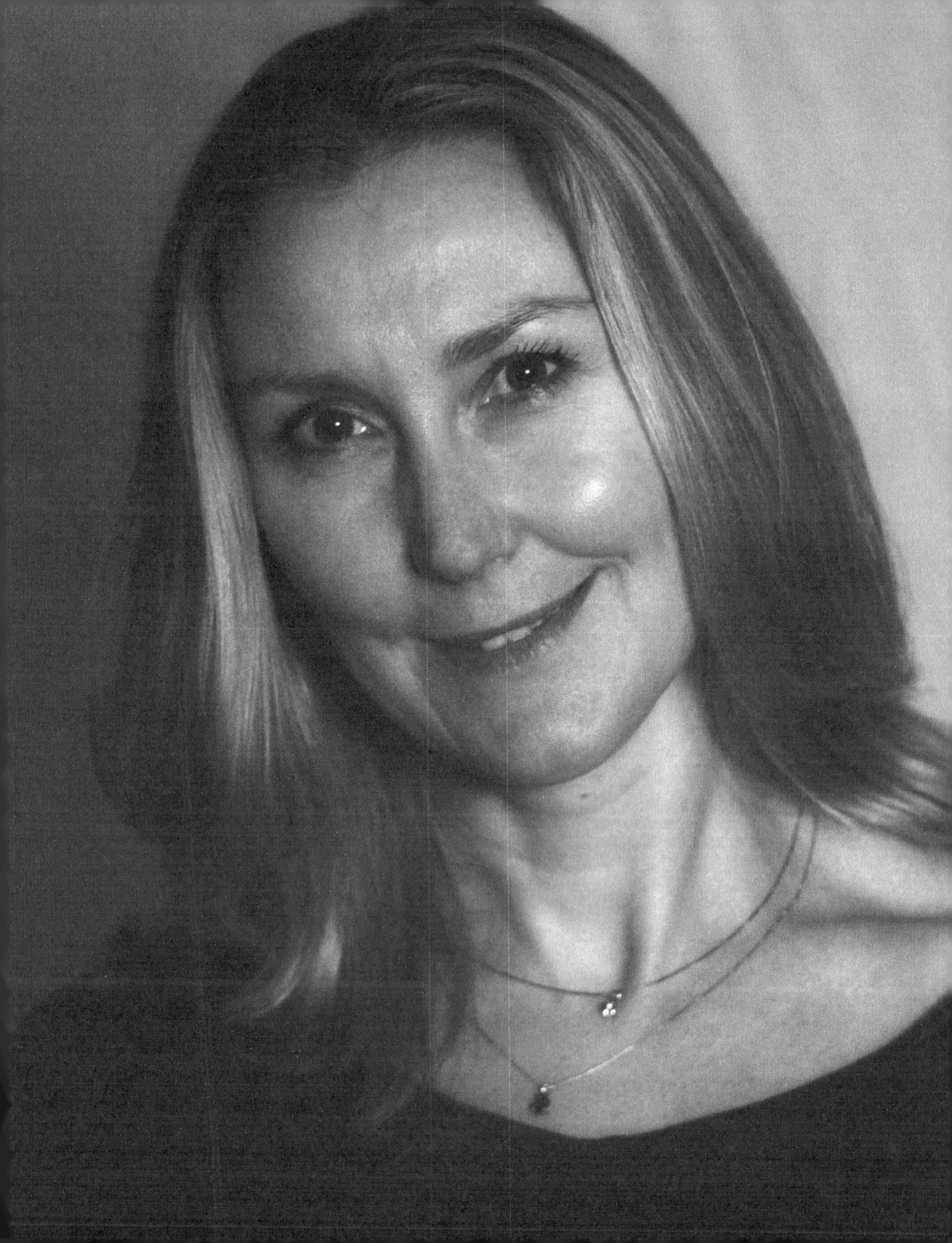

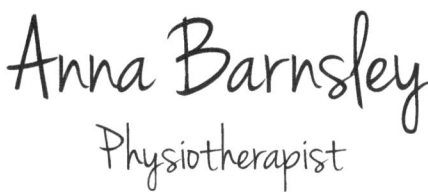

Anna Barnsley
Physiotherapist

As a physiotherapist, Anna Barnsley has explored and expanded her world through her work. From treating the England under-18s rugby team to working with amputees, to working in television, to being the tour physio for Take That, her journey has been far from run of the mill. Yet on meeting her, you are enveloped in the down-to-earth, genuine, nurturing and warm energy that she exudes. It was great to discover why she is so passionate about Physio.

I was introduced to physiotherapy by accident rather than design. While I was doing my A Levels, we were sent to do some community work, which took us to a centre with people who had learning difficulties. There was a physio there working with a little boy who had cerebral palsy. I watched as she turned this tight, angst-ridden child, into a fluid movable being and I was completely blown away.

I started a three-year degree in physio and whilst studying I had to work in the National Health Service, and then spend around two years as a postgraduate rotating around different disciplines. My first position was working with amputees in Essex to develop my musculoskeletal knowledge. The job was meant to be for twelve weeks but I stayed there for nine months. What was really interesting was that my dad is an amputee, who lost his foot when he was twelve. I was sitting with a couple of patients in the gym one day and the conversation led to me speaking about my dad losing his foot. This was the first time it really hit me that my dad was an amputee. He just got on with life, climbing the Matterhorn and the Monte Rosa, and is a huge inspiration. I never saw him as being different in any way.

As a junior physio you normally get experience from a number of different areas, so I moved on to work as a junior in a better teaching hospital. However, when I first got there I was placed in the outpatients department dealing with musculoskeletal medicine. I did rotation there for three months. Then I got a senior job based on musculoskeletal work. So, after graduating in 1995, I never worked in any of the other disciplines. There were many facets within musculoskeletal medicine and I got a very broad grounding in that.

During my first three months in the outpatients department I met an amazing physio, who inspired me greatly. She looked after a little local rugby team part-time, but got a job with a bigger club and didn't want to leave her team in the middle of the season. She put me forward because she knew I would love it and she was right. The first match that I ran for them was the first rugby game I had ever watched in my life. In rugby, the physio has to run on in the middle of everything, so I had to dodge players because I was not familiar with the way the game flowed. That was my first step into the sport and I worked my way up to looking after the England under-18s.

Physiotherapy

I am passionate about Physio because it changes people's lives. When someone comes to me in pain, whether it is a sports injury or a chronic back problem, it affects them fundamentally on every level – psychologically, spiritually and physically. To have that person in front of me, and know that I have the knowledge and tools to make them better, gives me a huge buzz. Everyone wants to know that they are great at their job and feel valued in what they do. So I make a difference in the life of my patients and they make a difference in mine, it is affirming for all of us.

There are various elements of physiotherapy that I am exploring at the moment. For example, there is some amazing work being done into pain mechanisms I find fascinating. This looks at neuro-physiology and where the concept of pain originates from, and layers that with the person's personality, life experiences and the way they process information. All of these factors contribute to their concept of pain. Often my patients need evidence of what is happening to them bio-mechanically. They want to know how muscular issues have led to the repercussions that they are experiencing, and you can take them on a further journey through other areas, once you have gained their trust.

My Work

My work is about turning a negative experience into something that has a positive outcome. Take chronic back pain, for example. On a physiological level it could be called a postural issue. So we could say that the person is overloading their back in precise ways, because of quite specific movements. We can change them bio-mechanically by loosening certain joints and treating the muscles related to the affected area. Then we can get them to do physical activities in order to offload the area they have been overloading. Ultimately, as a result of all those changes, their posture will be better, their health will be better and they will be both stronger and fitter. This is what occurs on the physical level, but it is also important to talk to them about what the back pain means to them in relation to their life experiences.

When a person has pain over an extended period of time, I aim to understand the deeper reasons for its manifestation. This will allow me to see if the issue is something that I can deal with quickly, if there are a lot of layers to think about, or if I need to refer them elsewhere. With some patients, it is important to get them to acknowledge that there may be other aspects contributing to their pain. They do not necessarily have to make drastic changes, but having the awareness would mean that they are listening to their bodies a lot more.

A lot of musculoskeletal physiotherapy is exercise based, which gives people a lot of control over their healing and pain. In giving them control on a physical level, it creates the space for them to think about what else could be contributing to the situation. I always aim to interact with the body on a very deep level in order to create lasting change, so I start by working with the person to activate individual muscle groups, allowing them to reacquaint and reconnect the brain with the body. For this process to be effective, they have to be fully engaged, which means getting rid of any distractions. It is about shutting everything off and just being with themselves. It might only be for ten minutes, but in that time they come out of their heads and really feel their bodies. They feel what the body does, how it moves and they spend time consciously nurturing it.

Being Open To Opportunities

A series of events led to me being involved in a football programme called The Match, in which celebrities played against former professional footballers. Jonathan Wilkes, a friend of Robbie Williams, was on the show. I worked with him for three years, so I got to know him quite well. Out of the blue one day, I got a call saying that Robbie Williams was in London and he had injured his back. He was supposed to be playing football the following week for Soccer Aid and needed help. Jonny had recommended me as a physiotherapist. I treated him at his home and on my second visit he asked me to be the physiotherapist for his 2006 Close Encounters World Tour. Within three weeks I had sorted my business out so I could leave it for nine months and went on tour. This was a most amazing opportunity. I grew up in a tiny little village with horses and cows. I did not have a television until I was around twelve and I spent most of my time riding outdoors, so I could not believe it. This was a huge privilege and led to me being introduced to Take That in 2010, and working as a physio on their Progress Tour in 2011.

My business just naturally started expanding to the point where I needed first one physio, then another, and then a receptionist. Before I knew it I had a team in place. I was bowled over with that process and carried on growing my business and utilising all of the opportunities I could. It was great for me at the time and I really learned from it. I loved having a staff of physiotherapists to nurture, but I also found running the business side of things frustrating as well. It got to a place where I was spending the majority of my time running the business, which took me further away from the hands-on element of physiotherapy that I loved so much. Now I have scaled things back down and only have one physio that works for me. I work closely with her, which is really nice. This way of operating works far better for me in my present life situation.

Everything that has happened in my career occurred at times when I was really ready for it. I am now in a place where I have a family and I am combining that with my business. Life in the end is all about balance and I feel exceptionally grateful for where I have been and where I currently am.

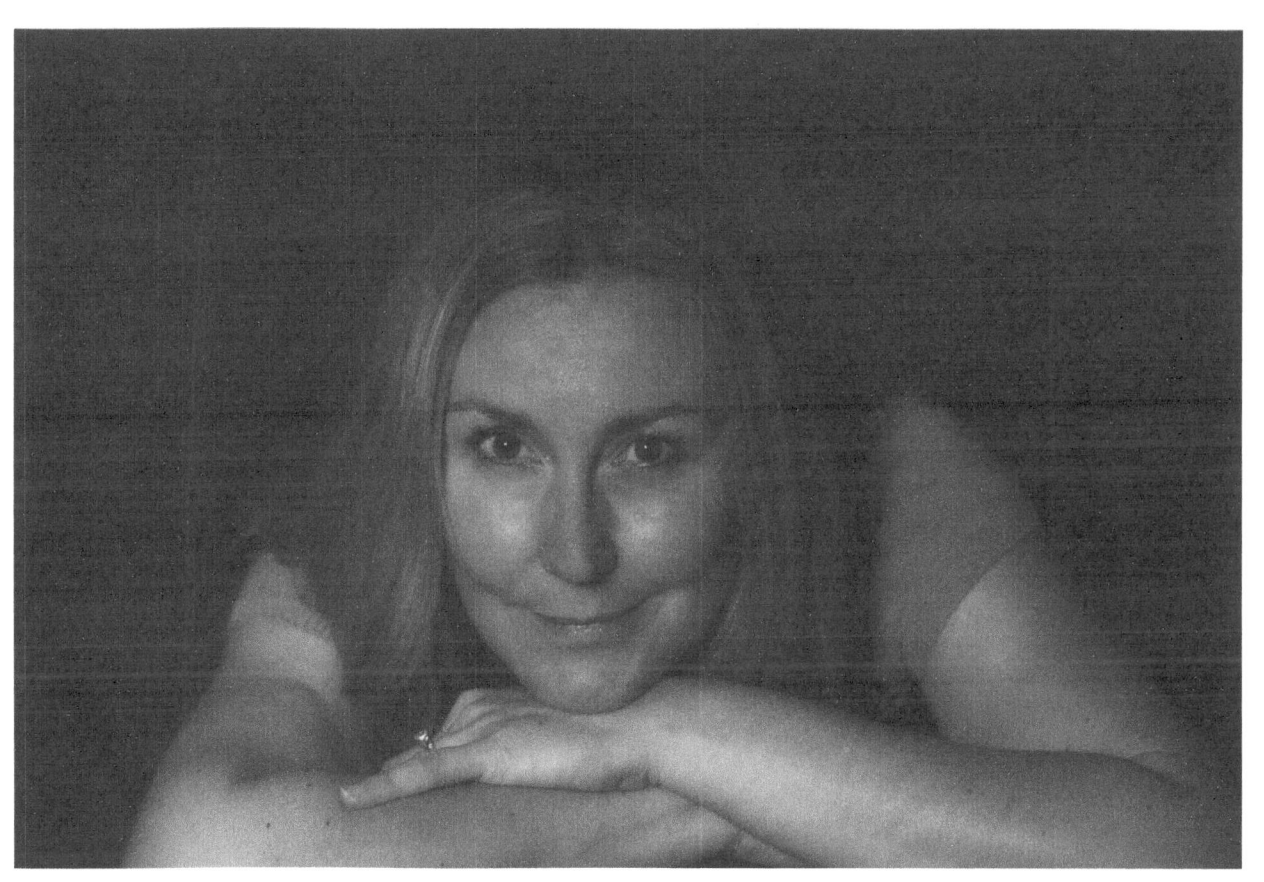

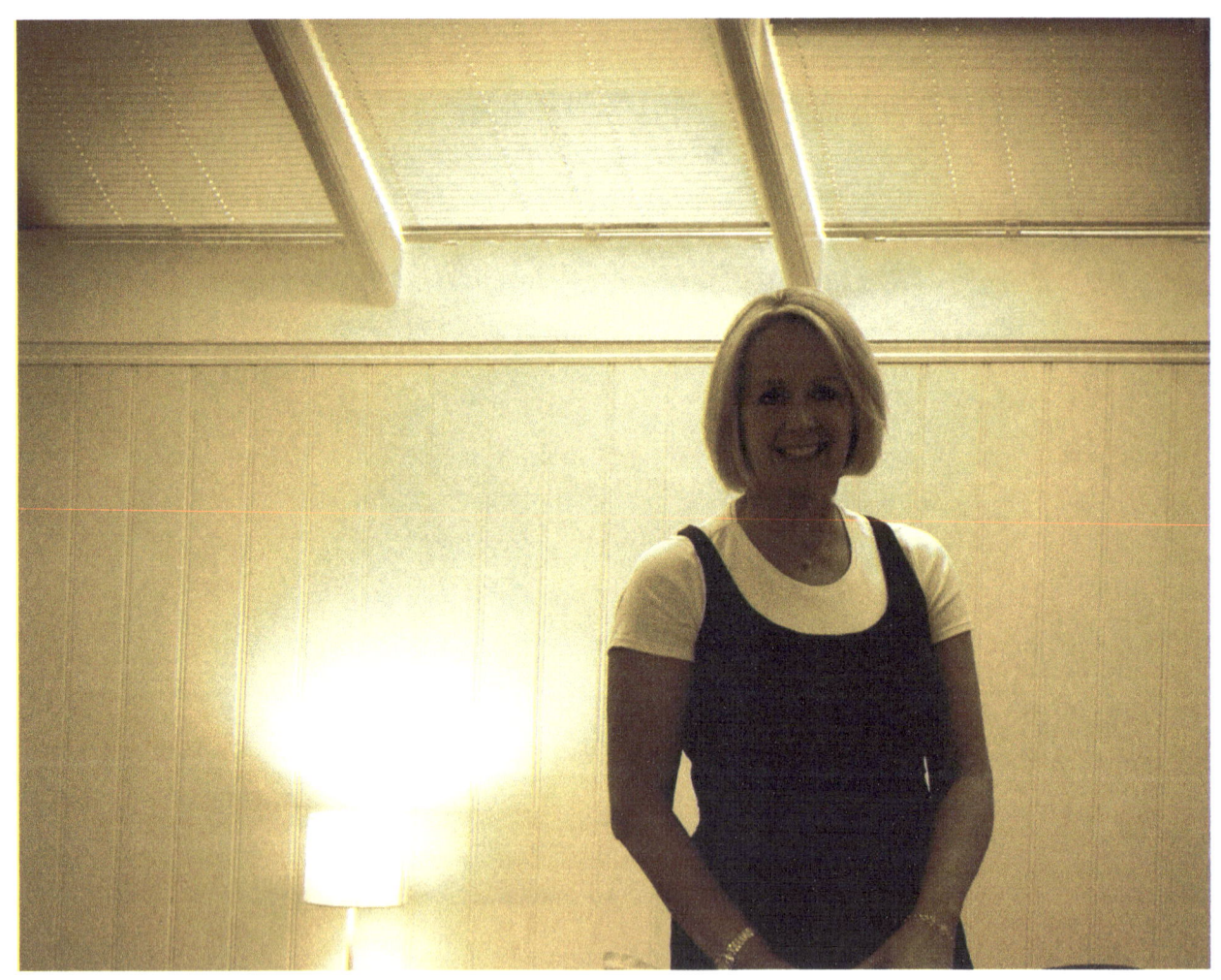

Christien Bird
Founder of The White Hart Clinic and Physiotherapist

While in conversation with Christien Bird I got a very strong impression that her motivating factors are her love of community and her passion for integrative health. These two things combined have seen her heading up a clinic of holistic and complementary medicine, where the emphasis is placed on providing outstanding health services within an informal, warm and friendly environment. It was clear that in her own field of work as a physiotherapist within Women's Health, her focus is very much on assimilating relevant information from sound scientific research, and communicating this in a manner that will allow women to make good choices about their health and their bodies. It was great to get an understanding from her on why support systems are so important.

At the age of seventeen, when I began to think about what I wanted to do with my life, my thoughts about my career were relatively random. Nonetheless, I always knew from quite a young age that I wanted to work with people. It is coincidental that my choice was physiotherapy because it could quite easily have been psychology. I was influenced by the logistics surrounding where I wanted to go to university and where my friends were going. But, in retrospect, what I really loved about physiotherapy was the combination of working with the physical body and the practical aspects of working in a really hands-on way. If I had to choose again, I would make the same choice.

Physiotherapy in a Hospital Environment

Once I began working with the NHS, I really enjoyed being a part of quite a big team. I loved the depth and variety of people I interacted with on a daily basis. It provided my life with such a rich tapestry in every sense of the word. However, there were challenges in that a large number of people remained unchanged by the treatments. A person's socio-economic demography can make a big difference to their well-being and ability to heal. So many people would come into the hospital in a low mood with a depressed outlook, which would act as an obstacle in the treatment of pain.

Scientific evidence supports the fact that a patient's mental state and the information communicated by the therapist, both way play huge roles in the creation of wellness. Additionally, research has shown that in the case of acute lower back pain, people who were treated straight away would have less of a chance of becoming depressed a year later. Sound reassurance can be a very active ingredient in a case where there is a painful situation and the patient does not understand what is going on. If treatment after injury is not immediate, their fearfulness can produce a belief system that there is something really wrong with them. Once this belief is set in place it can formulate a state of mind, where there is a high possibility of the injury reoccurring later on down the line.

The method we use to treat a patient and the way we diagnose their issue is important, but them coming in once or twice a week and being reassured that they are going to be ok, is the part that really matters. If someone is supported and cared for through that acute phase of their recovery, their belief system surrounding their pain is very different. The neural pathways that they form in response to the challenge of the injury will be far more conducive to health, compared to someone who has had to cope through it all on their own. Often this is what creates the difference between someone treated by the public health system with limited resources and someone treated privately with unlimited resources. The needs may be exactly the same, but the healing time would be vastly different.

My Passion for Women's Health

Musculoskeletal physiotherapy provides a broad landscape to a student. So when it came to researching and running my own clinic, I felt that it was necessary for me to narrow my area of work. There were not a lot of people specialising in women's health at the time, which was a motivating factor. Additionally, there is a lot of evidence-based modes of practice and research within this area, and since I am quite a linear thinker this really attracted me.

Musculoskeletal physiotherapy in general has really progressed within the last twenty years. However, because women's health has always been attached to the obstetric and the gynaecological world, there has been a lot more funding in place for it. This means that it sits much more in the medical field as opposed to the holistic world. The result is that there has been much more peer review literature, consensus and debates on treatment. Being a woman myself, I feel strongly about how women experience childbirth, what happens to their bodies post pregnancy, and their body's performance through the various stages of their life.

Providing a Support System for Women

A team of three of us are developing a health support system for women. We work quite closely with the community and are providing group support to mentor women through their various phases. Women's first experience of childbirth is completely new, so we give an opportunity for more experienced women to act as mentors. Most women will tell stories about how they felt that they were not assertive enough about their first delivery. Also, for many people, grandparents and parents are not readily available as a source of wisdom and information. However, with social media and other networks, we can put people in touch with each other.

I believe that it is important for women to have good information on the choices available to them. They may have choice in pain relief, but that is not really what a good childbirth story is about. Part of our work within the women's health team is in disseminating useful, well-researched information, and making sure that it is available within the community. For instance, at the moment there is very clear information that forceps delivery has an adverse effect on the health of the pelvic floor muscles. Data from thousands of ultrasounds have shown that, in many cases, the muscles are ripped from their origin. Once women have this information, they are more aware of what may happen. Eighty percent of women can have a normal delivery. If the baby really is reluctant to come out, then a caesarean may be a better option.

When a woman chooses to take a risk with her pelvic floor muscles, rather than have a caesarean, that is a real choice. If a woman knows that a combination of forceps, obesity and their age, predispose them to problems with their pelvic floor muscles, it may change the way they proceed with things. As it stands, the reason the information is not out there is because caesareans are expensive and forceps aren't. It takes assertiveness and being well-informed in order to make those choices. As a therapy team, it is important that we are a part of the voice that brings this information to women. Even if it is on a small local level, when there are a number of local voices put together, it can begin to act as a trigger which will eventually help to change the practice.

A Holistic Clinic within a Community

I have always been a great believer that work life and personal life should be quite close together, in order to keep things simple. Once I had my own children, I decided to start a really small physiotherapy practice and it has evolved and mushroomed into a multi-disciplined clinic with over twenty-five therapists working together.

I absolutely love the management side of running a small business. The clinical team is great and I am really confident that every therapist will go the extra mile for each patient that walks in. This makes me feel really good about what has been built here.

Whenever we ask customers how they would describe the clinic, the words informal, friendly and professional keep popping up. We are to the community what I would like us to be. I care about the community because I think, as people, we are hardwired to connect and interact with each other. I try to ensure that this level of connection is available within the clinic and amongst the therapists themselves. It would be a shame if people worked here just for the space, rather than because it was a place where they really wanted to work. Treating patients is a big part of what we do and can offer us great satisfaction. But working together within a great team adds a lighthearted contrast to all the hard work, which is fun. We put a lot of energy into every patient, so it is important to feel a sense of support from the work environment. This way of working has definitely been informed by the positive experiences I had when working within a hospital for the NHS. The White Hart Clinic is basically a community of therapists in service to the community.

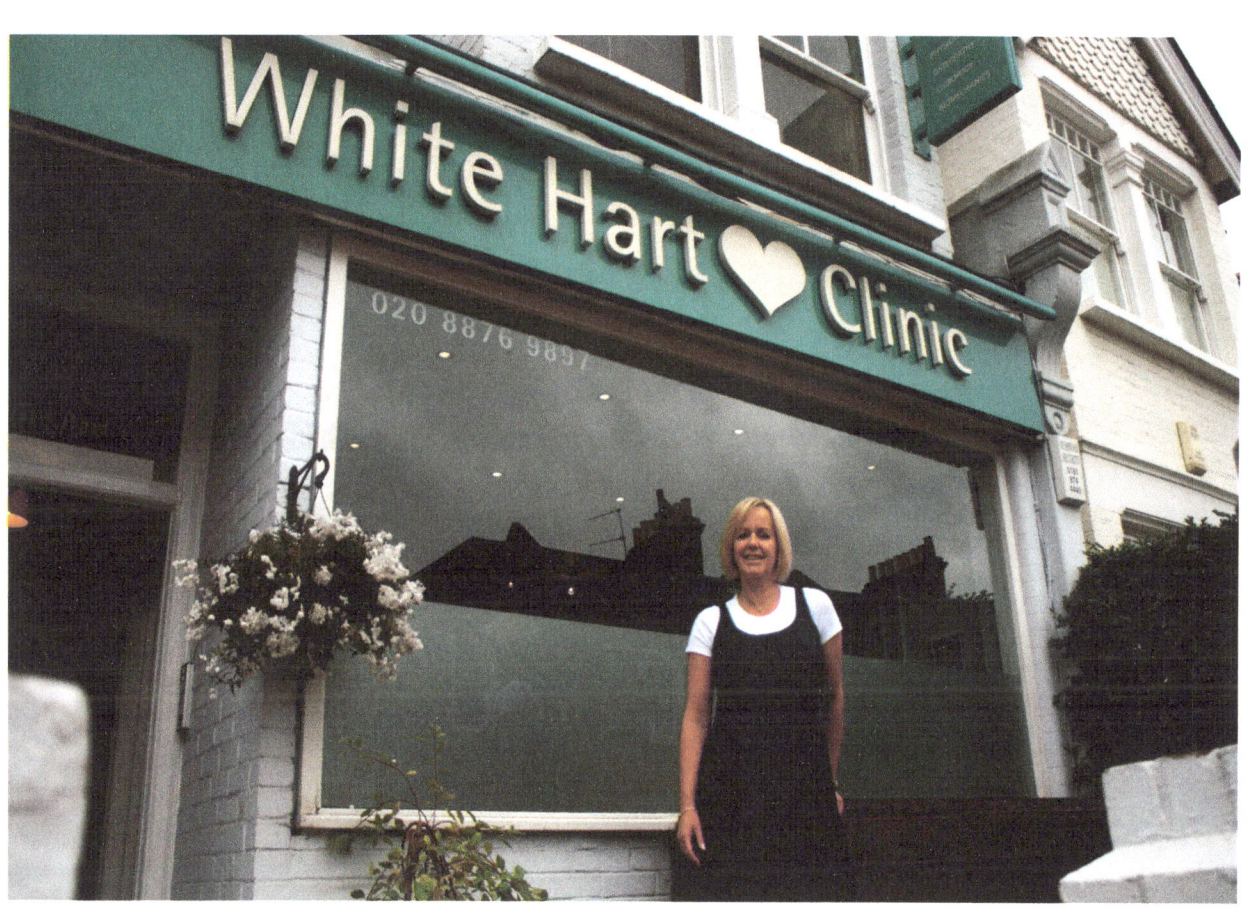

Mind

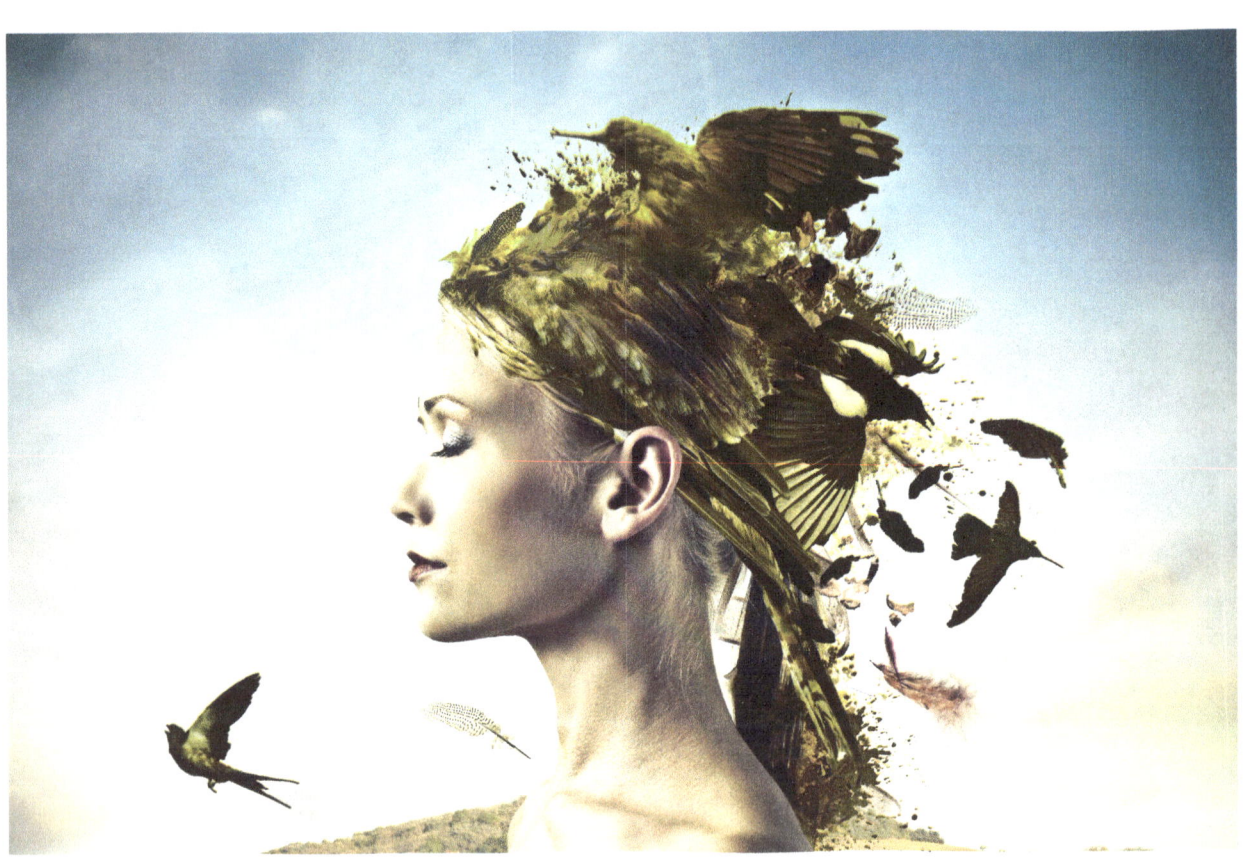

Treatments

Cognitive Behavioural Therapy

Neuro Linguistic Programming

Hypnotherapy

Meditative Practice

"Often it is not the situation that arises for a person that actually decides how they feel, it is their interpretation of it. The way we think is what really decides the way we feel."

- Christine Wilding

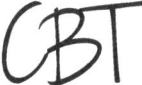

CBT

Cognitive Behavioural Therapy or CBT was developed through the merging of works by Aaron Beck and Albert Ellis. Two of the main areas worked on by the therapist are anxiety and depression. CBT first aims to find out what issue or problem the client faces and then, through a series of action-orientated goals, allows the person to create a shift towards a more enhanced, positive and optimistic way of being. There is an emphasis on being present, aware, and in the now, as a way to facilitate this shift on an even deeper level.

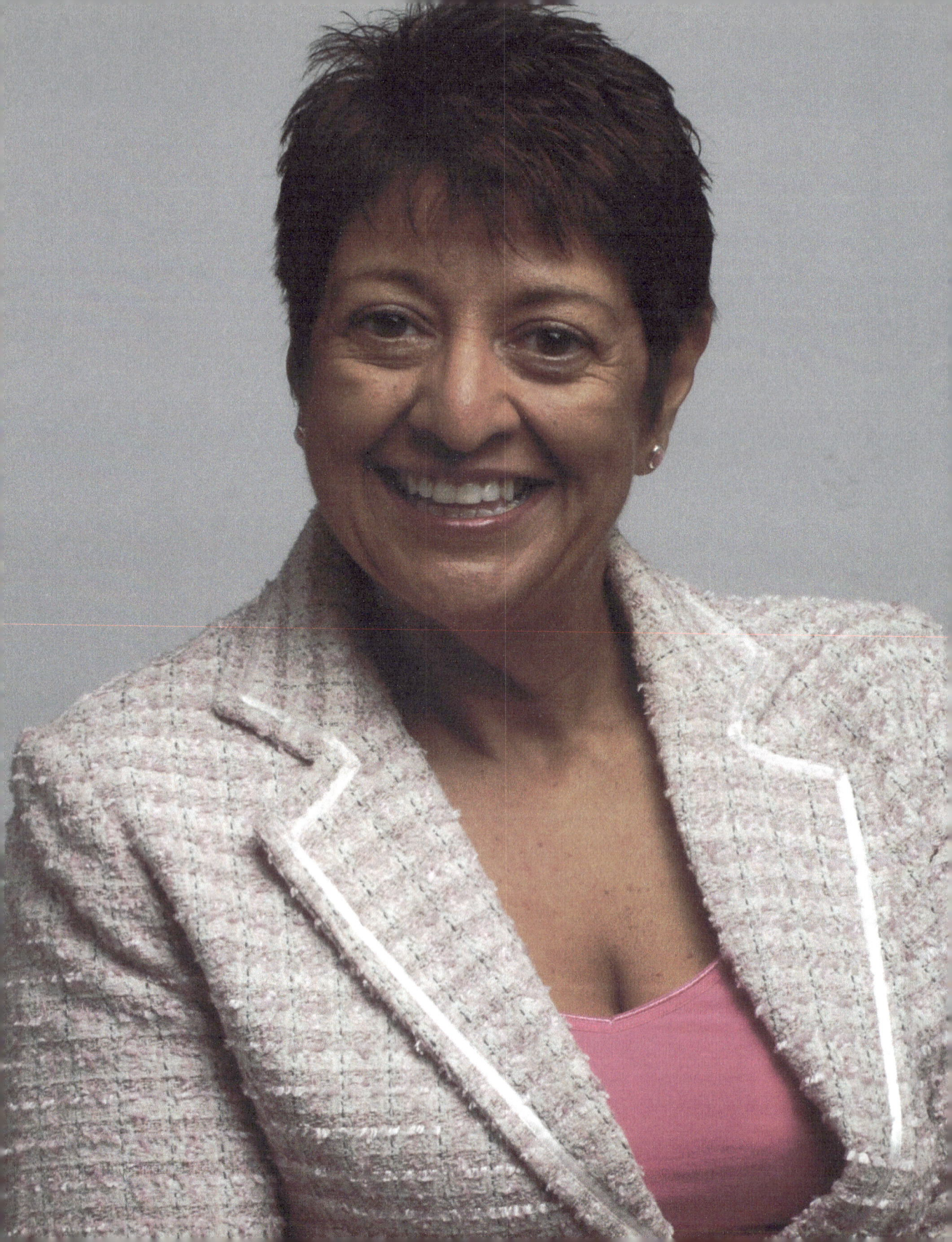

Gladeana McMahon

Cognitive Behavioural Therapist, Trainer, Coach and Author

Gladeana McMahon is what one could call a one of a kind work of art. She has a huge amount of energy and when it comes to the subject of Cognitive Behavioural Therapy (CBT) and Cognitive Behavioural Coaching (CBC), this energy has a great force of passion driving it forward. She has been in the field of mind work for 36 years and has had an influence in every possible area including, lecturing, TV presenting, motivational speaking, writing, therapy and coaching. It was enlightening to speak to her about the coaching model she co-developed based on CBT and how this model is being used to expand the field.

Personality wise, I was always that curious child who keeps questioning why. I was also very creative and quite lateral in my thought processes, so I was able to see connections where other people wouldn't. I wanted to be in the performing arts, but when I got to eighteen I had a confidence crisis. Although I got a place at the Royal Academy of Dramatic Arts, I began to panic and convinced myself that I was not good enough. Looking back now, I can clearly see that I sabotaged myself because, at the time, acting was my passion . When I left school at sixteen, my Asian dad and Jewish mother were both completely horrified.

Between the ages of sixteen to twenty-one there were copious amounts of jobs available. I went out and worked in a number of different and varying industries. I was very bright, a fast learner and adaptable, so I tried many different things because I had no idea what I wanted to do. In 1976, at the age of twenty-two, a friend rang me up from a youth counselling service and asked for my help to advertise a job, since one of my roles had involved running an employment agency. He described the job to me and I really liked the sound of it. I asked to be considered for the role and was successful. I started part time at first and four years later was working full time, while doing a three-year diploma course in counselling. It was evident to me that I had found the thing that I had been looking for. I was completely passionate about the counselling field and whenever I am energised by something, there is no stopping me.

The Journey to CBT

The first training I undertook was in Humanistic Counselling; however, in its practical application it never seemed to work for everyone across the board. In an attempt to bridge the gap, I then started a five-year psychodynamic training. But by the start of the third year I knew it was not for me. I then did a Behavioural course and followed this by doing CBT, and finally I had found the perfect fit.

Clients are incredibly wise and knowledgeable about themselves, in ways that I don't think we always appreciate. But the problem is that if you do not know what a door looks like, however much wisdom you have, you are not going to find it. CBT allowed me to help people to find the door to a different way of being. It was up to them if they wanted to go through it, but at least I knew how to help. Previously, it felt like I had been working in a very hit-and-miss kind of way. However, with CBT I felt that I had access to fantastic tools, strategies, theories and philosophies. I also loved the fact that it was a collaborative approach, so the client and I were working together to achieve the outcome, which felt like a truly empowering method. Once I was confident with the therapy aspect of my work, I wanted to supervise others. From there I became a trainer and author in the subject.

Cognitive Behavioural Coaching

I am accredited as a CBT practitioner; however, I also operate a coaching practice and together with Professor Steven Palmer, Windy Dryden and Michael Neenan, I developed a coaching model, which is based on CBT, called Cognitive Behavioural Coaching.

When I got into coaching in the early nineties I started off as a 'closet coach'. Coaching was not well known and therapists were very condescending about it. But the more I worked with the coaching model, the more I realised how effective it was. It had a preventative element, which could stop people heading down a path where they may eventually need clinical therapy. I also felt that coaching allowed me to work with people who were not distressed in any way, but who wanted to make the most of their lives.

Coaching has two main areas. There is executive coaching for individuals in organisations and the approach is about considering the needs of the organisation, as well as the personal goals of the individual. Then there is life coaching now called personal coaching, which is very much like being a therapist in private practice. It is an individual, one-to-one arrangement and it could cover a whole host of personal goals, ranging from work to emotional to lifestyle.

Coaching has come a long way since I started. You only need to look at the number of therapists who are training to become coaches, combined with the fact that coaching is fast developing towards becoming a profession for many in the field.

The Difference Between Coaching and Therapy

The difference between coaching and therapy lies within the client group that you are working with. A simplistic way of looking at this, is that cognitive behavioural therapy is for people who have therapeutic issues, so they may be depressed, anxious or distressed. Basically no one goes into therapy if they are happy with their lives. There is something blocking their way. In the therapeutic sense, we are dealing with the clinical population. Cognitive Behavioural Coaching deals with people who don't fit the therapy criteria.

With the model for CBC, the client is functioning well, but may want more from their lives, be it career-wise or personal-wise. Coaching is skilled based, practical and helps people to develop a solution from their own resources. It helps them with strategies to aid development and goal attainment. For example, in executive coaching, I might get someone who is a technical specialist, brilliant at their job, happily settled in an intimate relationship, with nothing that could be described as a clinical issue. But they may have been put in a position where they are now expected to manage people and find that this aspect is very different from their previous role. In a case like this, I would coach them in management strategies, helping them to develop the internal and external skills that they need to become a good manager. There may also be other aspects such as communication, emotional intelligence and unhelpful ways of thinking that also need to be addressed.

Equally, it could be someone who has to go out and give presentations. They may get positive feedback that their presentations are great, but spend the week before worrying about it and unable to sleep. This is not an unusual occurrence, everyone worries about something at some point in time. When someone comes along for coaching, it is more about taking what's good and making it even better.

In both these cases, we would coach the person in the areas that they would need to make changes in order to alleviate the need to worry. Cognitive Behavioural Coaching takes the CBT framework, which includes aspects of positive psychology and mindfulness and adds other more practical knowledge-based elements. So, for example, I have worked in organisations as a manager and so know what is needed to effectively manage people. This is information that the average person may not have had access to. They may need practical tools, training in specific areas and a different perspective or way of viewing the issue. As a coach, we help individuals to develop a way of thinking, feeling and behaving, which will enable them to be happier and more productive in their outcome.

The Therapist Behind the Therapy

When it comes to my work, I am embedded with a philosophy of excellence. Focusing on delivering excellence means you are in a hugely responsible position. You can make the difference to someone in a positive way or you can make them worse. You need to think of yourself as a neurosurgeon who has to work within millimetres. It is incredibly important for a therapist to respect this level of responsibility to the client. As a result, it is necessary to make a commitment to keep learning and developing.

Life is about balance and accepting that we are who we are. I will never be a retiring wallflower because it is not in my nature. When I am really old, I want 'Go Faster' stripes on my zimmer frame. As therapists we are also human, which is why it is important to work with others in your field and to get their feedback. I do not walk on water, there is no one in this world that is completely perfect, and those closest to the person you admire the most will say things about them in private, that they would never say in public. You could be good, fantastic and honourable, but you will always be human, and through it all that is a great gift.

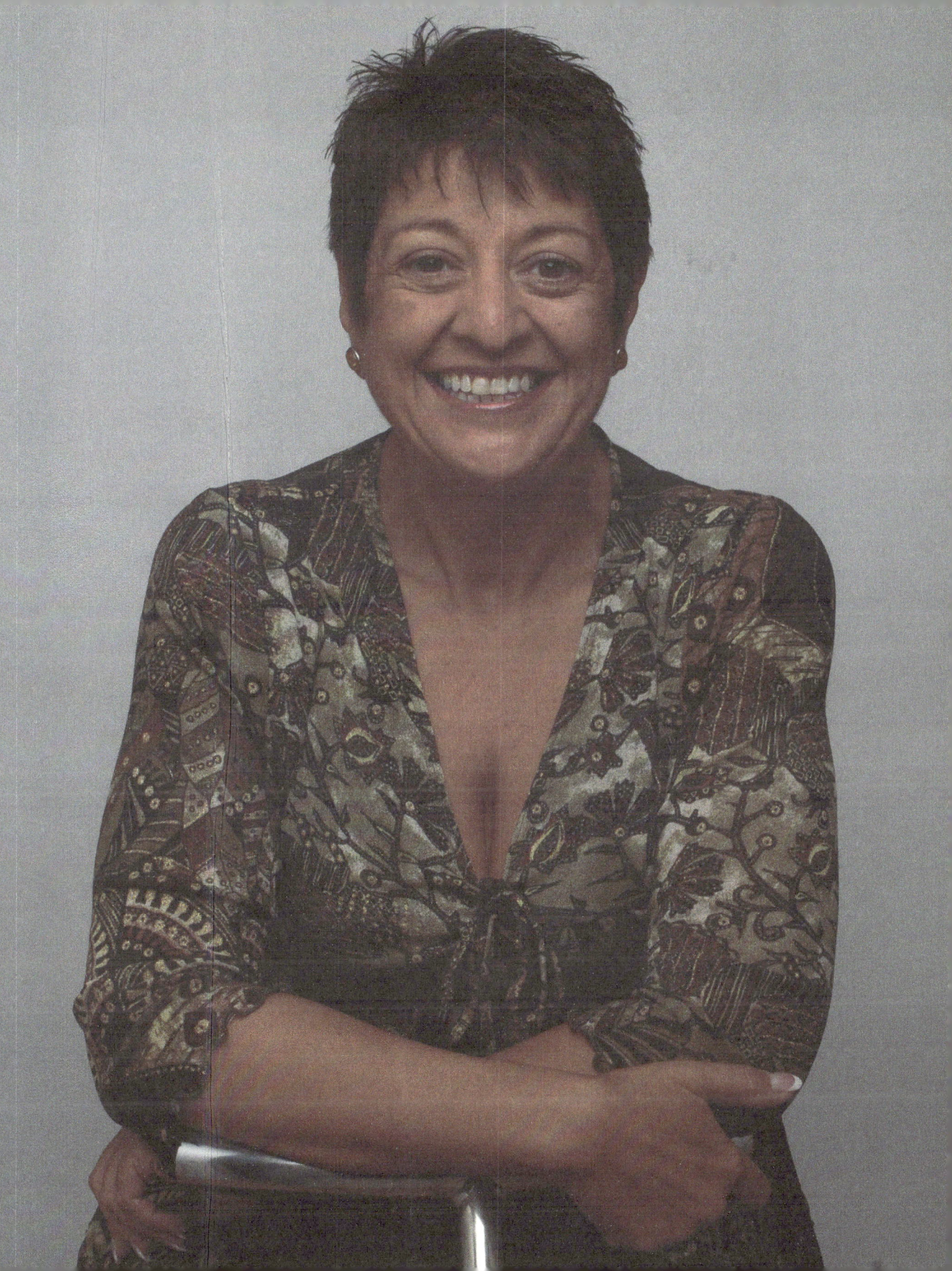

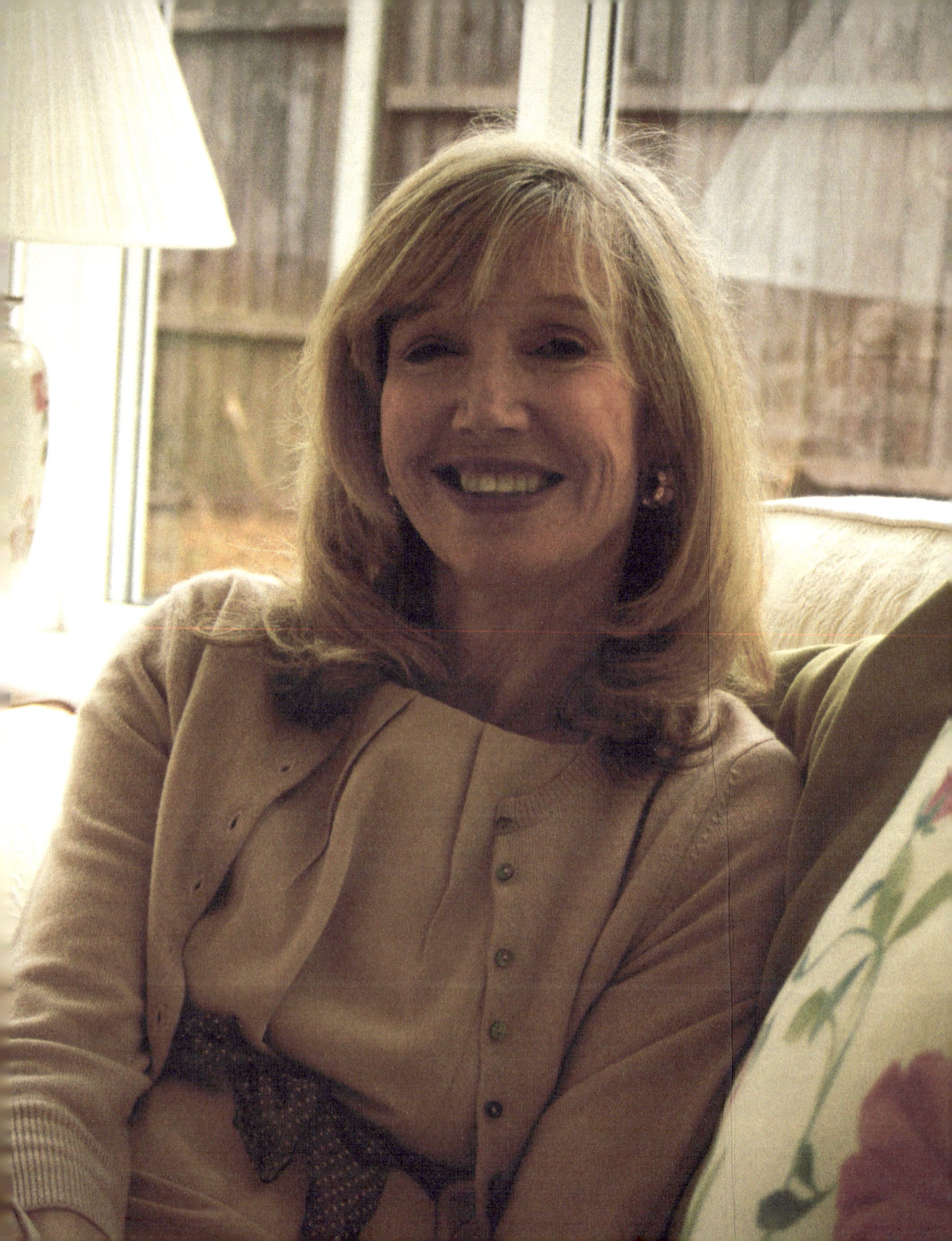

Christine Wilding
Cognitive Behavioural Therapist and Author

Christine Wilding runs a private practice and is the author of eleven publications in psychology, counselling and Cognitive Behavioural Therapy. She was so impressed with the change that CBT made to her personal life, she switched her career from Human Resources and retrained as a therapist using this approach. Through CBT she experienced and understood what it meant to take control of her choices at a time when she was completely unaware that there were options available to her. As she speaks about her work, you get the resounding feeling that for every problem we may experience there is a solution; we just have to open our view to the possibilities and alternatives.

My interest in people fuelled my desire to become a Therapist. My previous career was in Personnel and my studies within Human Resources contained a lot of psychology. So the psychological aspect of how we act and respond was already in my awareness. My introduction to CBT as a therapy came when I was diagnosed with breast cancer nearly twenty years ago. The treatment involved chemical therapy, which is known to cause depression in some cases and this is what happened to me. Luckily, I was being treated at the Royal Marsden and their clinical psychologist offered a short course of CBT to help with this side effect.

Twenty years ago CBT was not as popular as it is today. However, I loved it from the start. To me it was a psychological practice of common sense. So much so that one could quite easily ask the question, 'If it is just common sense, why is therapy needed?' But of course the more pertinent question would be, 'If it is just common sense, what prevents you from actually solving your problems?' This is where the therapy starts: working with the client to discover what their own perceptions of problems are and looking at whether a re-evaluation of both thoughts and actions could be necessary. CBT is very understandable, practical and solution-focused. Its effectiveness lies in the fact that it allows people to realise that there are options to every situation in their life.

CBT

Generally, I work to treat depression and anxiety. This can take many forms including social anxiety, health anxiety, phobia, Obsessive Compulsive Disorder (OCD), panic and work-related anxiety. Our options are often the first things that get narrowed when we are anxious or depressed. But often, it's not the situation that someone faces that will decide how they feel, it's their interpretation of it. The way we think is what really decides the way we feel.

CBT helps you to re-evaluate both your thinking and your behaviour. Sometimes there is a more balanced alternative to our negative thoughts and beliefs, which helps us to feel better and more motivated. There are also times when our negative thoughts are valid and this is when we help the client to move from their worry-oriented mode to an action-oriented mode. The basis of CBT isn't simply to disprove all our negative thoughts as being mistakes, but to help us to more accurately estimate their validity, and then think and act accordingly.

In a sense, CBT is an educational model that teaches the client to become his or her own therapist. A good therapist isn't going to find the answer to your problem for you, but they know how to help you to work it out for yourself. Instead of telling someone what to do, it asks the person to evaluate what they feel to be the right direction for them. It presents the person with a scenario and asks them what they make of it, which encourages them to be curious and to think 'outside the box'.

There are always a variety of different ways of seeing things, which may not occur to some people if they don't have professional help. If someone has social anxiety or OCD, for example, the thoughts and actions they see as helpful may actually be unwittingly maintaining their problems. A professional consultant is there to teach the client to tolerate anxiety, live with uncertainty and take risks. By doing this people test out their erroneous belief that harm or danger will come to them, and defeat it. The person will find that what they thought was going to happen doesn't, or if it does, it isn't as bad as they had envisioned. We take the focus away from the anxiety and work on the beliefs instead.

There are different treatment protocols for each of the various specialties, but CBT will generally help with any problem that you've got and it has the sound back up of being researched and audited with highly successful results.

My Work

I say to my clients that we're both experts: I have the skills and techniques but they have all the information about themselves. We work together to find out what's going wrong, why it's going wrong, what's maintaining the problem, and what we can do to resolve it.

Take depression, for example. I normally present clients with an image of having two different brains, one positive and the other negative. We all tend to have positive and negative feelings but, in general, a lot of our thoughts lie in the middle of these two brains. If we find ourselves drifting more towards negativity, this brain begins to work really hard for us. The more we think negatively, the more habitual this becomes. All of the evidence we gather supports our negative views and we discount the positives without realising it. The negative brain is working 24/7 and the positive, or optimistic brain, is on holiday, doing absolutely nothing. When we get to that point, we have no idea why we are thinking in a negative way, because it is so natural to us. Optimism is important in therapy. If you draw the optimism out and work at this, you're at least a third of the way there.

To get the rest of the way there, we look at setting goals. CBT is very goal orientated, so I would ask the person what their goals were and what was preventing them from getting to where they wanted to be. Clients often, when depressed, provide rather vague goals of, 'Wanting to feel happier', 'Not wanting to go on like this' and other similar suggestions. The therapist helps the client to define their goals much more specifically. It then becomes possible to work with clear examples of negative thinking and behaviours, which may be preventing them from reaching their goals.

The belief system that you are the most passionate about determines the way the world presents itself to you. This is usually very true of depression. However, there are different types of depression. Some experiences fall into the category of 'event specific', where trauma has caused the depression, and others can be termed chronic depression, which is less explainable as, on the face of it, there seems to be little wrong with the life of the sufferer.

Event-specific depression can usually be easier to get over as it is possible for people to recall a time when they felt more optimistic and to regain that type of thinking. With chronic depression, people cannot remember a time when they felt any other way and have no concept of how they might think differently. In this case, it can take longer to reach down to the person's basic beliefs on why they find life such a negative experience. However, even in such cases, CBT is effective for achieving recovery.

All of my experience with CBT, both personally and client-based, shows that it works. It is very satisfying to see people who come to me initially in complete distress, then blossom and flourish and go on to lead happier and more fulfilling lives.

The Future

Since its origination in the 60s, CBT has developed hugely and is continuing to change. One criticism that has been levelled at it is that it lacks a human approach and does not have the same kind of empathy that, for instance, Person Centred Therapy has, where it is thought that a sense of connection and understanding is enough to produce change. I have personally felt that compassion should have a big place in therapy and I think CBT will develop to bring this into its approach.

Additionally, there is now a discipline called mindfulness-based CBT. This not only challenges thought systems, but also addresses how we can begin to live in the present moment and be calm and non-judgemental within ourselves, making connections, with other people or with nature. So, for example, when we are out and about, we take the time to look at the trees, the sky and the birds, instead of the constant dialogue we have with ourselves, and bring all this into our lives. This sort of therapy is very powerful and very uplifting. It is necessary to be solution-focused, because if we're not we become victims, but I also like the idea of learning to be tranquil within ourselves.

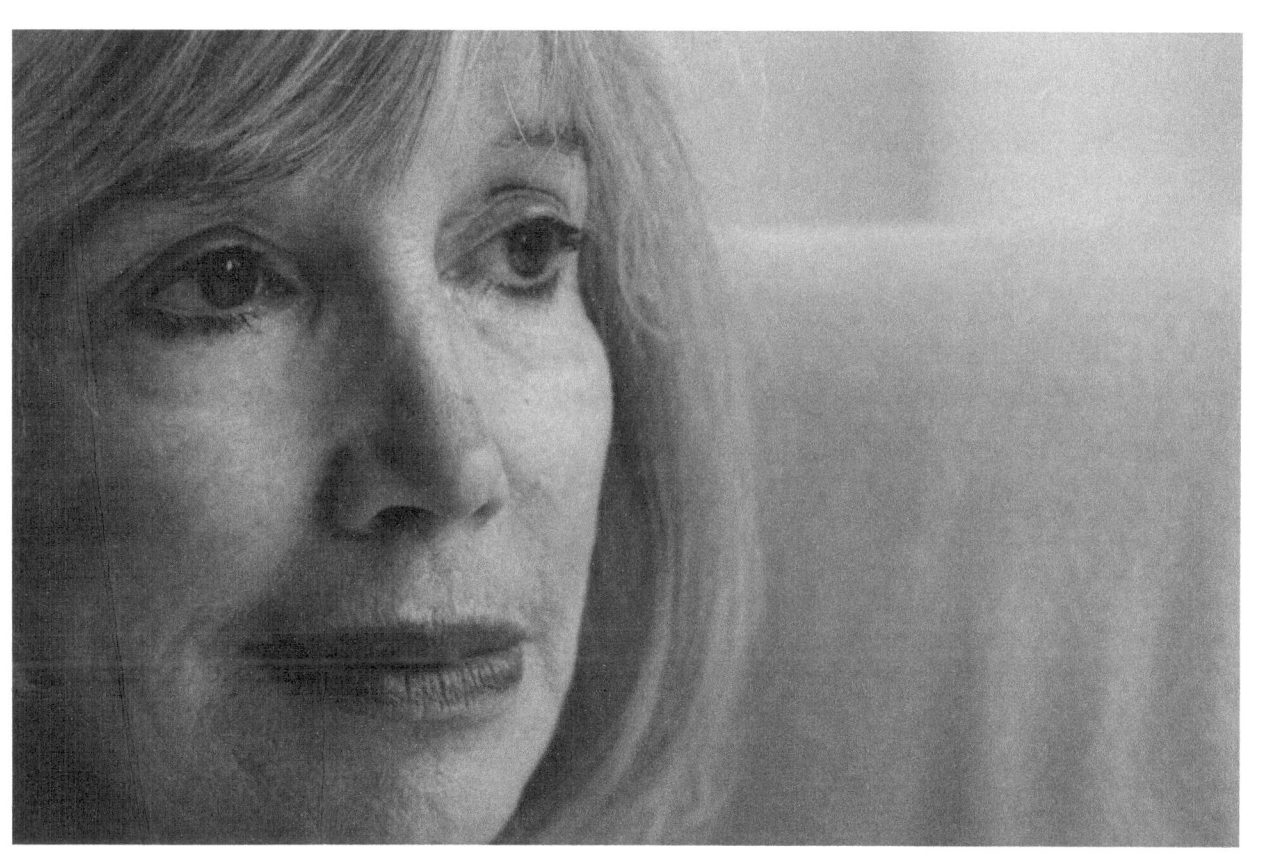

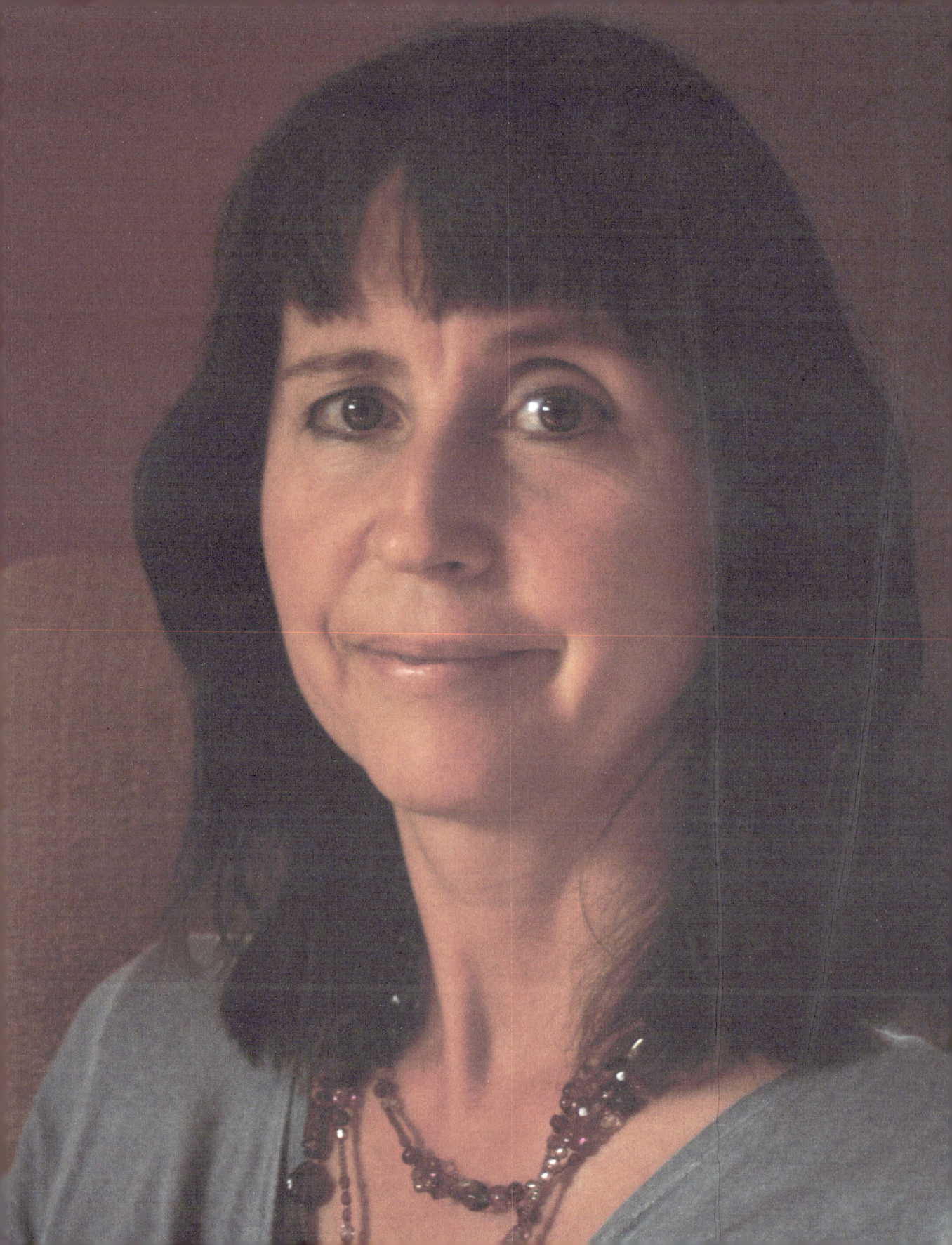

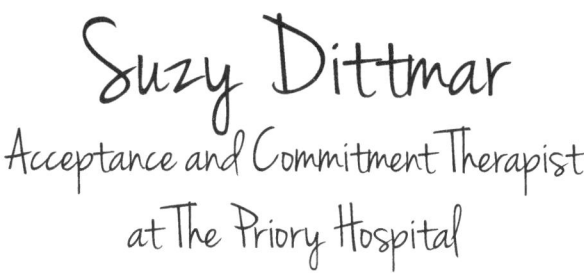

Suzy Dittmar
Acceptance and Commitment Therapist
at The Priory Hospital

On meeting Suzy Dittmar you get a sense of someone who is thoughtful yet playful. If you seem ambiguous, she will pose you a series of questions to make sure that she understands you perfectly. She takes pleasure in connecting to the hidden beauty that is found in seemingly simple things and finds simplicity in complexity. It was a great pleasure to get a snapshot of Cognitive Behaviour Therapy (CBT) from her and her place within it.

Although I am a Cognitive Behaviour Therapist, CBT has many different directions and strands. I would call myself an Acceptance and Commitment Therapist (ACT) I have always been very interested in thoughts; even as a very young child I was aware that there were different ways and levels of thinking. I saw that some thoughts could take the form of words written in your head or they may be little fleeting ideas that you have to hold onto, while other thoughts are more visual and create images in the mind.

I came to this work later in life by doing a course in hypnotherapy, then a Master's degree in CBT and, since then, I have been doing training courses in ACT. As I go along, I learn more, so I am just following my interests and instincts in order to discover effective ways to work with people.

Acceptance and Commitment Therapy

We all have things that we want to do in our lives. Even when someone is quite un-well they tend to be relatively clear on what they would ideally like to be doing more of. It could be that they want to connect with people, have more friends, spend time with their family or have a fulfilling job. People tend to know what is important, but they have thoughts and feelings that act as barriers and throw them off their path.

If we look at a lifeline, it may meander and go this way or that, but it will follow who a person is and who they want to be. However, they may have thoughts that say, 'I am not good enough' or 'I am not worthy enough, and will never be any good'. If they listen to these unhelpful thoughts, they won't even try to take a step forward, or will give up if they are not immediately the best. ACT is about helping people to identify what they value, what is important to them, and what enables them to move forward, despite their thoughts and feelings. During a session we may sit and talk in a therapy room or we may do mindfulness exercises.

The first time I do a mindfulness exercise with someone, I generally just invite them to close their eyes and become aware of what it feels like to sit in their chair. Noticing the physical sensations of sitting and just accepting them, allowing them to be as they are. Parts of their body will be comfortable and parts of it won't; all of that is fine, that is just the way it is. I will then get them to notice their breathing and really focus on that. The exercise is generally about sharpening the part of us that observes thoughts, feelings and physical sensations. So rather than being swept along thinking, 'I am this pain' or 'I am this feeling', it is possible to say 'I am having a thought' or 'I am having a physical sensation', of this or that.

ACT is about accepting what needs to be accepted. There is hardship and difficulty, and you should obviously do what you can do about that. But if you try to fight against the things that are inevitable, you use up a lot of energy and make yourself very tired, when you could instead hold them lightly and they will recede into the background a bit more. One example is chronic pain. You could constantly try to push the pain away, making it smaller in your head and getting angry that you have it in the first place. Or you could do a very paradoxical thing by inviting it in, holding it lightly and saying, 'Yes, you are allowed to be here'. This way it can blend into the background, giving you more time, energy and focus for the things that you do want.

My Work

I work at the Priory Hospital as well as having a private clinic. The addiction aspect is the part of The Priory that people are always familiar with because of the media. But the addictions unit is only a part of what goes on there. I work in the general mental health unit, where the majority of people require help with anxiety, depression, obsessive compulsive behaviours, eating disorders and so on.

The way that I see my work is, I am here, a human being, doing my own thing. I am climbing up my own mountain but I am by no means a perfect mountaineer. I will have my own challenges to work with sometimes. But because I am over here, I can see things that maybe you are unable to see on your mountain with it being so close to your nose. I may be able to ask questions or point things out that I can see from here, but I am not the expert of your experience because it is your mountain and only you can climb it. I can give people useful information about their issues and how these issues can manifest physically, but I am unable to tell them what they should do.

Sometimes I will have personal experience of what a client is going through and sometimes I won't. Some people's mental processes I just don't have, they are different to mine. I don't have to experience the exact same things as they have in order for me to ask questions that might help them. I can see that a certain thought might be unhelpful and I know things that a lot of clients don't know when they first come along. I know that everybody is soft inside and even the people who initially seem scary want the same things, but just have different ways of going about it.

Everyone has a vulnerable side; everyone just tries to live life in the best possible way. People may come across as very hard and callous, but once you go below the surface they are behaving that way because of some hurt they are trying to cover up. It is a strategy they have developed.

From a behaviourist point of view people are flock animals who do well when they have social connections, are part of a group and feel settled in their family, community or group of friends. However, when things happen and somehow that person is isolated or isn't connected to others, it may lead to behavioural patterns that are not very good for the people around them.

I don't work in prison hospitals and I have never worked in the forensic field. I work with people who are all really just scared inside to some degree. For the most part, they are not people who want to harm others. Generally, we all have an inbuilt mechanism where we want to be accepted by our group, but things can go wrong with that.

Putting ACT Into Action

I am someone who is able to point out an obstacle or blockage in a person's way of dealing with their thoughts and feelings. They may think that something is part of their path. For example, they may say, 'I am just not good at talking to people', to which I would ask them to look again and assess whether it could be an obstacle that may be overcome. I can provide questions and exercises that help people think and look at their experiences, rather than focusing completely on what the mind is telling them is going on. I help people to see that there is more to them than their unhelpful thoughts and painful feelings.

Rather than believing every thought that comes along, they are able, with a wise mind, to question whether the thought is helpful or not. Thoughts can be a bit like advertising: you would not feel the need to respond to everything you see in the media or on television. In the same way, you should be objective about your thoughts.

If the mind tells you it is nicer to sit in front of the telly rather than go out and dance, you could treat it like an unruly kitten and say, 'Come on kitten, I know you don't want to, but we are going dancing anyway because it is good for us in the long run and we are going to love it!'

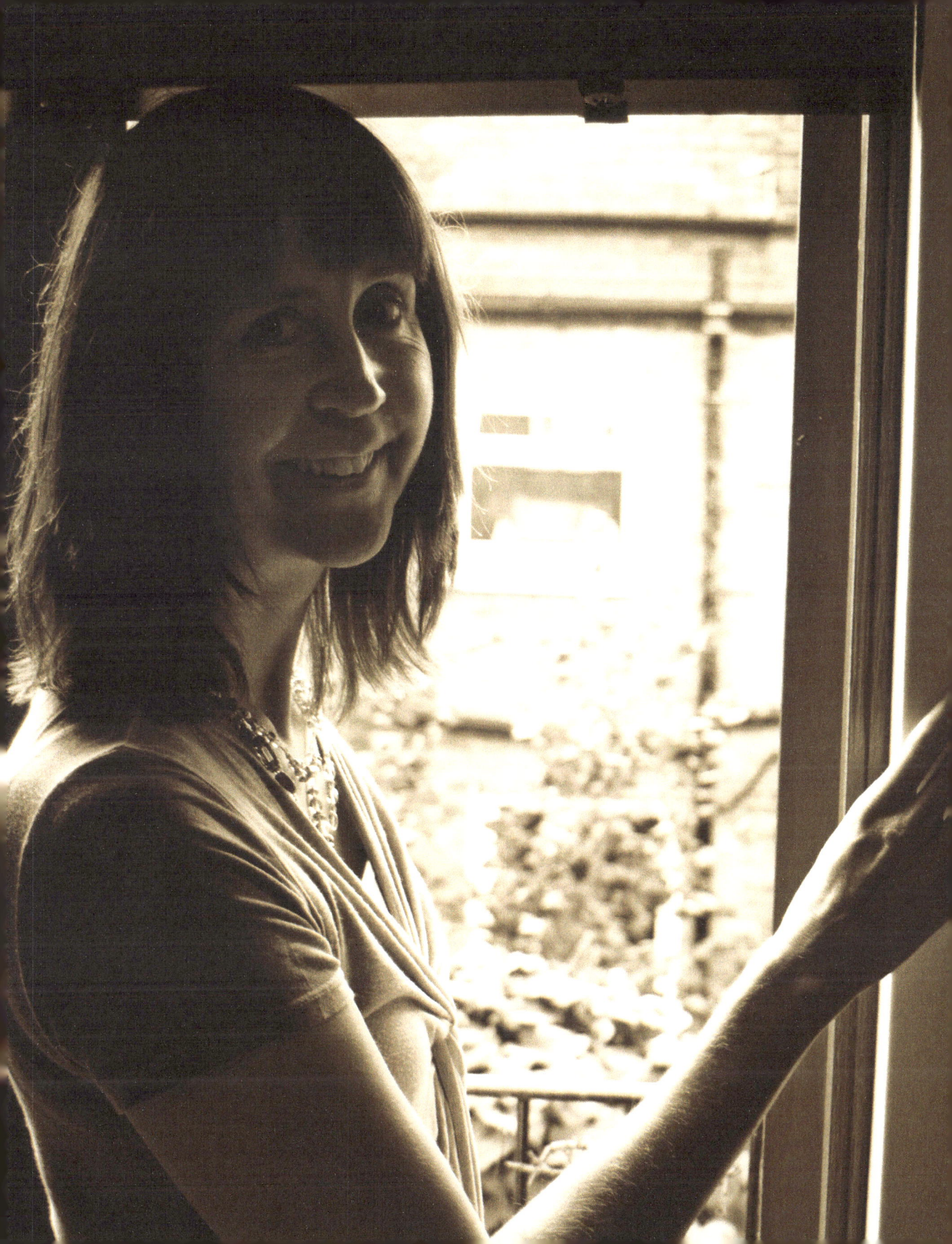

"We understand more and more, that all change has its root in the metaphorical landscape within. I work holistically with people to access deep change within this landscape, which in turn changes their rational understanding of themselves and provides for a better experience of the world around them."

- Nina Madden

Neuro Linguistic Programming

NLP was created in the 1970s by Richard Bandler and John Grinder from the United States. Neuro refers to the neurological pathways or the way that our nervous system responds to stimulation. Linguistic points to the language we use to create certain responses. Programming is about the learned behaviour that we portray as a result of our experiences. These three areas can be worked in an integrative way to create change, reach goals and expand life experiences. For example, by changing our behaviour and language surrounding something, we change our neurological response to it.

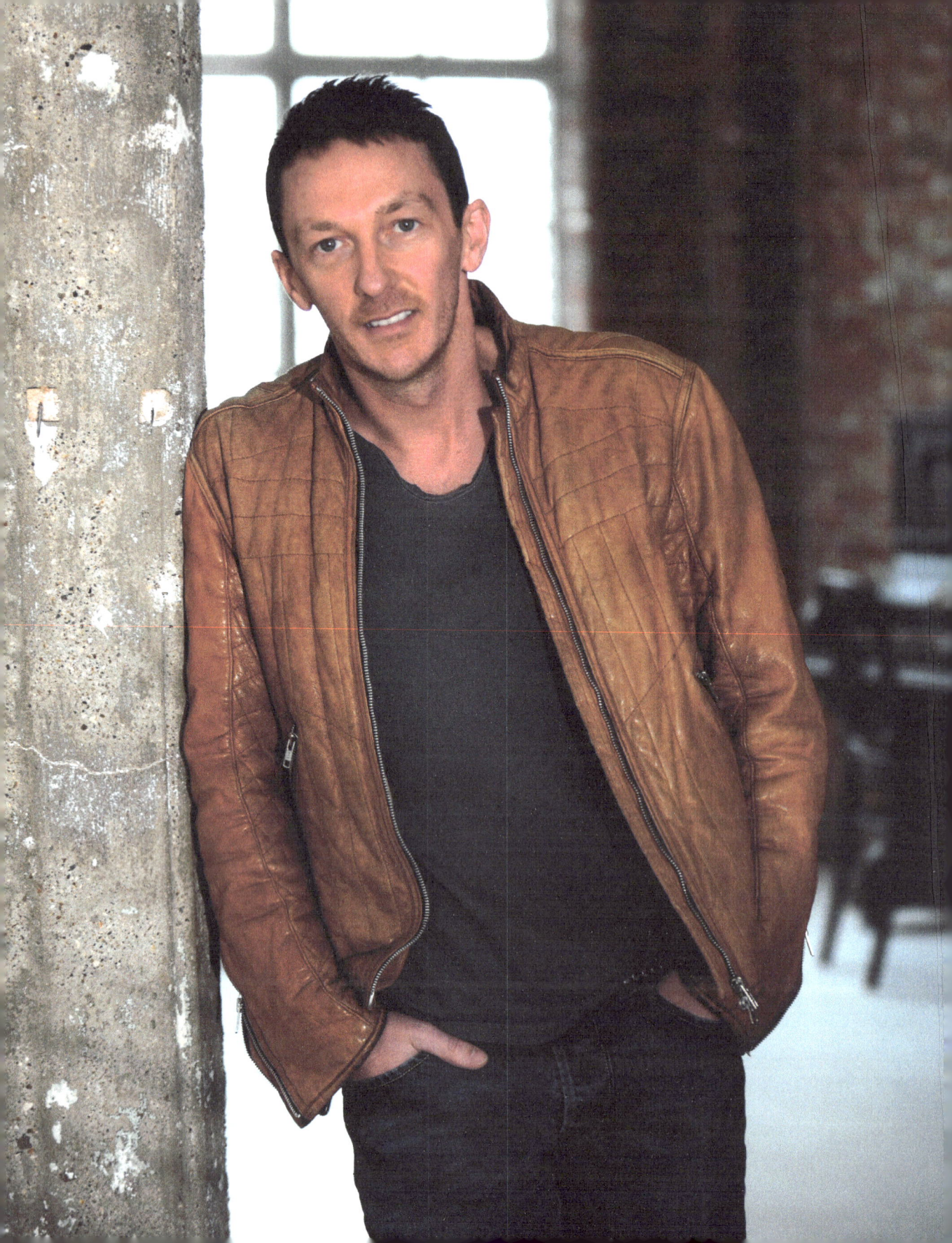

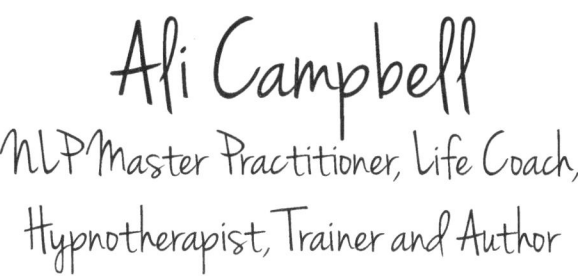

Ali Campbell
NLP Master Practitioner, Life Coach, Hypnotherapist, Trainer and Author

Ali Campbell is a down-to-earth Glaswegian with a cracking sense of humour. He is quite a force within the field of NLP, heightening public awareness of this modality and spotlighting his success through television, books, media coverage and workshops. He seems to have an innate gift of getting straight to the point and finding the most direct route to help others to change their minds and, as a result, change their lives. It was an expansive experience to get a view through his lens.

I had a phobia of needles, or anything piercing the skin, but I didn't realise it until somebody pointed it out to me, I just thought I fainted quite a lot. As a kid we went to see Romeo and Juliet with school and there was a scene where somebody was stabbed and I fainted. At the age of thirteen, I put that down to not having any breakfast and it being hot on the bus to the theatre. Later down the line I was at a party and someone put the film Pulp Fiction on and there was a scene of an injection and I fainted again. This time I put it down to having a little bit too much to drink and being tired.

Finally, I booked in to see the dentist for a check-up. I really hated dentists after a bad experience with one when I was much younger. I eventually plucked up the courage to go but when he pulled out a syringe to give me an anaesthetic I passed out. He was the one who informed me I had a phobia and suggested NLP and hypnotherapy as a way to fix it. I took his advice and not only was the problem fixed, but I was just blown away by how something so simple made such a drastic change to my experience. As a result, I did my NLP practitioner training and found out that I was actually quite good at it. Coincidentally, I was disenchanted with the corporate world I worked in at the time and NLP offered me a change of direction. I started very low key, working out of the same dental clinic where I discovered I had a phobia and everything built from there.

NLP

When working with someone using NLP, I would normally get them to access three memories – the first, the worst and the most recent. The worst memory is completely subjective, and generally people tend to have a good recollection of the first time something happened. There are NLP techniques that we use to collapse these memories. Phobias take no time at all to change.

.

Our interaction with the world is normally processed through our filters and our previous experiences. You and I could both go to the same party and have completely different recollections of exactly the same experience. We attribute importance to things depending on how we are pre-programmed and we create our subjective experience on the inside, often completely independently from what is happening on the outside.

We produce subjective experiences by using the building blocks of various states, including pictures, sounds, feelings, tastes and smells. Our brain automates how we react when presented with certain situations. So when our internal senses are stimulated by something outside of us, we interpret how we are supposed to react based on the filters we have in place. Mental filters give us certain feelings and create certain experiences within us. If something is perceived as being scary it creates a scary state, if it is perceived as being joyful, it creates a happy state. However, these states are totally changeable and, in exactly the same way that you can fall in love, you can also fall out of love. You can change your mind so that one day something can cause you great pleasure and the next day the same thing can cause you great pain. Nothing has changed on the outside, our perception is solely based on how we interpret it on the inside. NLP brings our attention to the fact that, by changing our perception we change our experience.

Deep-Rooted v Superficial Issues

The idea that some fears are deep and others are superficial, some things are easy to change and others are hard, is completely arbitrary and subjective in itself.

If you're stuck at home and you haven't left your house for sixteen years it is not a deep- rooted issue. Fundamentally, your fear is created by a thought. So when you put your hand on the door, a panicked thought washes over you that says something bad is about to happen.

We run our lives one thought, one decision and one choice at a time. As soon as you stop having that thought, you stop reacting in that way. It is no deeper and no more superficial than that. The innate nature of self is to be well, full and fulfilled. If someone is in emotional pain the sooner they stop that painful thought or series of thoughts, the sooner they stop being in pain. The plaster does not heal the wound, the wound heals by itself. The plaster just creates the environment in which it is safe to heal. This is quite a successful approach because you are seeing the person from a place of being well already, as opposed to seeing the phobia and focusing on them being ill.

Teaching NLP

The teaching aspect of my work came about after a particular conversation a couple of years ago. I had been really busy at the time and a lady sent me a heartfelt email about a personal issue she had. I sent a short reply back to her saying I was sorry to hear about what she was going through, but unfortunately my schedule was packed and I could not fit her in. She wrote an email in return saying that it was hard enough to be in her situation, but to also know that there was help, and not have access to it, was even worse. That stopped me in my tracks.

I made some space to go and help her and, within an hour, she had got the change she needed. But it struck me that even with the best intentions in the world, I could not be everywhere at once. NLP was something that had been taught to me, so I started teaching others, using the ways of practising that I had developed over time and found most effective.

NLP and Life Coaching

When it comes to coaching in the UK, people buy an outcome and will get a coach for that. This is different compared to other places, like the US for example, where people will be more open to going on an exploration. In this scenario the coach will help you live to your true values, find your higher self and discover the best 'you' ever. That type of coach in this country usually ends up back at their day jobs because they are financially broke.

Most coaches approach coaching from the perspective of what they can do to change the world. However, most clients will come to a coach for a specific reason with a personal goal in mind, so the two approaches are fundamentally different. My clients usually hire me to get a result. We do not go on an exploration, nor do we wonder around the forest and look at the trees. We have a destination that we are walking towards. We will quite often get to places where the person feels stuck, usually as a result of programming, limiting beliefs and phobias. It may be that they are in a job that is far from ideal and would like to change, but are fearful of making the shift. They may be terrified of public speaking or are continuously self-sabotaging. It is essentially the things that cause them to be in their own way. We use the coaching to get a view of what the issues are, and then NLP to create the release that is necessary to allow them to move forward.

My Work

The way I see my work is that each person is like a spring and over time they get stretched. The tension in the spring does not come from the thing that is creating the stretch; it comes from the spring wanting to go back the other way. Release comes when you realise that it is not a scenario that is pulling you out of shape, it is your thoughts about what is going on that create the problem. A spring does not take years of therapy to regain its shape after being pulled, it just snaps back naturally to where it needs to be, that is also the way we are. As practitioners working with others, our belief that clients are well needs to be stronger than their belief that they are not.

I often get asked what the favourite part of my work is. Without a doubt it is when I look into the eyes of the person in front of me, and we both know that there has just been a shift in their thinking, which means they are never going to be the same again. I am reminded of the phrase, 'It is only work if you would rather be doing something else'. I can honestly say that there is absolutely nothing I would rather be doing.

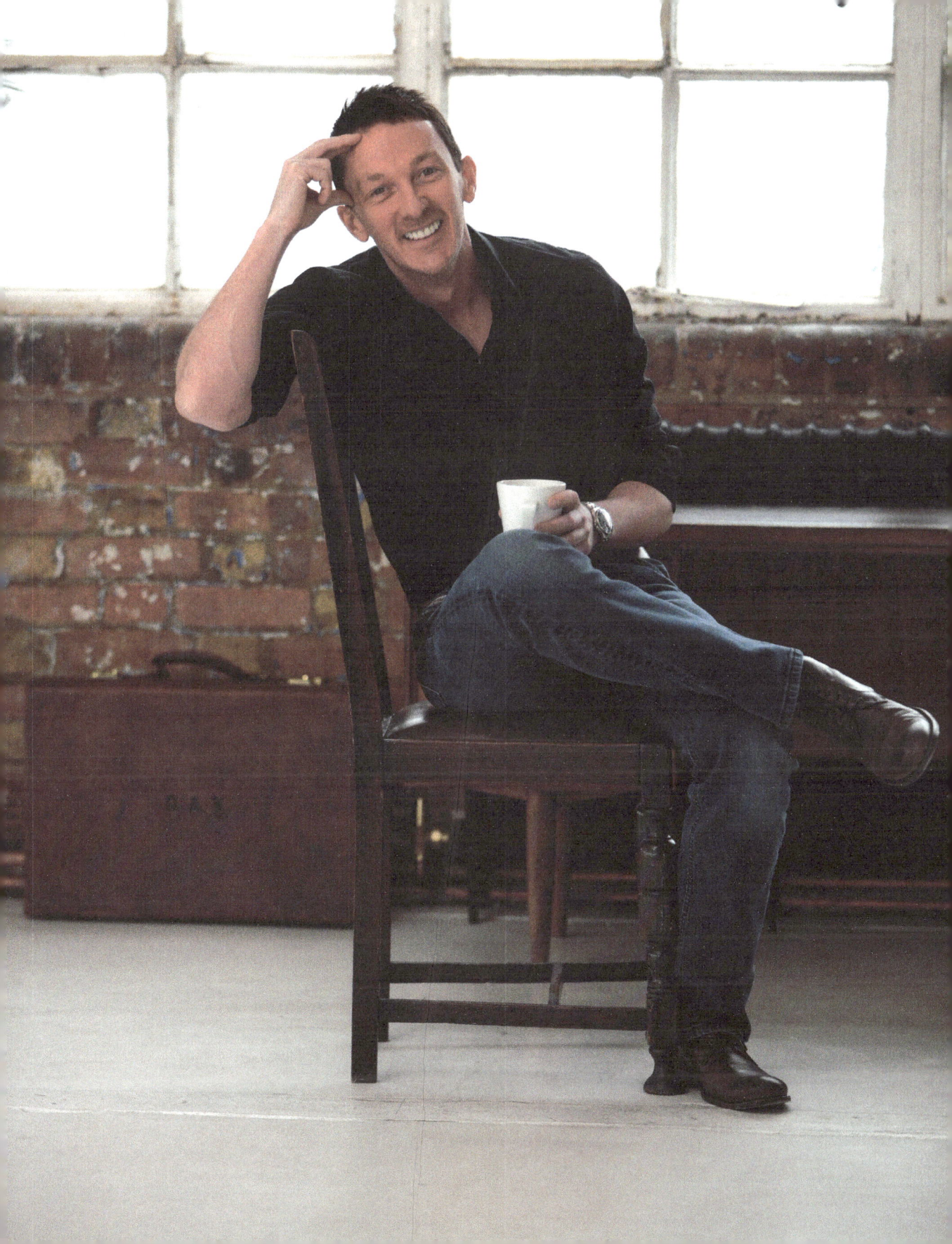

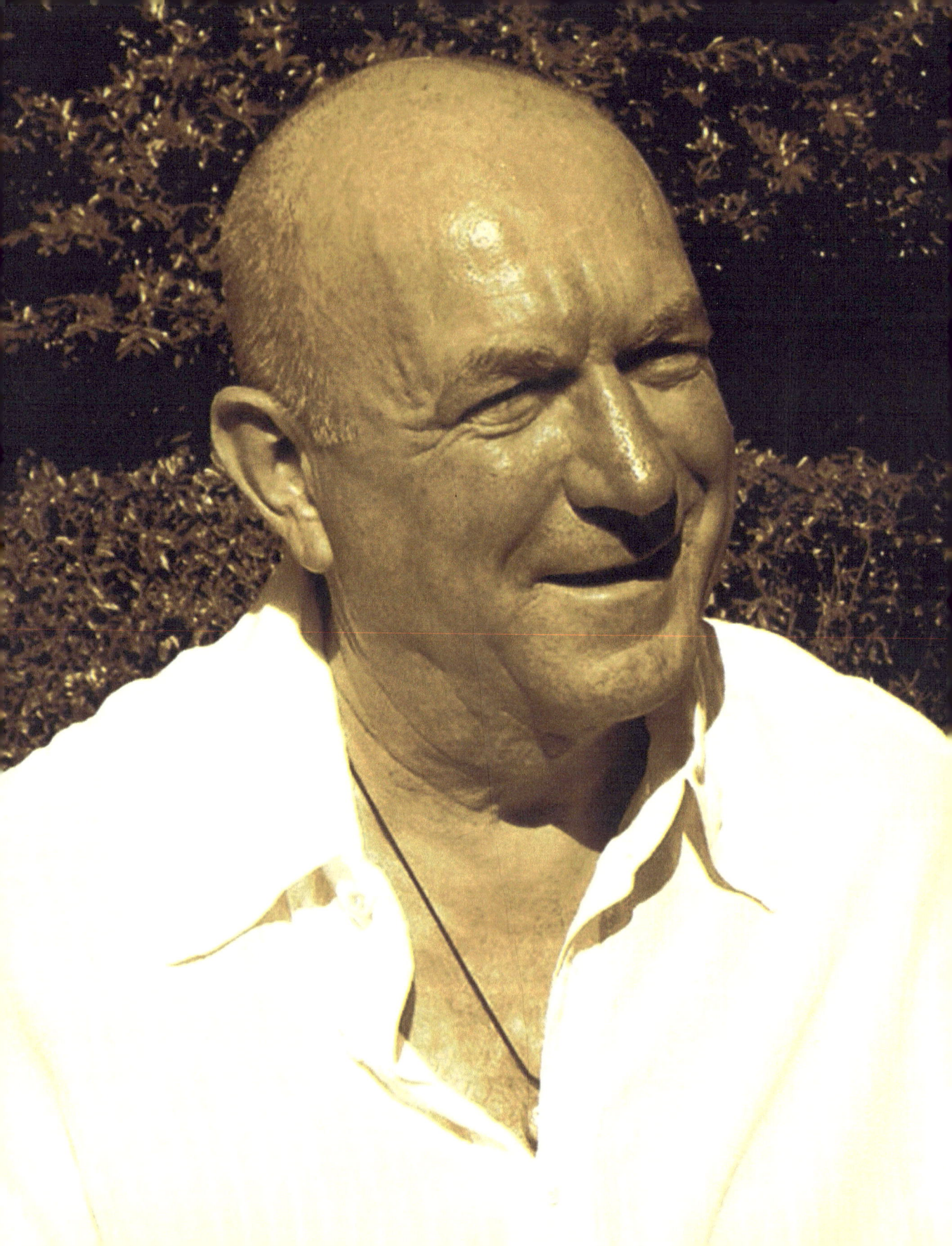

Ed Percival
NLP Master Practitioner, Life Coach and NLP Master Trainer

I got the distinct impression during my conversation with Ed Percival that he works to meticulous standards. So much so that Richard Bandler, one of the co-founders of Neuro Linguistic Programming (NLP), has awarded Ed by personally issuing him with the sixth master trainer certificate. Ed has spent a large part of his working life helping others to achieve goals, high performance levels and enhanced life experiences. During our exchange the term 'not easily bought' sprung firmly to mind, as I got the sense he was very clear where he ended and I began, holding quite firmly to those boundaries. As a result, I got a very fair and clear picture of what NLP really means to him.

Coaching is something I started when I was twelve years old. The first year class at our school could not have basketball sessions as there was no one to lead them. I asked the PE teacher if I could be the leader so that they could play and he agreed. I really enjoyed the experience and being a coach has continued throughout my life, from managing 120 people at Hoover by the age of twenty-one, to currently acting as a coach for individuals, trainers and teams. I believe that coaching is about preparing my clients for the future and, as a coach, I am always looking for things that work and are effective. In my experience NLP works.

I discovered NLP in 1986 through Frogs Into Princes, a book written by Richard Bandler and John Grinder, published seven years earlier. I found the content quite extraordinary and I was readily able to apply the ideas being presented. This spurred me on to read a bit more about the subject and I did Richard Bandler's one-year programme between 1995 and 1996, which was the only one-year programme he ever did and was attended by 120 people. After taking Bandler's course on Design Human Engineering, I was asked to assist him on his training for trainers and in 1998 he gave me the sixth master trainer certificate.

NLP

NLP was first created by Bandler and Grinder for people in therapy because, in the late 60s and early 70s, a lot of therapists were not making any progress with clients. People were generally in therapy for years, but Bandler and Grinder found that there were certain therapists who were getting results and made contact with them in order to find out what processes they were using. Since then things have moved on and most people now teach NLP as a way to enhance performance.

When I first started teaching NLP to practitioners and master practitioners with Colin Blundell, we wanted a model that would give them a clear understanding of where they were when working with clients. We developed the training around the concept that NLP is a state-driven modality. The concentration at the heart of NLP is either on the state that you are in, or that you can get your client to enter into. To access states we use specific language patterns to either put people into a trance state or alternatively bring them out of a trance and into a more conscious state. It is essential at the start of the session to have an outcome firmly in mind. This means being really clear about the goal that we are aiming to achieve. Other areas to focus on are behaviour, which takes into account how an experience is being processed by a person; relationships, and how these are dealt with; and strategies that are used or actions that they take in order to get things done. Keeping all of these areas in mind allows the practitioner to get a clear view of what is showing up for the client and what they need to do in order to get results.

NLP is a modality rather than a therapy. If I call myself a therapist this makes the assumption that you are not well and that you need therapy in order to get well, which is quite limiting. The NLP practitioner ought to have enough of a range to be able to turn people around who are a bit down, as well as cater for people who want to improve their particular skill set. So it does not simply serve one thing or the other, it is a modality which can inform anything that you do. So, for example, a skilled nutritionist can use NLP to get people to follow their dietary advice, become more accurate in their counselling and be more committed to the programme. It has been described as a meta or overriding modality, meaning that you can use it to inform anything that you do.

Changing States

If you are only focused on people's thoughts and beliefs you are missing out on eight tenths of the work. I do not want to downplay the importance of changing people's belief systems but there are a lot of other parts that would multiply the effects you are getting. If you are getting good results, just by changing belief patterns, then placing your attention on changing the way that people experience life and the way that they process their experiences as well would have a huge upward impact on the results that you achieve.

NLP enables state-driven change. So, for example, if a person is finding it hard to get into a good learning state and I am only working with them on changing their beliefs, then change is highly unlikely to occur. It would be like trying to push water up a hill. Whereas, if they can change their experience of reality, it would make changing their belief a lot easier.

Does NLP Make For A Better Person?

NLP makes a person more effective at what they do, rather than making them a better person. Suggesting that someone would become a better person by doing NLP would have dangerous implications. Becoming a better person to me is living to a higher set of values, and NLP is much more superficial than that. If someone has NLP practised on them, it is not going to make them a more moral person, whether they are a practitioner or a recipient.

My understanding of NLP is that it is a state-driven modality rather than just a belief system modality. You can tap into a person's state without having to access their beliefs. There are language patterns that can drive people into a less conscious state, where hypnotic suggestions made can override their personal belief, or into a more conscious state, where hypnotic suggestions can be actioned by them.

Practicing NLP

I think that it should be necessary for all NLP practitioners to integrate their own experience of NLP before they begin practising on others. There are a lot of appalling NLP practitioners out there who have a low level of understanding and collect NLP processes like stickers or scout badges. However, they do not have the elegance or the integration to make proper use of these processes. In cases like these, the practitioner would often say that they have identified the client's problem and know what needs to be done to have this problem fixed. I call that NLPing on people. It is very disrespectful and unskilled and it gives NLP a bad name. My approach is that I want to sneak up on people and do the work without them noticing. They walk away from the session feeling like they have just had a conversation and, all of a sudden, the entire world has changed.

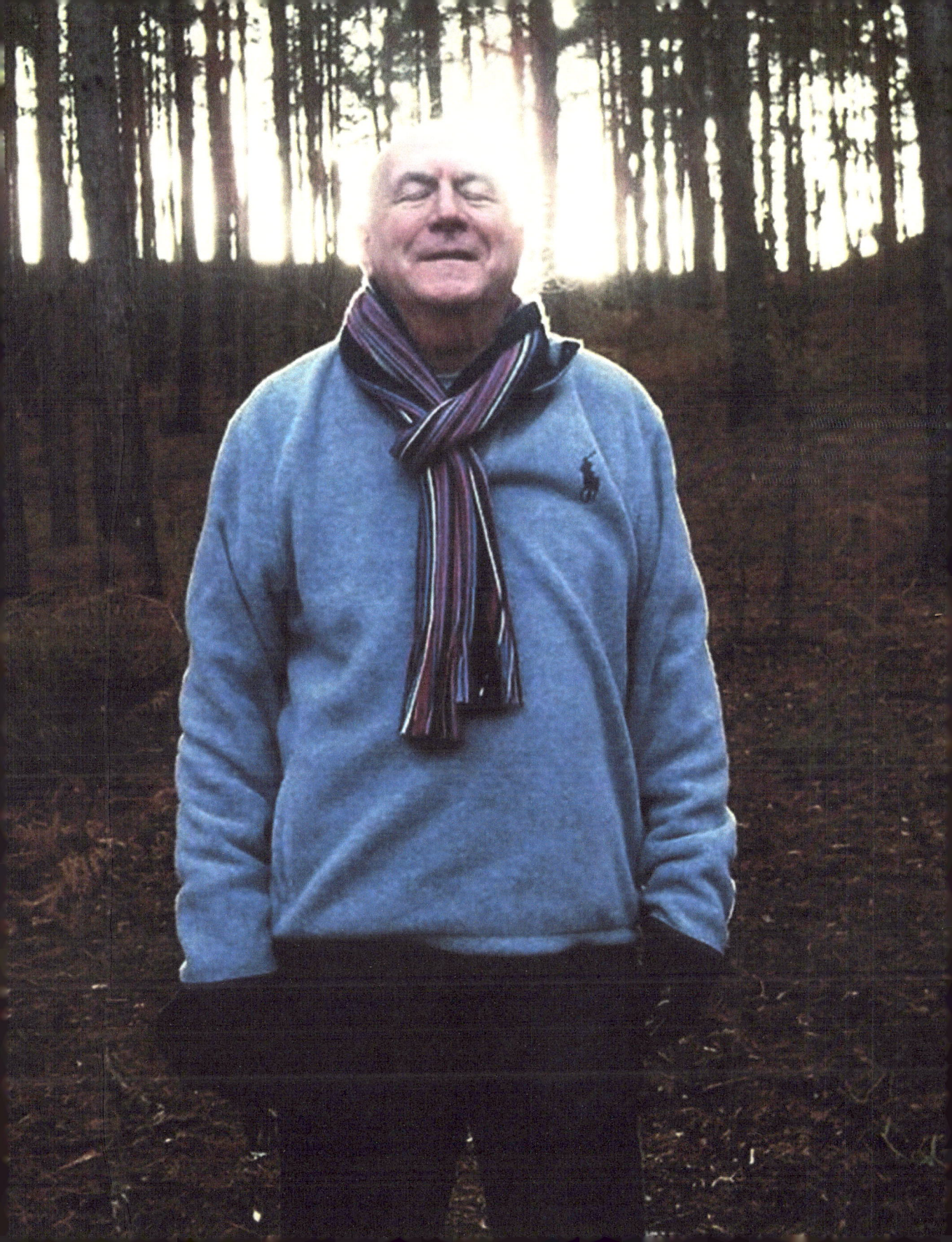

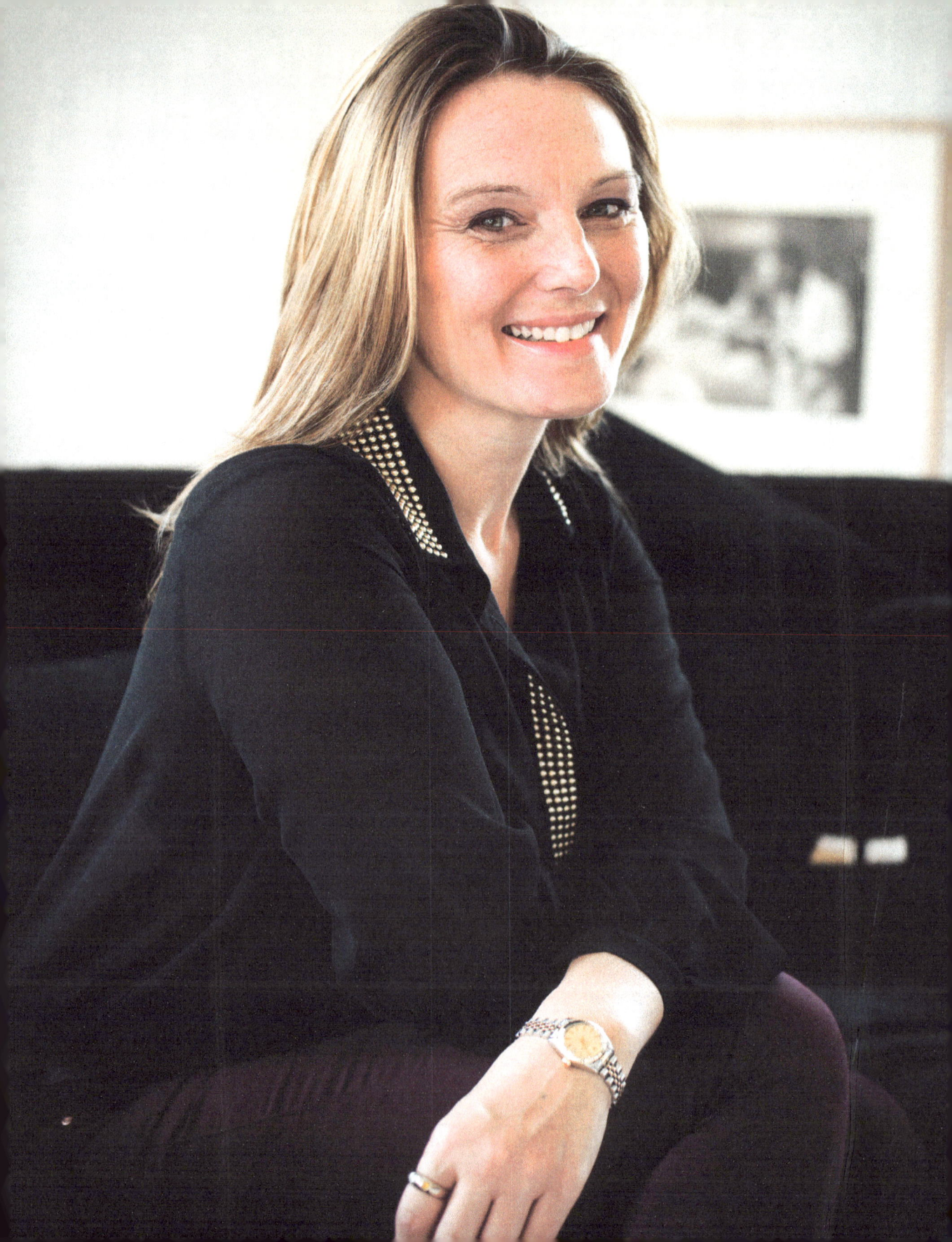

Nina Madden
NLP Practitioner, Hypnotherapist, Life Coach and Teacher

Nina Madden, who is half Irish and half Swedish, is one of life's intrepid explorers. The creative impulse has always been a source of great inspiration to her. This has seen her travel the world and immerse herself into the fabric of varying cultures, arts and communities. Growing up in a very academic family environment, Nina is thorough in her understanding and knowledge of her field of choice, human transformation. She has combined all the ingredients of her journey in life, to create an exceptional cocktail of alchemy. It was a joy to talk to her about NLP and its power to restructure and renew the mind.

My interests have always been in psychology, literature, the human condition and art. I have also invariably been fascinated by the bigger questions of 'Who am I and what am I doing here?' I went through some difficult challenges in my own life and as a result my development as a therapist has been organic. NLP was instrumental in pulling me through a tough and painful occurrence, so I got a first hand introduction into how helpful and useful it could be.

In terms of my background, I come from a family steeped in the world of academia; however, this did not hold much interest for me. Instead, I was interested in Art and travelling the world. Laos and Thailand became my home for eight years and I set up a business there as an antique art dealer. What drew me to the world of antiques was the story behind the objects. Each art piece had a spiritual, cultural and historic story to tell and a full life behind it.

On moving to London I began a completely different chapter in my life. I was hungry to study and did two masters in contemporary art and critical theory, and wrote about the articulation of trauma within narrative memory. I was also interested in the poetry of Paul Celan whose language breaks into fragments, and the Columbian artist Dors Salecedo, whose work has a suffocating rather than narrative feel. When we experience trauma, language is inadequate and simply cannot envelop the experience, so often we feel that it fails us. This is where my journey began in focusing on the mix between trauma, therapy and art.

My Work

Because of my own life experiences, which were difficult at times, I have a lot of empathy with the life situations of others. Once you have hit rock bottom yourself, you are able to trust that, no matter what a person is going through, there is always a possibility for them to get out of it. Helping a client release the effects of a painful or negative experience and letting go of the angst they have been carrying around, in some cases for years, is a very uplifting thing to do.

I hear my clients and the people around me like music. Just like a song, a person has a base beat, which is their underlying beat. Sometimes my work is about helping them to change that beat from negative and fearful, to positive, expectant and confident. The therapist always has to keep their awareness on their own base. This means focusing on the message that they are sending out to the client. The focus of the therapist is key because the message that the client emanates with, could be distressing. As a therapist I tune into the base of the client and, in doing so, our two beats can make for something interesting and transformative. This allows the client to move into a different internal dynamic of space and sound.

NLP

I came to NLP through life coaching and was introduced to it by chance. I met an NLP trainer who said that I should come on his course. I had a positive hunch about him and just went with it. He taught in a really out the box sort of way and I had a few very big personal breakthroughs during that week. I came to the realisation on the course, that I had some beliefs in place that were holding me back. Using the NLP tools that I learnt, I was able to get rid of them completely. With the transformation of my thoughts came a strong physical shift, and I knew instantly that this was powerful and that it was something I wanted to progress into. NLP reorganises the way you think about things and once you expand your understanding everything changes in the way you move forward.

Within NLP and hypnosis, we previously referred to unconscious and conscious elements of the mind. These concepts are obsolete now and we understand, more and more, that all deep change has its root in the metaphorical landscape within. I work holistically with people to access deep change within this landscape, which in turn changes their rational understanding of themselves and provides for a better experience of the world around them.

Facets of the Mind

I like to think of the mind in terms of a huge ancient library containing loads of books, and in the centre there is an old cabinet with index cards, referencing all these books. When the mind presents a particular topic or problem, you go to the index card and pull it out and then you realise that there are many different books all on the same subject, and all in different parts of the library.

In real terms, this means you may have a metaphoric representation of an issue, where the connections are more abstract. You may have a conceptual representation, which is triggered by certain types of language and words. You may have an embodied understanding of the issue, which means you are triggered on a physical level and all these varying ways or representing the issue have to be addressed. You may try to rationalise a loss or rejection, but if you still feel the pain in your body, still experience yourself metaphorically as all alone, surrounded by emptiness, no rational talking will create lasting change. This is why operating on your deep metaphors is so much more powerful.

Many times therapists like to think of there being a core belief or a core problem, because that makes it nice and clean for the therapist. But the reality is not always so clear-cut. The human mind is more akin to a matrix and my work with one individual often takes me to many places in time and space.

Developing My Work

My clients come from all walks of life. Working with so many different people is a gift. It is very enlightening and humbling to be invited into people's lives on such a personal level. I love my one-to-one sessions with individuals and, informed by this, I am now developing an enhanced NLP programme that brings the latest discoveries in neuroscience into the NLP syllabus. This is a very unique course within the UK.

Additionally, I also offer training and development workshops in NLP. These advanced workshops take aspects of NLP, puts a spotlight on them, expands them and explores them to their ultimate possibility. My plan is to do more by way of writing as well. The future will contain books on subjects to do with the mind, our emotional self, who we are and what our place is within the world. NLP is a very creative explorative discipline, the founding concept is an attitude of curiosity. We are always investigating what is happening with the person and what is going to make the transformation for them.

My Business

I draw a lot from my life experiences when it comes to my work. During my time living in Thailand I learned a lot from the culture. There was a real kindness in interactions with the people and a soft element to the energy. I learnt early on in my time there, that in order to be successful in business, connections and friendships were paramount. When you learn to instil kindness in each connection that you have with each person you come across, your business becomes naturally successful. This way of thinking definitely informs all areas of the work I now do.

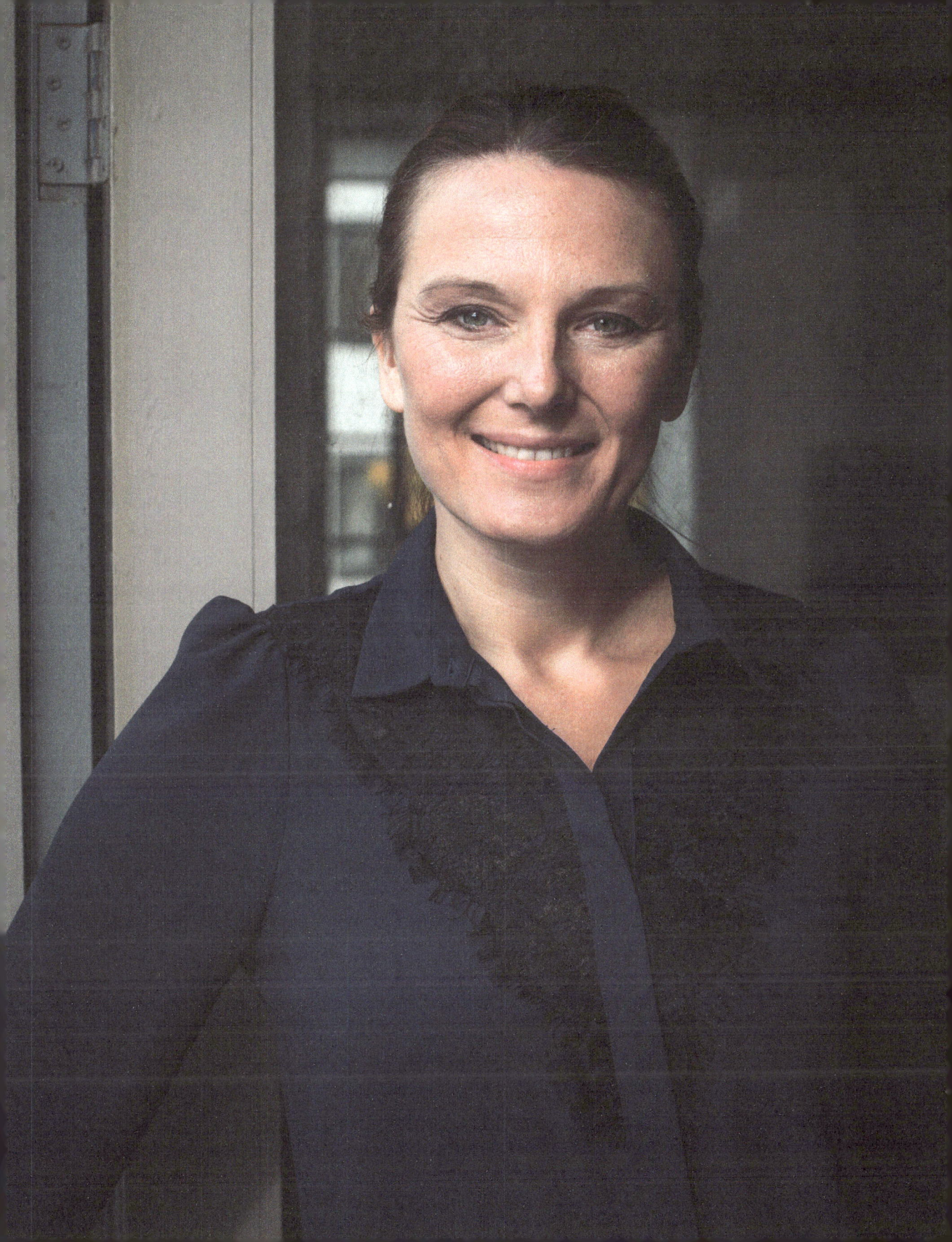

"It feels great when I am able to help people clear away their masks, so that they can operate from a more authentic place. It is about building their self-worth and self-esteem to really learn to love and take care of themselves. The aim is to get them to the point where they know they are enough. It is important for them to be courageous, brave and strong in that conviction."

- Jacqueline Hurst

Hypnotherapy

Hypnotherapy works by putting the subject into an altered mental state or trance state, which creates a heightened response to suggestions. Hypnosis can be used by a therapist to produce changes in thought patterns, behavioural patterns and emotional responses. These changes can be translated into helping the client to break habits, such as smoking or erratic relationships with food, leading to obesity, bulimia or anorexia. It can also be used to induce relaxation at times when there would normally be anxiety or stress, which makes it effective in the treatment of phobias and physical symptoms of stress, including skin conditions.

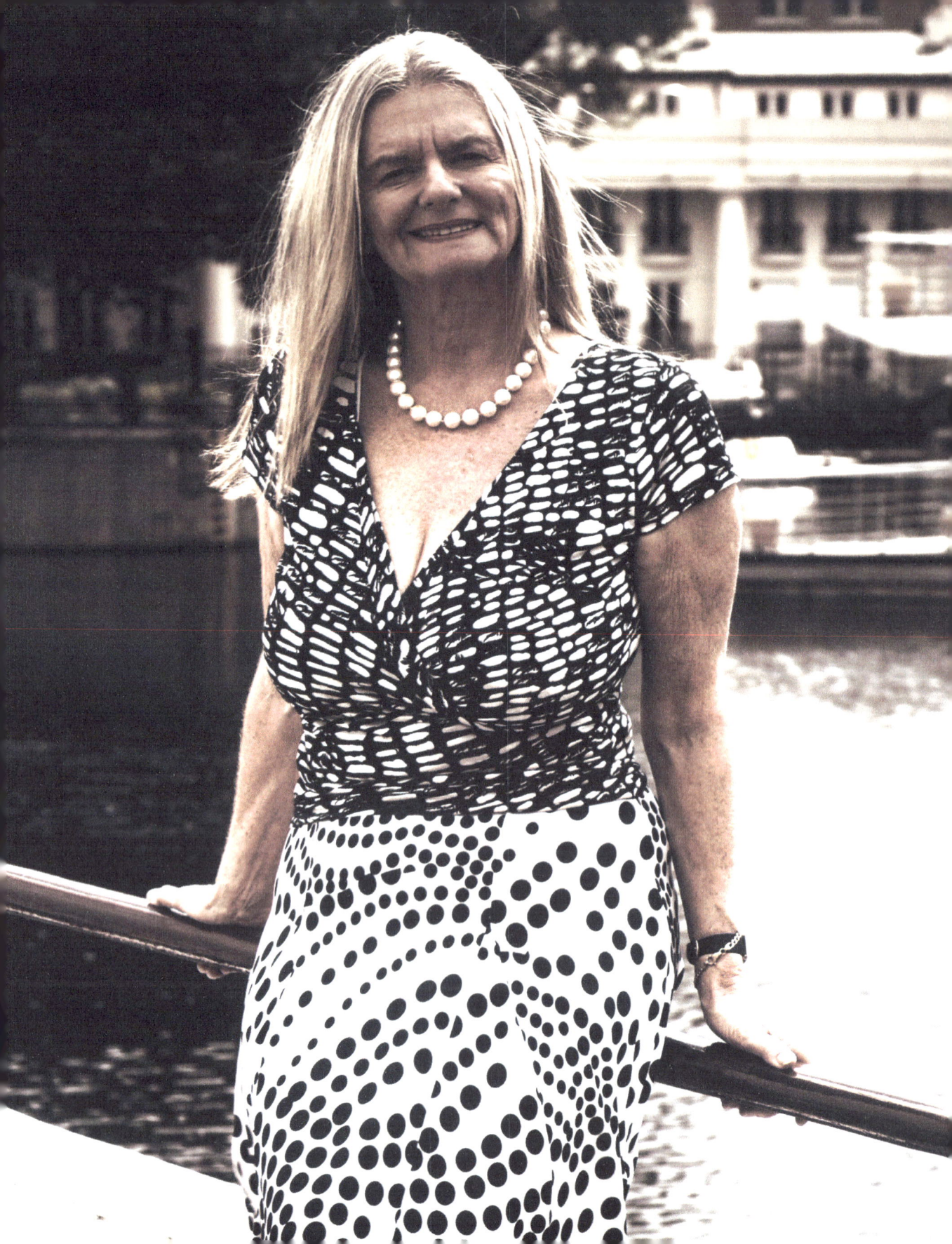

Valerie Austin
Hypnotherapist, Author and Teacher

Valerie Austin started her practice as a hypnotherapist in 1989. She had always been interested in the subject of hypnotherapy from a scientific viewpoint, but when a car accident left her with debilitating memory loss, it offered her an effective cure. This spurred her to become one of its most avid pioneers in the UK. She was one of the very first people to bring hypnosis into the hospital environment and, through her outstanding courses, seminars and media coverage, has been responsible for educating people globally on the power of trance and the subconscious mind in creating lasting transformation.

I have always been fascinated by hypnosis and when I was told I could not be hypnotised, this added intrigue. I am non-visual and, as people are usually asked to visualise, someone who is unable to see mental images is just told that they cannot be hypnotised.

Generally, hypnotherapists do not know how to work with people who are non-visual, but non-visual people do have knowledge of what they are being asked to visualise and know what it looks like. These people do not even realise that they are non-visual unless they have been tested. I have been testing people's ability to visualise for 20 years. Funnily enough a lot of accountants tend to be non-visual in my experience.

I believe that visualisation starts in childhood. When someone is unable to visualise, it is because they may have had an accident or have not used this ability for whatever reason, and over time it disappears. You can sometimes succeed in getting some people who are non-visual to be visual through hypnotherapy. I personally have not done it because I have never needed to.

My Personal Introduction to Hypnotherapy

I had a car accident which left me with a 24-hour memory for about a year and a half. In an attempt to unearth someone who would be able to help me, as it was a problem, I ran a story in one of the newspapers that said that I was getting married in Hollywood, and added, 'Would the bride remember her husband?' I was eager to find a cure for my predicament because I had stopped earning money after the memory loss.

As a result of the article, I was contacted by an American hypnotherapist who was travelling in the UK. He offered to treat me when I came to the US and the hypnosis cured me completely for around a year and a half. But then I had a highly stressful period, where my parents died and various other challenging things occurred, and I reverted back to a memory loss. However, whereas before I had a 24-hour memory, I now can only remember the last two weeks. People I interact with generally do not notice this because the more they ask me questions, the more I can access the memory. But without being asked it would just disappear and my mind would be an absolute blank.

The positive part of having the memory I do, is that I live very much in the moment and do not dwell in the past. This has enabled me to put together a hypnosis technique, which is a unique way of talking to the subconscious, and was devised because of the memory loss. It is teachable, excellent and has a high success rate across the board.

My Work

I currently charge £5,000 per client for one-to-one sessions and I only see a handful of clients a year. My main goal has been to bring my work out to others through courses and conferences. When I first started out working as a hypnotherapist in 1989 I targeted smokers and the results were black and white, they either stopped smoking or they didn't. Everyone around them knew when they stopped and they themselves were so proud that they would tell everyone. All of this provided a good source of word of mouth marketing. My clients used to consist of a third smoking, a third weight issues and a third everything else. In the early nineties I worked at The Priory Hospital, dealing with disorders and various really complicated issues. I was the first hypnotherapist brought into a hospital and was commissioned to work together with a psychologist.

The main thing that I am interested in now, and I never thought I would be, is cancer. A friend of mine, who is anattorney, had level four cancer and was given a 15% chance of survival a couple of months ago. Fortunately, she was not given radiation or chemotherapy before the operation. We worked with hypnosis and her diet and the tumour shrank by half. This has now gone to level two and she has been given an 89% chance of survival, which is a huge achievement.

Defining Hypnosis

There has been a lot of controversy over explaining what hypnosis is. The best explanation I can give is that it is like a daydream. You go into a form of trance, which acts to switch on the subconscious mind, and is similar to switching on a computer. You are then able to talk with the subconscious, while the conscious mind looks on. The trance state is a bit like giving the conscious mind a tranquilliser. It is still there, but it is not as active.

I teach the skill of regression within my course. This means fishing to find out what the source of the problem is, and then dealing with it from that place. The issue that the person is struggling with is not an inherent part of who they are, so it can be termed a virus of the mind. When there is a repetitive problem with depression, alcohol or relationships, it can be easily compared to a virus within a person's mental state.

Hypnosis and Beliefs

Does hypnosis work primarily with belief systems? The answer to that would be yes and no. The reason I say no is because the virus is usually a result of trauma. In a traumatic situation your consciousness is quite busy and is not operating effectively as a filter. As a result, it has let faulty information into the subconscious. Your belief system comes in after that, because this faulty information speaks as your voice and you trust it.

Hypnosis and The Mind

To me the mind is like a computerised robot. Its main job is to make sure you are happy and get what you want. But from time to time it gets a virus, which stops it from functioning in the same way because it now has a disruptive force within it. This is a normal occurrence, we all have traumas at some time in our lives. If we have not had trauma in childhood, it will have a stronger impact later in life. This is because in our younger years, painful situations can be a source of strength. However, we interpret them differently as we get older. Most of these viruses can be eradicated just through hypnosis. When hypnosis is used in the right way there is no need for anything to support it. This is because it will do the job just on its own.

So many things are possible with hypnotherapy. For example, under hypnosis it is possible for someone to have a major surgical procedure and not have anaesthesia. It is not something that people would generally want to do, but it is possible. I studied with a doctor who did many operations using hypnosis in Ireland and one of them was an amputation. He was in the accident room and there was a constant flow of people in and out. Using hypnotherapy techniques was made easier by the fact that when people are frightened, they are generally more open to hypnosis. This highlights the point that hypnotherapy is not dependent on the person being in a relaxed state.

The Future

Hypnotherapy at present is getting integrated and mixed with so many other things. As a result, its effectiveness is often diluted or lost. I find this frustrating at times, but I do not fight it. I just keep on with my work, both teaching and doing conferences. My aim is to teach with excellence and keep what I teach, for as long as I can, as pure hypnosis. It does not mean that the people on my course have not learnt about other things, and that is perfectly alright, but when they come to learn with me, they are learning undiluted hypnotherapy.

It is so amazing what hypnotherapy can do and it shocks you each time someone leaves the session transformed. It could be something like being able to eat vegetables for the first time, whereas previously they had a phobia. Hypnosis is really rapid in the way it works. Some people may need a few sessions to clear their consciousness, but when hypnotherapy works it does so in an instant. This is why it is a constant source of fascination for me, I never stop learning and never get bored.

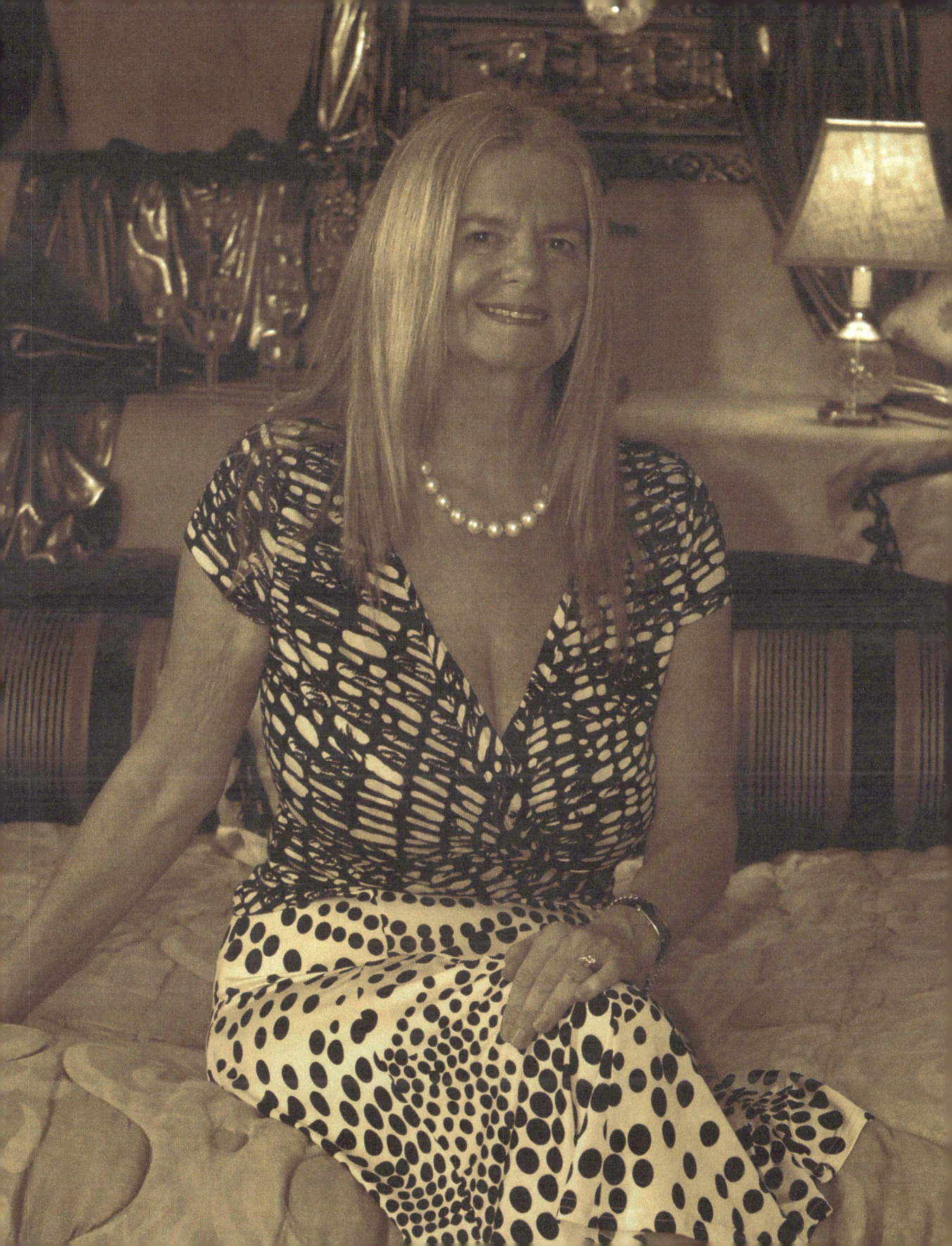

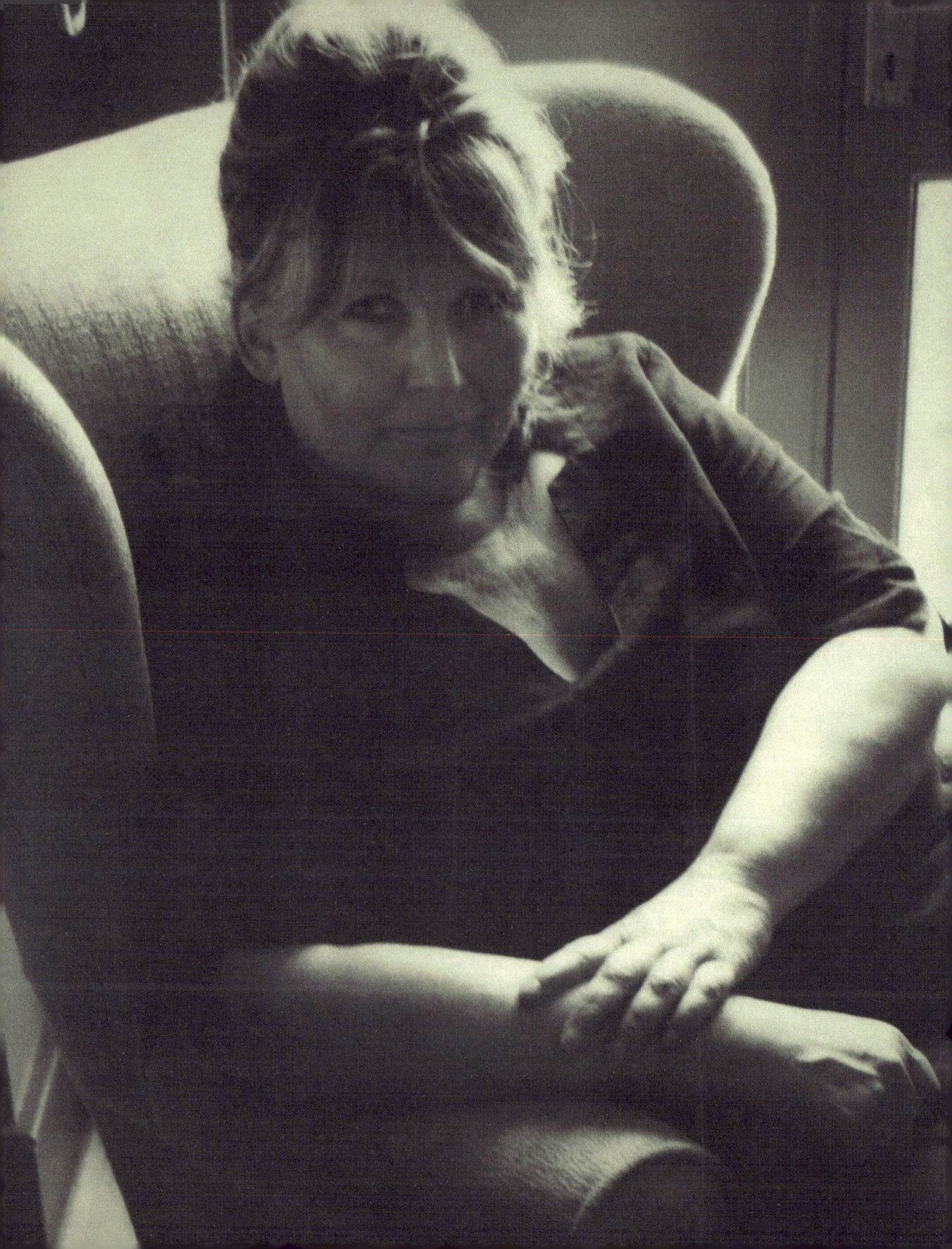

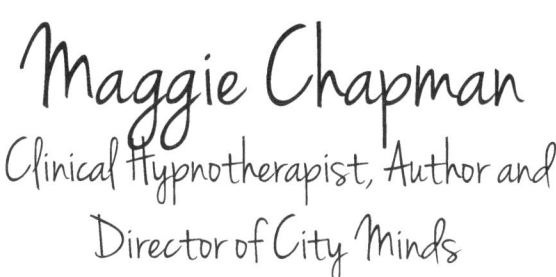

Maggie Chapman
Clinical Hypnotherapist, Author and Director of City Minds

Maggie Chapman was drawn to working with the mind from the age of 16. Although there was a detour into the world of Business and Accountancy, she is now back where she feels she belongs: working on transforming and expanding the human experience through thought and belief systems. She is a leader in the field of Clinical Hypnotherapy and is also involved in training others to a standard of excellence through her company City Minds.

I started off, when I was 16, doing voluntary work in a secure unit of a mental hospital called Netherne in Surrey. We were just a group of teenagers who were going in and talking to people who needed to be interacted with on a social level. While I was there I met a number of severely psychologically disturbed people and I cut my teeth on that experience. From then on, I knew I wanted to be involved with the mind in some way and so I took a psychology degree, but hated it. It seemed to me to be very much about academic study and theory, as opposed to people. I think the way a psychology degree is presented now is much different to how it was back then.

I decided that I would do a business degree instead and went into accountancy. I enjoyed numbers and was good at the job, but my heart and soul was not in it. As time progressed, I became interested in retraining and returning into the field of working with the mind. So I started a counselling course. Very soon after that my family was involved in a massive trauma, which catapulted things forward. I went on to study trauma counselling, which helped me to understand all different forms of abuse – physical, emotional and every other level.

At the time I was also working on a voluntary basis with physical disability and the emotional side of disability, while researching various different courses, and came across Clinical Hypnotherapy, which seemed to make the most sense to me.

Clinical Hypnotherapy

Clinical Hypnotherapy is about how the mind can have an effect on not just our bodies and the way we behave, but also the physical symptoms and illnesses we produce. Accessing the mind and effecting change through hypnosis became fascinating to me and it fitted in with everything I had ever experienced in own personal life.

I learned how to train other people and became a lecturer in Clinical Hypnosis all around the world. Then I got involved with creating a Master's Degree in Clinical Hypnosis and developing the course, so that it could be recognised and respected as an intervention. Laterally, there was the whole Cognitive Behavioural Therapy (CBT) explosion, so I studied CBT. In my practice I integrate Transactional Analysis, CBT and Clinical Hypnosis.

The key to this process is that it enables someone to look after themselves. It is empowering, goal directed and action orientated. It is very much about accepting that you are where you are, looking at how you can get change, and giving you strategies that will help you. So ideally, it's about getting someone up and running within a period of time.

I get a huge kick out of knowing that what I do can make a difference. It is immensely satisfying. I have knowledge that, when shared, makes someone's life better, particularly the knowledge of how we biochemically disrupt ourselves. When we are disturbed by emotions we are out of homeostasis. Hypnotherapy brings awareness and gives you the tools and strategies to bring yourself into balance, so you are not disturbed by the world and the people within it. This gives you a sense of control, which means that biochemically you are at ease, and you think and behave in a way where you access your potential. I find it quite exciting.

Influence

Albert Ellis has been a major influence to me for sure. He was one of the founders of Cognitive Behavioural Therapy. In my opinion his thought processes were incredibly clever. It is also humbling the work that he did. He came up with a psychological theory that fits with each and every person's human experience; it must have been so meticulous and painstaking. He is definitely to be applauded.

I am a strong believer that learning comes from experience. People make conscious judgements and beliefs based on their experiences. I take exception to the broad brush of the personality type. Instead, I think that there is a physiological type that you are born with and your environment then influences that. It reminds me of that wonderful saying by Buddha, 'Your thought informs your deed. Your deed informs your habit. Your habit hardens your character. Be mindful of what you think.' There is no character trait;

All behaviours come from a thought. A belief is a thought that you have evaluated and decided to live from and act out. Everything that has manifested itself in this world started with a thought, so healthy thoughts are the way forward. It is just logical.

My Journey as a Clinical Hypnotherapist

I feel blessed to have a very intense level of curiosity within my nature. But the knowledge that I have now has changed the way I think, feel and respond in the world, without a doubt. I would probably have been hugely reactive if I hadn't gone on this journey. Whereas, because of my curiosity and the path that I have taken, I have been able to make sense of myself and this learning is still continuing. The older I get, the more humbled I am by people and knowledge. It is quite fascinating; I don't think I will ever have all the answers to anything.

Some people are born with the creative ability to play music, others to draw or write. I just had this gift of inquisitiveness about the mind. I remember as a small child wondering if everyone saw colours the same way I did, or whether they saw them differently. I have always been fascinated by how other people think of the world. Being human is an intriguing experience, as is the development of knowledge to understand how much of our behaviour and thoughts are driven by chemistry, and how much by conditioning.

Clinical Hypnosis and Being Human

I stepped away from working with the mind and managed in the world, but it was never satisfying. My own personal trauma fast-tracked the whole process and got me into the work I now do. On some level, as much as I wish the trauma had never happened, it opened opportunities. I gained a greater understanding on what it is to be human, but it was at a huge price. It is a hard balance in my head, but I do understand that somehow a door opened and, rather than becoming a victim of my trauma, I was able to do something with it, which is a more helpful way of being in the world. It is something that is quite innate within me I think.

If you think about it, in trauma work you have the victim and you have the survivor. If you viewed an incident as if it was done to you, and you had no control, yet it ruined your life and you stayed thinking like that, you will remain in that space. However, if you could think differently about that trauma, you can use it to create something that is really quite remarkable. You can gain and grow from it. That is part of my job, to take the victim which you have been, and help you come through to a place that is transformational.

A lot of the old Eastern knowledge, particularly Buddhism, is very much based in Cognitive Behavioural Therapy. We can draw inspiration from Buddhist philosophy when we are imparting what we know scientifically, but need to present it in a way that people can understand. Buddha says, 'Life is difficult!', which I challenge slightly, if I dare. The truth is, life is difficult sometimes, but life is also amazing sometimes. Life is not difficult always, otherwise we would all just give up. Life can also be filled with the magical.

Our experiences are always transient and changing. When I look at life as difficult, that is an unhealthy belief to hold. Which is why I take issue, because if your belief system is based on, 'Life is difficult', you will see life as difficult, whatever happens. You have already informed your perspective, therefore you are not able to see all the amazing possibilities. The other limiting belief is that life is not fair or life should be fair. But life is as it is, and it is fascinating in all its shifting changing moments. The human mind has a potential that is unlimited. If we take care of our bodies and our minds, the possibilities are infinite and I find that very exciting. I am just saddened that I am not going to be around 500 years from now to see what happens in this remarkable world of ours. I am so curious.

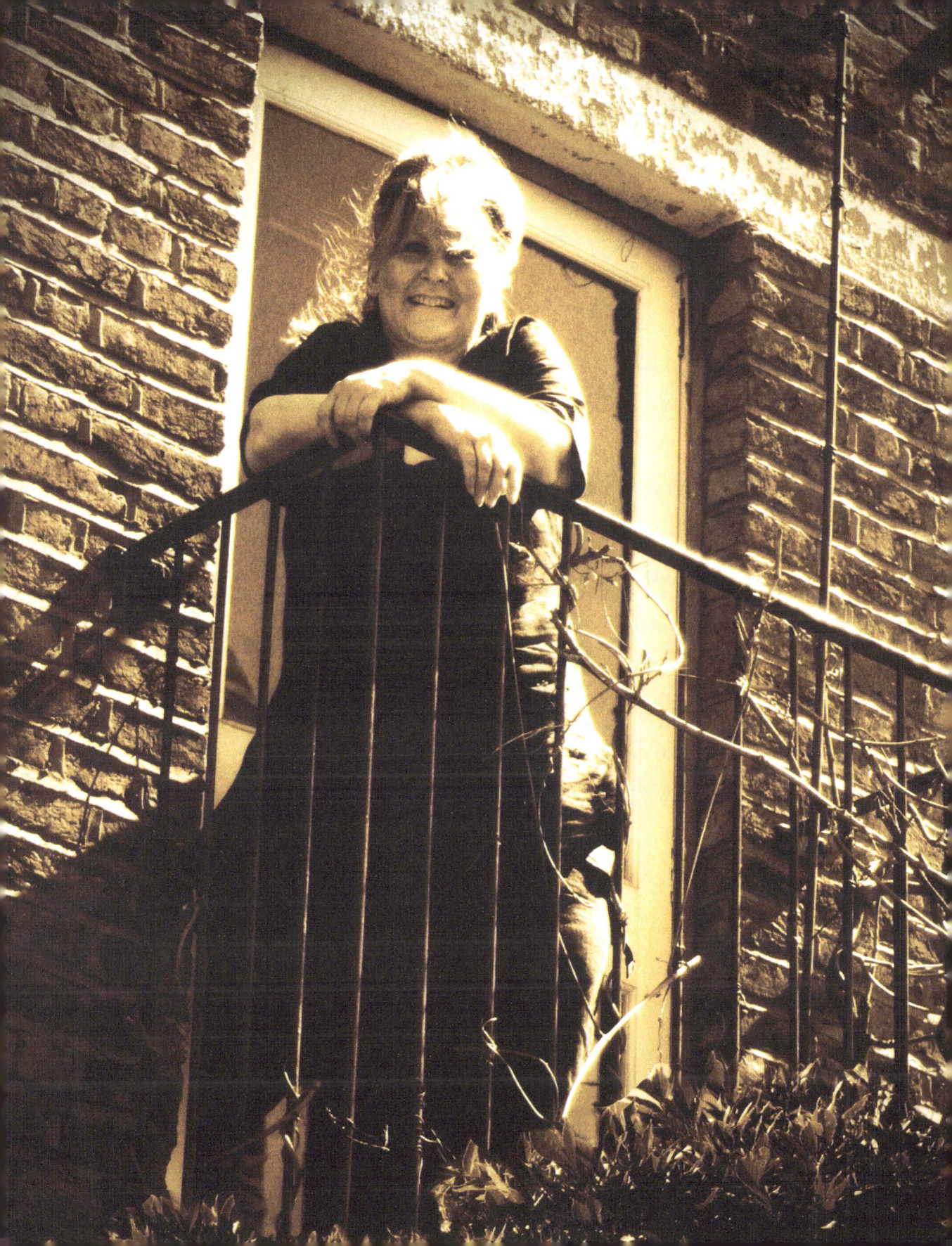

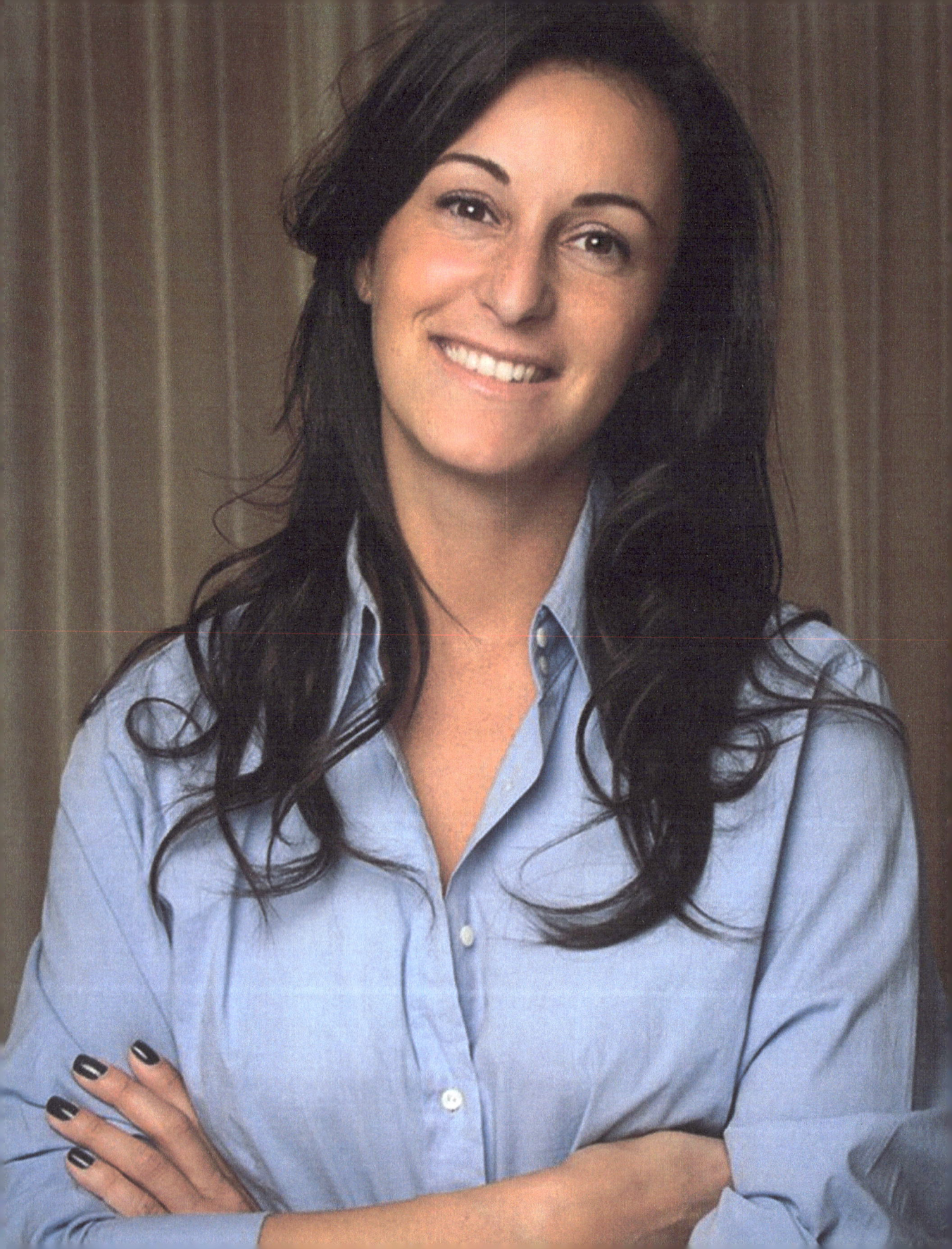

Jacqueline Hurst
Life Coach, Weight Management Coach, Clinical Hypnotherapist and NLP Practitioner

Jacqueline Hurst is what one could call a very wise woman in a young body, whose early years were lived on a fast track. Her teens and twenties were an intensely personal study of emotional upheavals, physical addictions and the painful aspects of being human. The person on the other side of those experiences is heart-based, empathetic, grounded and incredibly savvy. She has learnt her craft as a Coach, Clinical Hypnotherapist and NLP Practitioner, from the very best within the industry, and is determined to offer her clients the highest level of excellence through her mix of therapies. It was a real insight to speak to her of her journey.

My own experiences brought me to this work. I grew up with financial wealth but very little emotional guidance or stability. I became a drug addict from the age of fifteen, right through to the age of twenty-five. During this time I had cocaine addiction, anorexia and bulimia. I went through divorce, depression, anxiety; you name it, I had done it. At twenty-five I had a break down and was on my knees ready to get help. I tried everything available to me, including Alcoholics Anonymous, Narcotics Anonymous, NLP, hypnotherapy and life coaching. I was a sponge, soaking up as much as I could. Going through all those processes meant I became someone who is free of addiction, free of issues surrounding my body, free of anxiety and I got through my divorce. After all the occurrences during that period, the suffering, the hell and the suicide attempts, I completely get it when someone comes to me in real pain. I have been there, felt that pain and come through it.

Out of all the modalities I used to get well, I worked extensively with hypnosis as a way of accessing the subconscious mind and healing the past through regression. Also, a lot was achieved through NLP, it really challenged my thinking and was life changing for me. Additionally, simply talking to someone who would listen and understand me was hugely helpful as well.

The Journey

I think that a big part of my success today comes from the fact that when someone sits in front of me in emotional, physical, mental and spiritual pain, I truly get them and

I think that they understand that I get them, it creates an energy flow. I know from my own experience that it was all very well people having PhDs, diplomas and doctorates, but if they had not been through a major emotional challenge themselves, they wouldn't really get where I was coming from. That is what propelled me to becoming a therapist and doing this work.

I believe, without a doubt, that there was a purpose to all the challenging experiences I have gone through in my life. In the beginning, it seemed like such a tough road and I felt like I was never going to be well again. There are people who have never touched cigarettes, drugs or alcohol, and have no problems with food or relationships. They just seem to float through life. Then there was me who took completely the wrong path on everything. But looking back now, I know that everything that happened was right for me.

One of the things I have discovered is that there are so many facets to being a therapist. Some people are not able to work with intensity from a therapeutic standpoint. They may just gently engage with therapy, in which case I make the therapeutic session gently engaging. Also, it could be that the person is more interested in my work as a life coach, and they are looking for personal expansion. However, if they are on their knees and broken, it is a completely different ball game. You have to gauge where a person is and no one teaches you that at school. I really know that this is the gift my experiences have brought me.

It feels great when I am able to help people clear away their masks, so that they can operate from a more authentic place. It is about building their self-worth and self-esteem so that they can really learn to love and take care of themselves. The aim is to get them to the point where they know they are enough. It is important for them to be courageous, brave and strong in that conviction. I try to teach this as much as I can. Challenging people's limiting beliefs is always good fun!

I found that when I was on the road to getting well myself, some things were really powerful and some things weren't. I think that is what you have to gauge with a client. On my first sessions with people, I will do a lot of homework and groundwork. If I feel hypnosis is the best way forward, I will test their trance level before we work with hypnotherapy as a modality. With some of my clients it may be that hypnotherapy is not as effective as another mode. However, more often than not, I do use hypnosis, using parts therapy and combining this with coaching models and methods. Hypnosis goes back to go forward and coaching deals with the present time, as opposed to the past. Both have wonderful benefits.

Giving an example of how it all works, parts therapy is based on the surmise that we are all made up of different emotional parts. Let's say you had a problem with food and you just had to eat all the time. Consciously you know that this is not ideal for you and it is not what you want to do, but something keeps clicking in your mind and saying that you must do it. There begins a battle between your conscious versus subconscious minds. Your conscious mind is about 10% of your entire mind: your physical senses, all of your internal dialogue, your reason, justification and logic are all held here. But the problem with the conscious mind is that it deletes, distorts and generalises certain things. On the other hand, the 90% subconscious mind is where you hold your memories, your learnt beliefs, your learnt behaviour and your automatic responses. The subconscious has a huge influence and it is a part of the mind that does not lie, it records and files away your emotions or your various parts.

The majority of the time we are acting out of a subconscious memory and not realising it. To give another example, imagine you are three, and you are sitting in bed and you see a really big spider run past. You may jump and get a bit of a shock because it is quite unusual, but you are not frightened at this point because you don't know what it is. You then call your mum and dad and show it to them. As soon as they see it, they both start freaking out. In that moment you learn to fear it. As you get older, if you see the smallest of spiders, subconsciously your response will be to freak out.

With parts therapy we will work to explore why you were triggered to have that particular fear. When you are put in a trance you will be asked, what you have got invested in this problem and what part needs you to have this problem. Whatever your answer may be, we will then switch it to a more beneficial association. We will recalibrate your brain with parts therapy, so when you have certain feelings and emotions you will link it to something more positive and useful to you.

The Artist

I really work with my heart. Work wise I don't take things personally and I don't walk out of my office holding people's problems, but I really do give my absolute best to each and every client. I have never looked at this as just a business, so it has never been about how much more money I can make or how many more people I can see in a day. It was always about the main aim of 'how can I help?' I think this work comes with a certain level of understanding that we are dealing with people who are not very well at the moment. They need love, care, compassion, kindness and empathy. It does not mean dive in their pool and swim with them, it just means truly understanding their issue and helping them to see how to change in the kindest and gentlest way possible. That to me is extremely important.

The Future

I have been approached to do a lot of things and there have been opportunities in the world of television. But I love what I do here, it is really personal and I work with really amazing people, from the very top to the bottom and it is enlightening. I have no desire at present to turn that into a product and a brand.

My own journey has been immense and I really understand the level of strength that has come from it. I have been clean for ten years now, but when someone has had past addictions, people always label them and say that they are going to be an addict for the rest of their life. I just wasn't going to put up with that. I did not want a label, I did not want someone to say to me, 'This is who you are!' The strength and the courage it takes to go through the first year of being clean is like no other. When you go through something like that, trivial things are no longer important. They say only six or seven percent of people stay clean, that is a really small number. But if you get your mindset in the right place, things can change. Holding that space for people to discover their own strengths and truth is really powerful thing to do with my life.

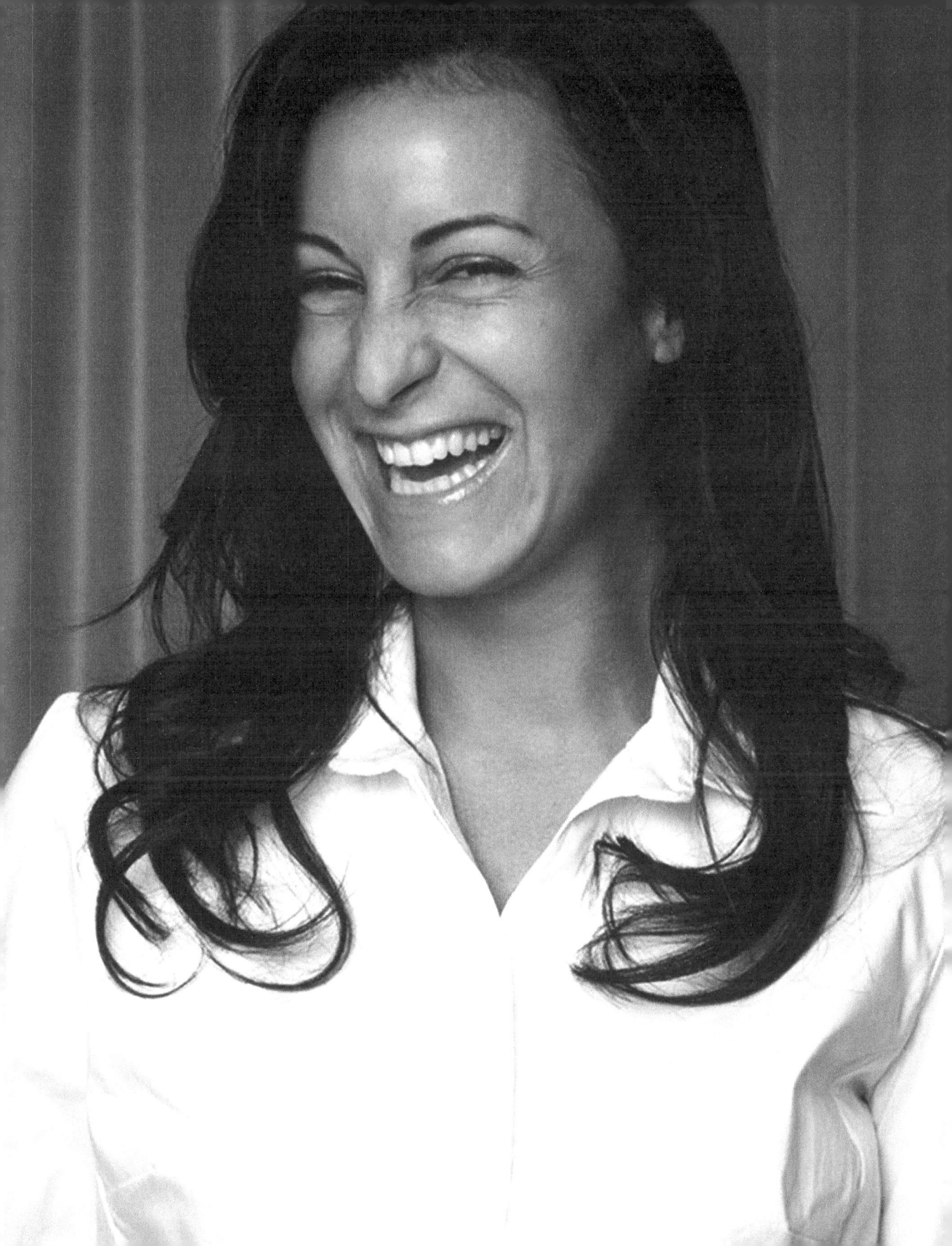

"If we are present and aware enough we each come to a place where we share a centre between us. From this space we are able to relate to each other with clarity as we are connecting through a higher perspective."

- Anja Saunders

Meditative Practices

When the mind is in a relaxed, yet alert, state our ability to respond to life is greatly enhanced. This Meditative section takes three very different practices and looks at them through the viewpoint of three remarkable individuals. Teresa Hale of the Hale Clinic talks about how important it is to create a firm Mind/ Heart connection. Chris Gaia speaks about mindfulness, which puts a focus on being present and being in the now. Anja Saunders speaks about creating a sacred circle so that the meditative experience can be shared with others. Together they give us a rounded take on why stilling the mind can bring us vivid clarity.

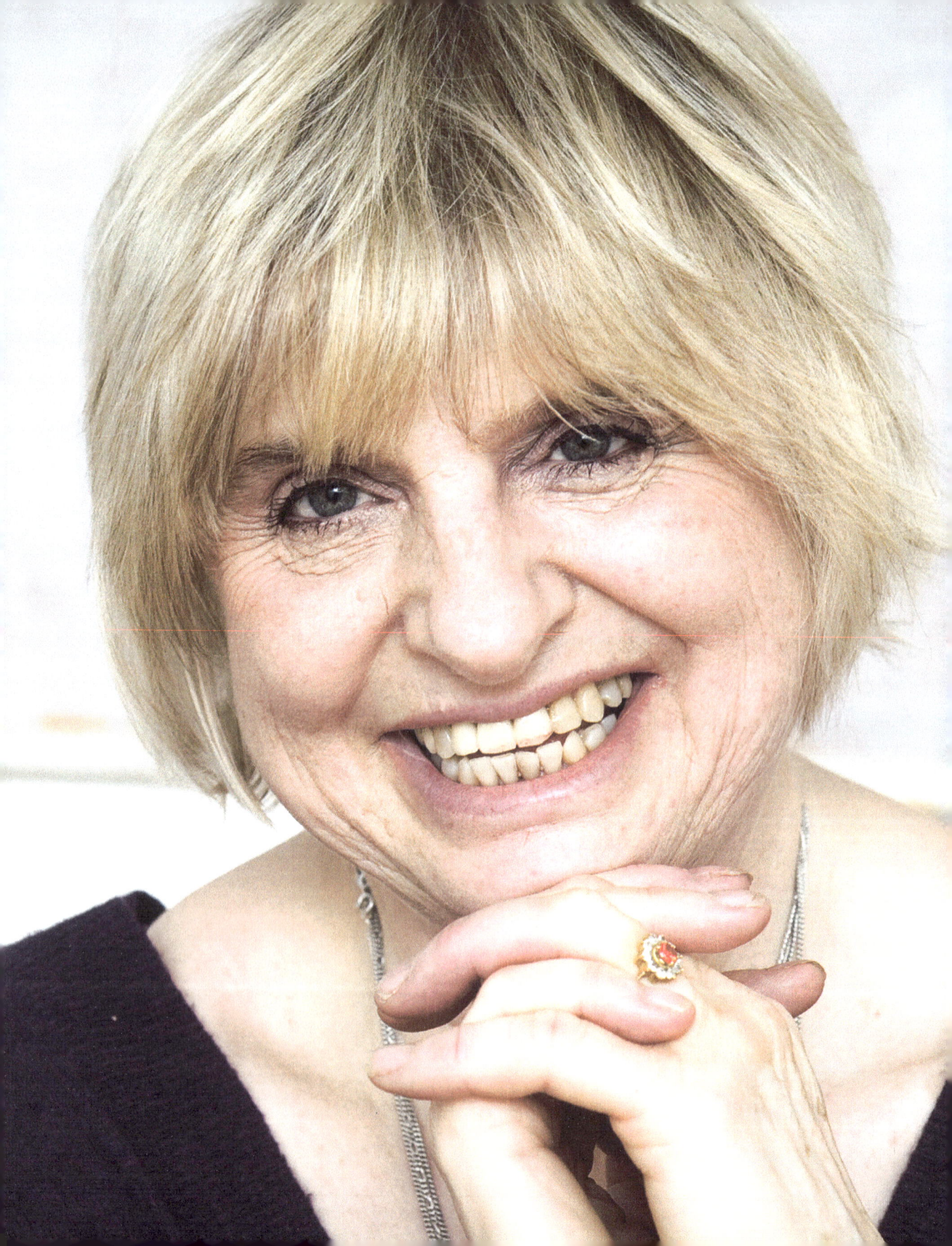

Teresa Hale
Founder of the Hale Clinic, Author
and Teacher – Atma Kriya Meditation

Teresa Hale founded the Hale Clinic in Harley Street, which was officially opened in 1988 by Prince Charles. She has been at the forefront in pioneering the integrative nature of Complementary Medicine. Her personal journey into Natural Health started as a yoga teacher and has over the years shifted to becoming a teacher of the meditation practice Atma Kriya. Her current quest is to facilitate a stilling of the mind in order to align her students to their hearts, their paths, their inner beings and their divinity. It was a pleasure to get her perspective on the importance of a meditation practice.

I studied philosophy and economics at university, but I felt that something was lacking in academics. When I discovered yoga while travelling, I knew I had found the missing link. Certain postures provided a feeling of ecstasy and connected me to my body in ways that I could never have imagined. I trained to become a teacher and once I stepped onto this path, I realised how expansive the road ahead was. For example, it is important to have a meditation practice alongside yoga to deepen the connection between body and mind, and a good diet is necessary in order to keep focused. Good core muscles are also needed to support the spine, so that the person can sit freely.

It was evident that other forms of natural therapies would allow people to have a greater connection to themselves, which would ultimately broaden their experience of yoga. So the idea came about to offer various types of complementary medicine modalities under one roof. I started The Hale Clinic with an osteopath and an acupuncturist and the whole thing evolved from there. I was lucky to have a lot of support from the Prince of Wales and the Royal Family, which helped to move things forward. The support was critical at that time, because it was a period when orthodox medicine would have liked to see a ban on complementary medicine.

Meditative Practice

As a yoga teacher it became clear to me that the more a person is willing to explore their depths through meditation, the greater their ability to connect to their soul.

Connection to our soul means connection to the divine aspects of who we are. The meditation practice I teach, puts people in touch with their heart and the love inside of themselves. Once we really understand that we are the source of our own love, it takes away the feelings of neediness and desperation that can underlie our connections with others. In order to bring this quality of love to our reality, we have to calm the mind and link with the heart. Through meditation we are given the key to tap into the unlimited aspect of who we are. This is impossible through the boundaries of the limited mind.

During a session I am always guided on what to say and what to do so it is important for me to get out of the way and allow the process. This requires both openness and non-judgement on my part. The way that I teach meditation, takes the form of either private one-to-one sessions or group work. I see a lot of business people privately, which is quite interesting. In some ways people from the business world are great to work with, because there is a need in their daily life to be very focused, which they bring to the meditation practice. Problems arise when they get caught up in stress, usually as a result of fixating on trying to control everything. My role is to show them how calming the mind can help them in their lives and their work.

Atma Kriya Meditation

I teach a spiritual meditation called Atma Kriya. Atma means self in Sanskrit and Kriya means awareness. I teach a simple course over a period of eight weeks, which is powerful, deep and transformative. Often people fluctuate between high and low points in their life. Atma Kriya is a way to bring peace to the mind and connect to the heart. Transformation is the end result of stilling the mind, because this state has the ability to fast forward people into exactly what they are meant to be doing.

Atma Kriya is devised to teach people specific techniques. When we look at Atma Kriya from a spiritual perspective, it is an exceptionally gentle way of purifying our energy. I have had students on my course who started off unableto assert themselves and through doing the practice became more assertive. People end up saying that they want to change their friends because they are now seeing them in a different light. Or they may find that they now want to do a different job. One of my students went from managing a successful modelling agency to becoming a nutritionist. A lot of insights come when the mind is calmed and everyone expresses this in their own unique way.

I always ask people what they feel at the end of every meditation practice. They say things like they feel more relaxed because they feel in touch with their heart. Grief may come up that they never knew they had. Some people even express that their experience was one of anger. All of these responses are good because it reveals any underlying areas that need to be released or illuminated.

The Inclusiveness of Meditation

You can talk about peace endlessly, I can tell you some great philosophies on peace and give you really brilliant books to read, but you have to be able to feel it in order to truly experience it. This is how even someone who is an atheist, for example, can come to meditation because it has nothing to do with faith or belief, it is about how they feel inside.

I sometimes have to change the language I use, based on the person I am with. So for some people I would not use the word soul, I might instead say superconsciousness or inner self. I may replace the phase 'connecting with the Divine' with 'creating an oasis of peace and calm'. In the end they are just words. What is important is that the person taps into their feeling. I think a lot of business people feel that there is something lacking from their lives. They may enjoy making money and there is nothing wrong with this, but they need to have a contrast that brings an awareness of who they are.

One of the main benefits of meditation for business people is that it brings a greater level of awareness and understanding. By going into the heart they are able to perceive more. The greatest issue for people in corporate business is the element of letting go of the need to control everything. In letting go they become more fluid, which creates space for them to work in a more expansive way. It is possible to be successful financially, yet still be detached from it all.

Energetic Being, Physical Body

The body is the temple of the soul, so we do need to look after it, yet we must be able to detach from it as well. In our western society the body is generally perceived to be the only reality; however, the truth is that we have another identity and reality beyond the body. Additionally, a personality is necessary to function in the world, but we need to align this to a source of sound guidance. The mind is limited in what it can understand, it will never be able to see the full picture. If we identify fully with it we experience a sense of having a void in our lives. We then search to fill the void in human relationships or in ambitions and achievements. When we connect to the divine aspect of ourselves or our superconsciousness, through meditation, we are satisfied. We can be in the world, enjoying the finer things in life, with the complete knowledge that we do not need these things to feel good about ourselves.

People get concerned about how to be in touch with their heart and still be in business. Just because you are in the heart does not mean that you do not use discernment. You would not shove your hand into a fire because you know what the result of that would be. Likewise, if you had someone in front of you who was a rogue, you would withdraw. The difference is that when you are heart-based, you would be less inclined to get into judgement, anger and emotions. It may also be the case that once a person gets in touch with themselves through meditation, they become really detached and they do not want to be a business person any longer.

Once we are aligned to our own hearts or dharma, we immediately find our greatest satisfaction. We then have the opportunity to find our inner truth and live in an authentic way, being guided by our highest perspective. This is what meditation is all about.

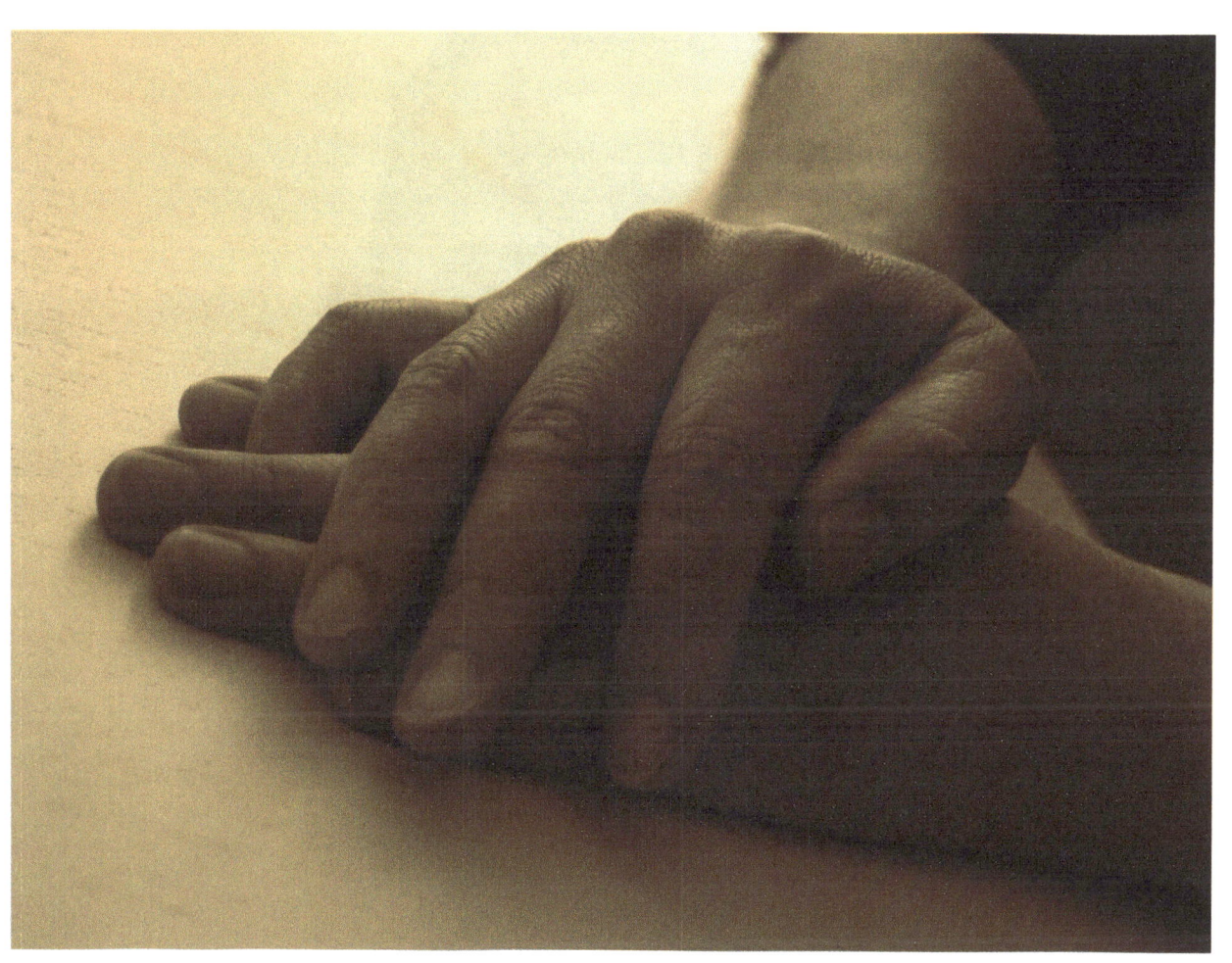

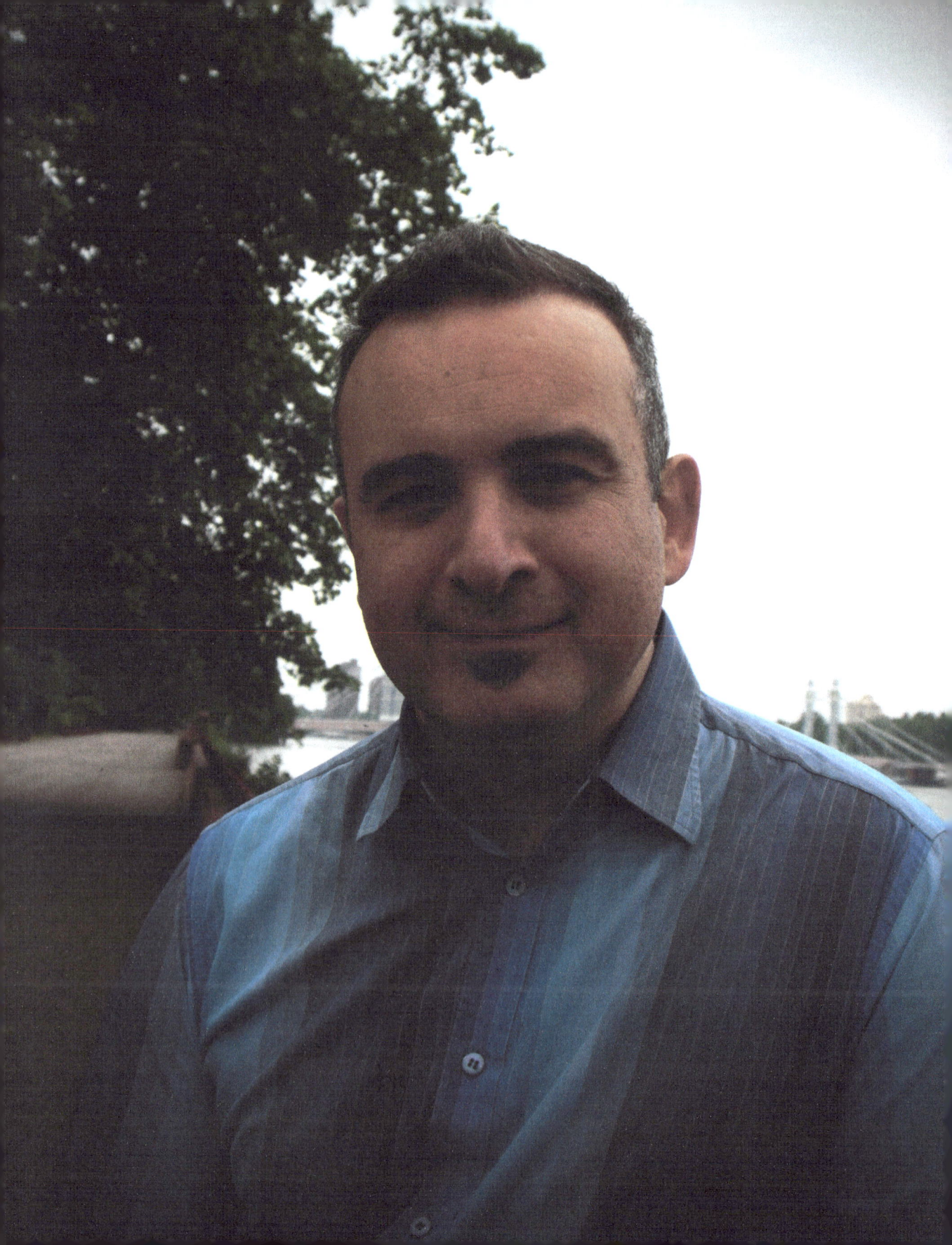

Chris Gaia
Mindfulness Teacher and Osteopath

My conversation with Chris Gaia was quite fascinating. On the one hand he has a deep understanding of Buddhist spirituality and has spent a considerable amount of time on meditative retreats in the Buddhist monastic environment. On the other hand he has a linear, medical and evidence-based understanding of the world of osteopathy. It is no surprise then that he teaches mindfulness, which straddles both the scientific and the subtle. Through a candid, genuine and warm character, he provided a vivid image of mindfulness and the way it has impacted his own life.

I have always had an interest in meditation and Buddhism, which drew me to go travelling around Asia. I ended up throwing myself in at the deep end with an intensive, silent ten-day meditation retreat in Thailand. It was both hellish and heavenly and as my journey continued I kept getting drawn back to that powerful experience. I ended up going back and doing about seven more!

On coming home to the UK, I went into a five-year degree in osteopathic medicine. There was a dualism in the two practices, with my meditative practice being at one end of the spectrum and the osteopathic practice being at the other. I always said that I wanted one foot firmly in something that was scientific, testable and solid, and the other to be in something quite opened and more exploratory.

I think science is really fantastic because it has a great way of testing and researching theories, which adds validity to a given practice. But it also has its limits because it presumes that everything is measurable in the same way, which in reality is not the case. Some things, like the intuitive, subtle knowledge and instincts that some doctors have, are immeasurable. The mindfulness revolution is really interesting because, to a large extent, it is bridging the gap between that which is scientific and quantifiable and that which is intuitive and immeasurable. This has made it acceptable across the board as demonstrated by the fact that Jon Kabat-Zinn, one of the greatest advocates of mindfulness, was recently in Downing Street giving talks on mindfulness to cabinet ministers.

Meditation

When I started off meditating I was not mature enough to appreciate it fully without my own agenda. In Thailand it suited me to meditate because it gave me a strong identity as a traveller and Buddhist. I knew I wanted to be an osteopath on my return to the UK, so I spent a lot of time centring myself through yoga and doing meditation retreats in monasteries. What I have always aspired to do is to embody the stillness of the monastery within myself. I still have regular meditation sessions and I still have a regular personal meditative practice. In the retreat environment I spent a huge number of days in silence. My life's work in a lot of ways has been to bring the peaceful retreat experience and feeling into the hectic London environment where I live. I have found mindfulness a perfect way of doing this.

Mindfulness

Jon Kabat-Zinn has been a huge advocate, pioneer and teacher of mindfulness. He developed Mindfulness Based Stress Reduction (MBSR) as a biomedical scientist at the University of Massachusetts Medical School in the US and is also a practising Zen Buddhist. He discovered a way to help patients, especially in cases of both chronic pain and heart disease, where doctors had reached their limits in terms of what they could do medically. He requested that the worst cases be sent to him. He had devised an eight-week course in mindfulness for them to follow. Mindfulness has strong links to Buddhism even though it is wholly secular in the way it is taught. Buddhism in a lot of ways is very down to earth and quite scientific in its approach, which has made it accessible to a wide range of people. It is completely experiential, so it gives people a set of very straightforward tools, which can be applied to their daily lives and it removes the spiritual or esoteric aspects from the equation.

My Work

It is evident that you are the greatest expert in your own experience. Someone can give you the tools and the means to do the work with mindfulness, but ultimately, it will be your experience. If you came to me and said you wanted to do a mindfulness course, my first question would be, 'What are your expectations?' Many people see wisdom as being something outside of themselves and would like the 'wise person' to somehow install the wisdom into them, while they remain passive. In reality this is not possible. The first step to wisdom is to recognise that the seeds are within us.

As a teacher, people can project a lot onto you and much of it is a fantasy. I don't always have a perfectly mindful life, I can get upset and angry just like the next person.

We are all human beings with the same tendencies to love and hate, laugh and cry. We all have wisdom and folly. Often we project our own concept of goodness (or badness) onto others. When we start to own our dark side, as well as our wisdom, we can use both to propel us further down our path. One of the most important aspects of mindfulness is creating a real awareness and acceptance of where we are right now. We might not be perfect but we are 'perfectly' as we are!

The act of teaching well is about embodying the things you talk about, being present, walking the walk if you like. I think ultimately mindfulness is about truly seeing and accepting the reality in front of us right now. This is how we gain an understanding of our interconnectedness. Understanding how interconnected we are is important. Someone made the cup of tea I am drinking at the moment, someone planted this tea, another picked the leaves, shipped it out, milked the cow and someone brewed it for me, there may be a hundred people just in one cup of tea. So the reality is that we cannot get away from our connections to others, individualism is a nice idea but it is not reality. When we start to see this we automatically create peace and nurture between each other.

Mindfulness in Real Life

There are so many facets to life, pleasure is an inevitable part of life and so is suffering. Mindfulness teaches us to once again recognise the wonder of life, the beauty of a winter's sunset, the touch of our partner's hand, the taste of a fine meal, normal stuff we often ignore. Conversely, it also teaches us to face the unpleasant, rather than closing off and distracting ourselves. Often it is the more difficult experiences that need our care. When we start to acknowledge the inevitable hardship of life, as well as the inevitable pleasure, we stop the painful struggle against the way things are. This saves us immeasurable extra pain.

Compassion is of the utmost importance here. I had a lady on twitter recently who contacted me because she kept getting into a very angry state. In the past when she became really angry she would either allow it to consume her or she would attempt to push it away or repress it. The experiment I gave her was to see what would happen if she simply held the feelings of anger as gently and kindly as she would a baby or an injured pet. She was just to observe it, without needing to change it or get rid of it and watch what occurs. She reported that she learned more from doing this one thing than she had from all the grasping and pushing away she had done so often.

From my own personal experience of watching my thoughts, feelings and physical sensations (even if they are unpleasant, unwelcome or unskilful), I find that bringing acceptance and kindness to them has a rather transforming effect. We hold our experience within a compassionate awareness, in the moment, allowing life to be just as it is. We sometimes try to control our lives and our experience and, if that way of being works for you then brilliant, but in my opinion we just end up banging our heads against a brick wall. How about coming into harmony with the way things are? Relaxing back into not having to change anything? Stopping the war, if you like..

This is the level of acceptance we need to have with ourselves and the things that life may present to us. Mindfulness allows us to cultivate that kind and loving embracing of who we are, just as we are. This poem by Rumi says it better than I could.

THE GUEST HOUSE

This being human is a guest house.
Every morning a new arrival.

A joy, a depression, a meanness,
some momentary awareness comes
as an unexpected visitor.

Welcome and entertain them all!
Even if they are a crowd of sorrows,
who violently sweep your house
empty of its furniture,
still, treat each guest honourably.
He may be clearing you out
for some new delight.

The dark thought, the shame, the malice.
meet them at the door laughing and invite them in.

Be grateful for whatever comes.
because each has been sent
as a guide from beyond.

-- Jelaluddin Rumi,
    translation by Coleman Barks

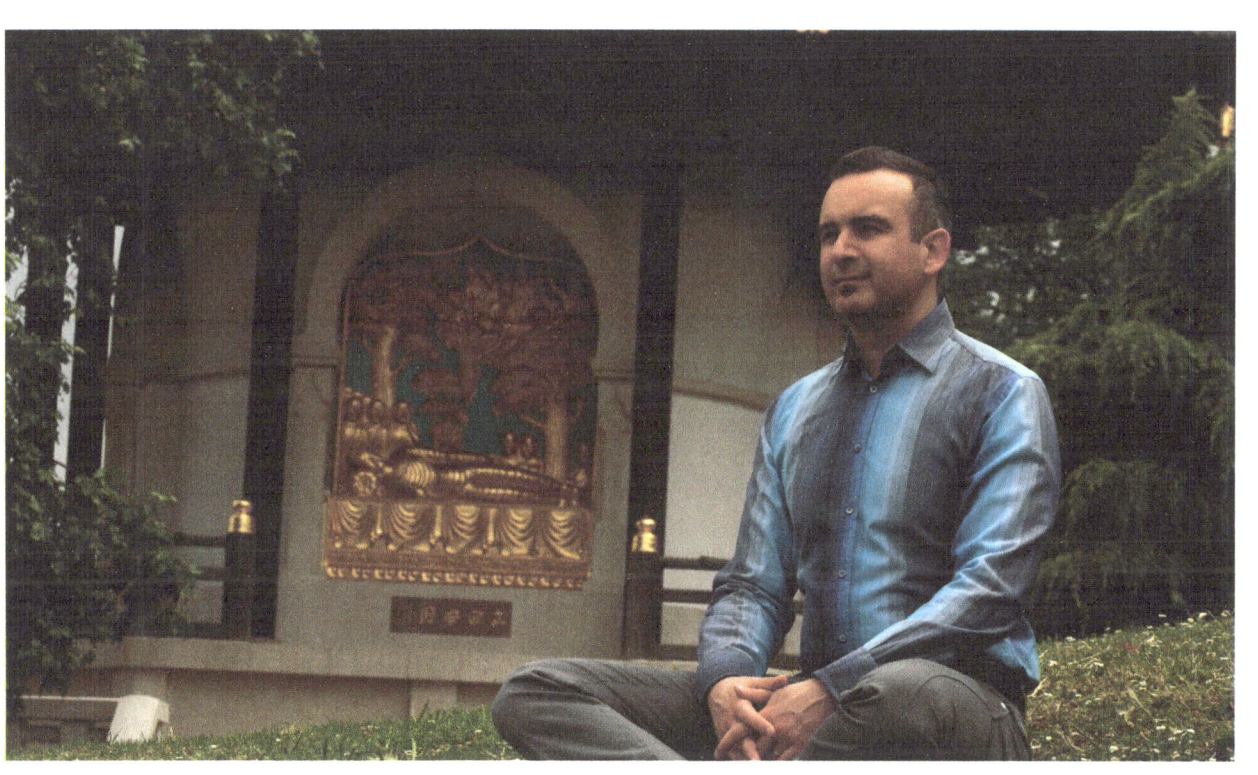

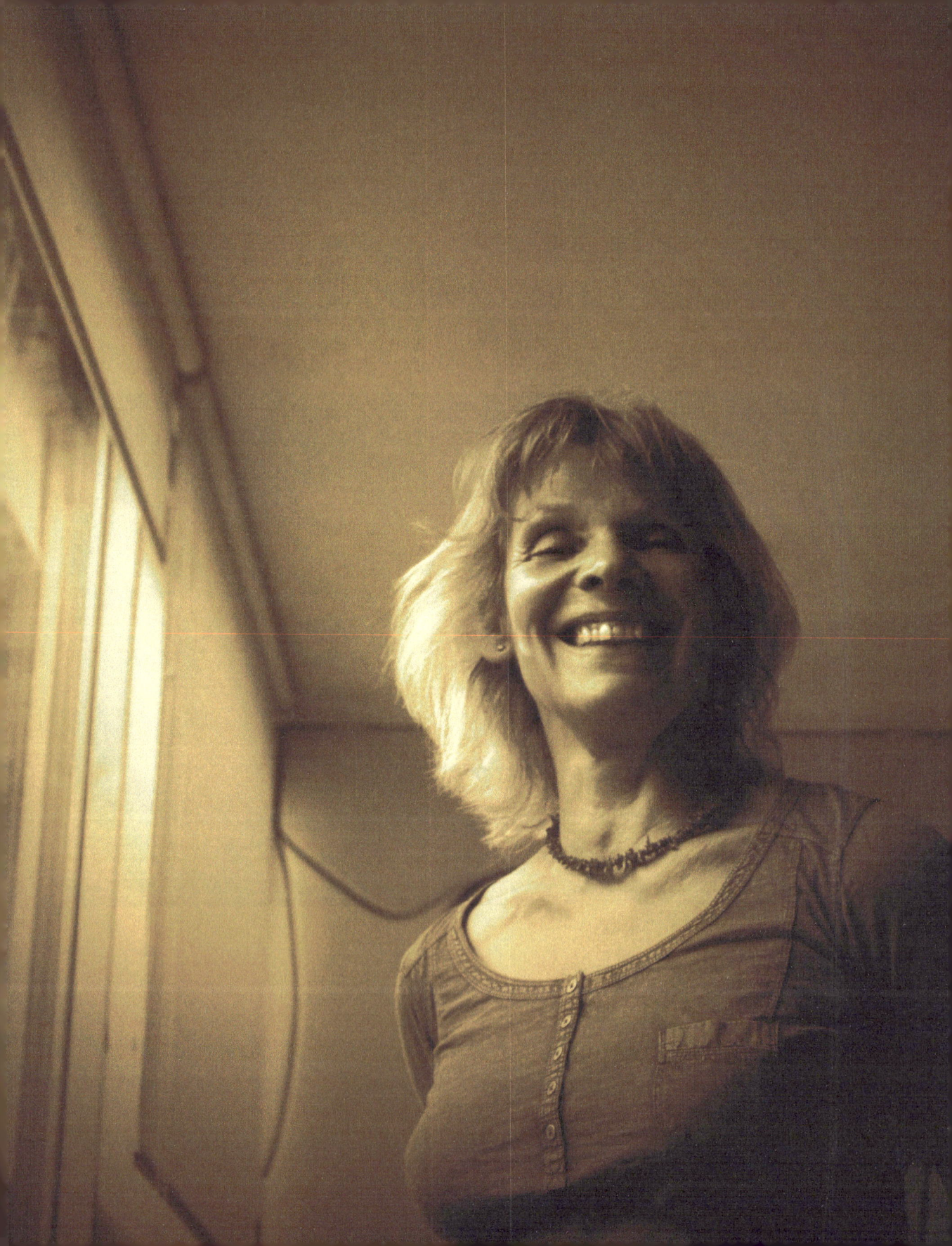

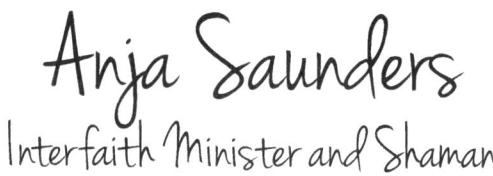

Anja Saunders
Interfaith Minister and Shaman

Anja Saunders is an ordained minister who is Dutch by descent and follows a shamanic spiritual path. There are many aspects to Anja's work, and she holds various circles where people can connect to themselves through an intent. These include circles for healing, love, resolution, contemplation, sound, movement and release. Whatever the context of the circle, the common ground between them is their meditative nature. They invite people to reflect, explore and open their awareness to the wisdom that lies at the core of their very being. It was this meditative nature of her work that I was interested in when I chatted to Anja. What unfolded in our conversation was a journey to the heart of what it means to create a circle.

I started out in theatre as a puppeteer. This eventually brought me to a study of movement in France. My teacher, Etienne Decroux, was an extraordinary man, who was in many ways more of a philosopher than a theatre maker. His approach was to focus on the essence of movement and expression, rather than the overt gesticulations and changes in facial expression that can often encompass theatre. He brought our awareness to the subtle shifts that occur in the movement of expression. It was through his teachings that I really began to understand myself spiritually and energetically.

I began to realise that my attraction to theatre lay in the fact that, through it, I could experience the magical. This magic was very tangible when I opened myself up to it and could be shared with other people, so that they experienced it as well. You can feel it in the moment when the focus is held so strongly you can hear a needle drop, or those times when the air is filled with excitement and the buzz of electricity. These poignant feelings brought with them a sense of aliveness that opened me up to all the layers of my being. However, although I was drawn to these profound elements of theatre, the world of entertainment did not create a match.

It became clear to me that theatre was not the medium for the experience I was seeking, and the healing arts were much more compatible. I became an Alexander Technique teacher and later I opened up a school for massage. Both of these opportunities brought a huge amount of expansion to my life, but were limited because they only really catered for a therapeutic situation. I began to look at how connections could be made beyond the therapeutic sense, which led to the development of my circle work.

Meditative Circles

Healing does not need to be confined to one-to-one situations, instead we can create a space for others to find their own way of being. I call it a circle because in essence what is being created is a holding vessel for an experience or a deepening awareness. Each circle contains a centre and this is where the Spirit resides. Everyone is at an equal distance away from the centre and, as such, equally contributes to the spirit. Each circle created is unique because, once a connection is made, the energy of each person begins to circulate to make up the whole.

In a meditative circle the focus is always kept on the central point, because the centre holds the highest concentration of the energy. This then creates a wave structure, where the centre radiates out to the edges of the circle and, much like a wave in the sea, it hits the shore before returning back to the centre. For this to work best everyone in the circle keeps an awareness on the centre. It is important that the diversity within the circle is fully honoured and every individual must be viewed with the same level of acceptance and openness. At the same time everyone is part of the circle, which creates a sense of oneness.

Central Intentions

Before the start of the meditative circle we set an intention of what we aim to bring to the centre of the circle. It may be a focus on healing or it may be an expansion of our understanding. Whatever the intention we choose, it is important for everyone who forms the circle to have an intent because it helps us to focus. The centre in itself needs nothing; it is always full, no matter how the circle moves. However, we need a focus that we can come back to. In all the time I have spent making circles, leading circles and holding space for circles, the central intent is what I keep a focus on and keep returning to.

Being part of a circle in this way is deeply nourishing, providing us with acknowledgement and recognition. I think we have an intrinsic understanding of this, which allows for a sense of something being relaxed within the core of our being. We get a homecoming feeling which then creates an opening in our awareness. Once this space has been created, neither the mind and its constant chatter, nor the world and its constant distractions hold any prevalence. We let them rest a bit, allowing ourselves to come to our inner truth. The beauty of the circle is that we can do all this together

Becoming An Interfaith Minister

When I had my massage school there was no time to focus on anything else. However, once I moved on from this I had some space. Information on the interfaith seminary crossed my path at this time, so I went to an open day and for the entire day felt really connected. We were asked why we had chosen this path and why we had chosen this time. I got clear and positive answers from myself in response and felt enthusiastic about committing to the two-year process; it was beautiful to explore the various world religions and to be on such a great path of expansion and development.

We asked ourselves during the second year if we wanted to go forward to ordination, which meant that we would be able to write our own vows to honour and serve spirit. We were told that as we developed it was possible our vows would change. The process of formulating such an oath was extraordinary. Additionally, we stood up with another sixty people and made our deeply powerful core statement. In my case, ordination brought to me the elements of circle sharing, ceremony, healing and ritual. I hold ceremonies, such as funerals, weddings and blessings, and offer meditations, contemplative circles and talks, as well as spiritual guidance, rituals or quests, and guidance walks in nature.

Meditative Practice

If I had to define meditation, I would say it is a way of letting go of what obscures the self, our true nature, so that we can come to Self with a capital S. My work enables people to connect to the spirit and essence of who they are. Shamanism is at the heart of my practice and informs my expression. For example, in one of my meditative practices I organise twenty-four-hour mini quests where we sit out for the night.

We usually meet as a group, create a sacred space and set the intent, with each individual being there for the process. I then go out of sight but remain there holding the space. In the morning I pick everyone up and we have breakfast together in order to share and process our experiences.

During one of my own personal mini quests, I remember sitting out in the night and my intention was to expand my understanding on what it meant to get in touch with nature. The outcome I was presented with was that in everything there is a nature. This was a meaning of the word 'nature' that I had not thought of before. It made sense to me because, when I was doing puppetry, I would take whatever object I was working with and find out how it moved in space and how it could best express itself. Things could have much in common and yet still be very different in nature. Nature expresses itself in various ways and it is always a profound experience when we take the time to notice the real nature of something or someone. This requires us to listen deeply and express our truth. If we are present and aware enough we each come to a place where we share a centre between us. From this space we can relate to each other with clarity as we connect through a higher perspective and through meditative practice we let go of what is hiding the self.

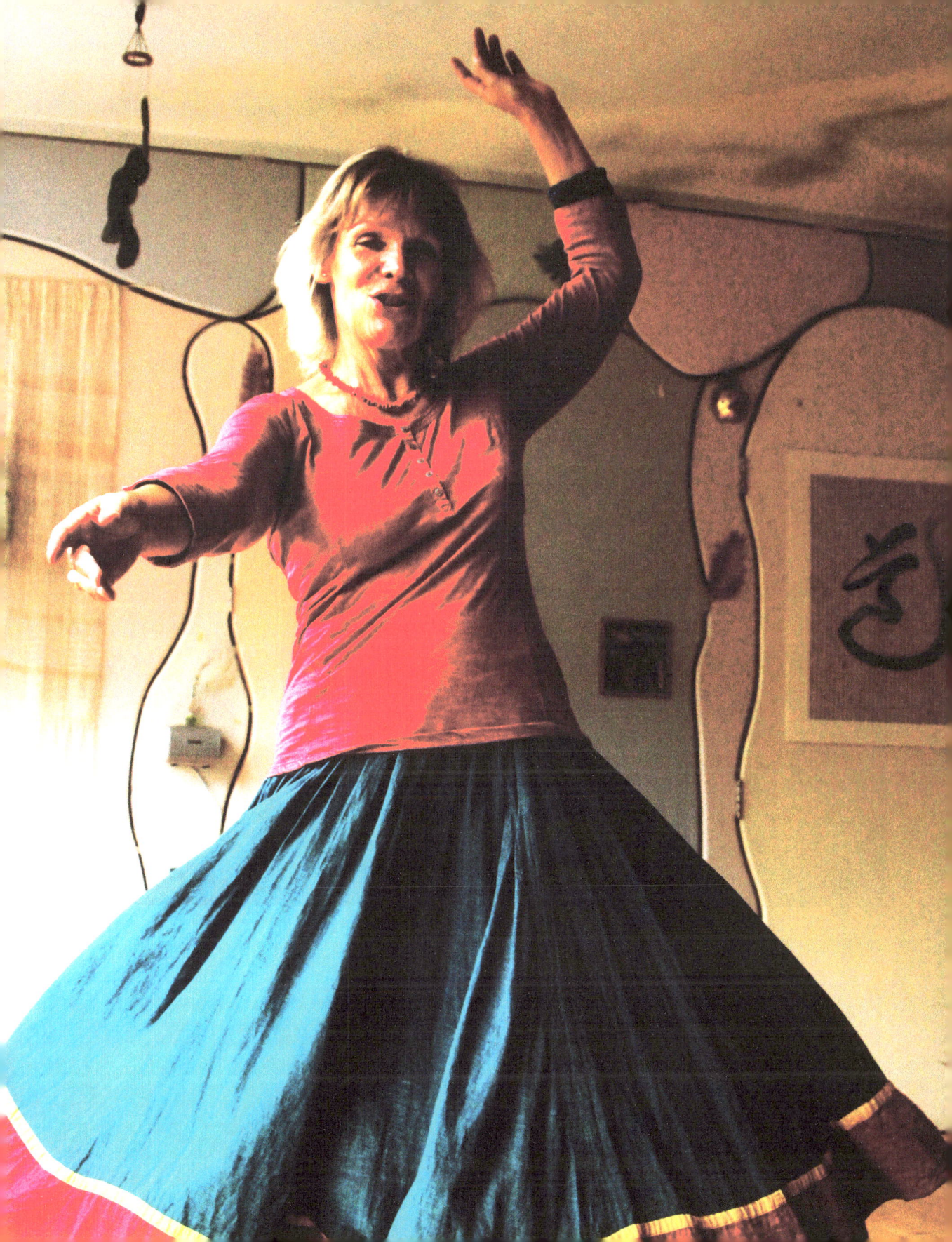

Energy

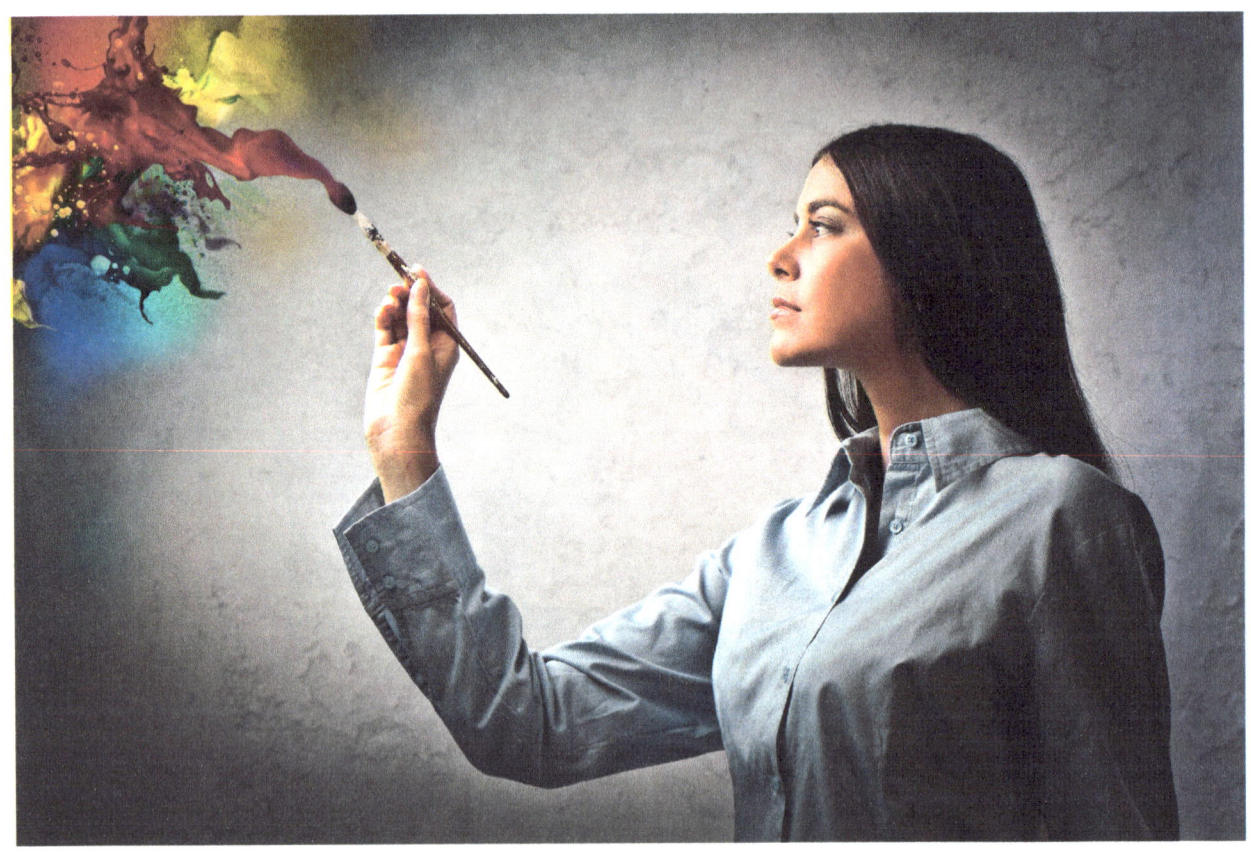

Treatments

Yoga

Energy Work

Sound Therapy

Acupuncture

"In New York we had ten thousand people doing yoga all at the same time. It was the most amazing experience, imagine Central Park with ten thousand people altogether singing mantras. Oh my God, that really is powerful!"

- Maya Fiennes

Yoga

Yoga originated in India and has strong connections to both Hinduism and Buddhism. The philosophy behind the practice is to bring about a union of body, mind and spirit. The postures themselves reduce stress, release tension from the body and can be used therapeutically to alleviate a number of health issues by making the body stronger, increasing the flexibility of the spine and increasing circulation throughout the body. There is a deeply spiritual aspect to yoga, which is sometimes left out in western practice. However, whether it is used philosophically or simply physically, yoga's effects on balancing the energy cannot be denied.

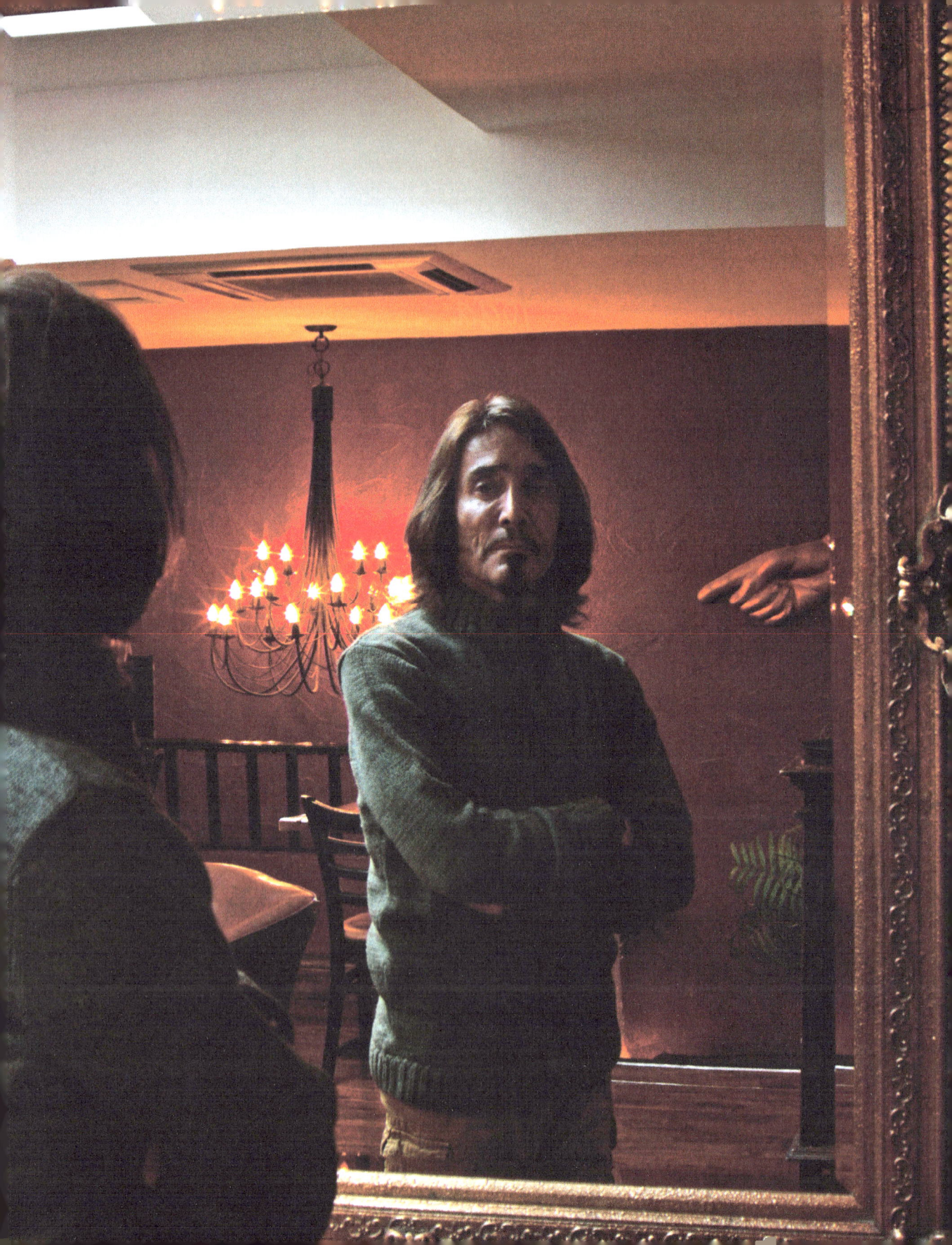

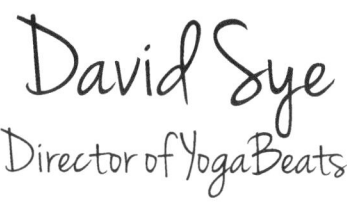

David Sye
Director of YogaBeats

The phrase that popped into my head at the start of my conversation with Yoga Maestro David Sye was 'uncompromisingly beautiful'. His quest is to live fully, truthfully and fearlessly. There is a deep understanding within him that love holds the key to opening the door to our connectedness to life. I met him to speak of yoga and the work he has done to promote unity between the Palestinians and Israelis in the West Bank. However, what unfolded was a dialogue on the meaning of living a life in awareness, in a state of presence and complete consciousness.

The West Bank

My interest in wanting to make some kind of difference to what is going on in the West Bank arose after I was influenced by an experience in Bosnia. I got caught in the war there, my passport had been stolen and I was on the run from the military police. I started teaching yoga in exchange for food. Because of the battle, all that was available to eat was cabbage and stale bread. This was when I really discovered how highly adaptive the body is, it can cope with almost anything. Even with such a limited diet I was extremely healthy during the time I spent there.

I got back to the West and, as a result of my time in Bosnia, I noticed how indulgent we are. If you are starving you quickly lose the need for gluten-free foods and tofu. It became clear to me that the body is like a child, all that it really requires is our love and care. When we take all the tribal fear-based rules out of the way and treat ourselves with love, we feel balanced within. We may not always get approval from others, but we feel right about ourselves.

The level of conflict that exists in the West Bank drew me there because my heritage is Jewish. But when I hug my brothers and sisters from Palestine, I don't feel that I am a Jew and they are Muslim, we just adore each other, we are human beings. Everyone says there is a border between Palestine and Israel, but I don't see it. In the work that I do, my interest is not in yoga. What I really care about is evolution and, by virtue of that, maybe I can share something with others.

Yoga and Our Evolutionary Journey

To me yoga is simply a doorway to consciousness. I don't want to do anything in my life unless it is conscious. The payoff to living consciously is indescribable. It's beyond words; you can't explain it to anybody, it sounds foolish and stupid when you try, but it feels extraordinary. I love yoga, I love the asanas, meditation and pranayama aspects of it, but a lot of yoga schools promote elitism, it is about people showing off how bendy they are and boasting of being vegetarian since birth. If yoga does not lead to compassion for yourself and for others, it's a waste of time.

As a yoga teacher, I am often going around offending a lot of people and I am very happy to do that. Not because I want to create controversy, but because I want to wake them up. We live in a world where people ask the question, 'How do I know I should love you before I know you?' The answer to that question is, if you don't love a person you will never know them. Your ego has to die in order for you to love. You can always recognise when the ego is present because it is hallmarked by seriousness. All the great masters are lighthearted and bursting with laughter.

I use yoga to break people out of their conformity and make them feel good. One of the things I learned in the war was that you don't know how long you have to live. We think we have an idea, but this may be our last moment. So there should be a celebration of who we are right now. Don't leave it until tomorrow, do it right now.

The Surrender of the Ego

When you have positioned yourself with your ego, you become very impatient with life. In losing your position, there is surrender and you say, 'thy will be done' rather than 'my will'. In that moment, there is no investment that someone should behave in a certain way to gain your approval or make you happy. Surrender in this sense can, at first, feel very much like death to the ego. Christ called this process heaven on Earth, Buddha called it Nirvana, and Abraham the Promised Land. They were not talking about some place up in the sky, what they were referring to is this world. As soon as the ego surrenders, this is heaven on Earth.

While it is true that we need the ego to function in this world – in essence it makes you who you are and me who I am – it is important that we are mindful as to what we are aligning it to. When we have a huge investment in an outcome, then we have to be really careful of the ego as it can convince someone that spirituality is a good idea, because it will make them a load of money. That's when you get all the fake gurus, all the various forms of yoga and metaphysical messages, which then get marketed to hell and cost a fortune to attend. People spend a lot of money to go to these things because everyone said they should, but they walk out scratching their heads, wondering what it was all about. It leads to nowhere.

Many would describe being duped as a painful experience and, the more pain you have, the luckier you become. When people come to me for therapy I always tell them they are lucky they are in pain, because the next step is letting go of what is not working. The ego itself will tell you that there has got to be a better way and, as soon that happens, the perfect book will fall off the shelf or you will bump into someone who can help you.

All the masters say that the ego is only thing that stands between you and the enlightenment that follows you through every lifetime. It is the animal side of us, which has created an insurance policy to make sure that we get fed. However, it comes from a place of worry and, in the end, the worry becomes fearful. As soon as you relinquish the fear you begin to truly live.

Influences

My greatest influence has come from my teacher Clara Buck, who was exceptional. For example, when she was ninety she went backpacking in South America. She always told me to burn the candle at both ends and take no security. She used to say, 'If you want to surrender, live dangerously. Do the undoable, live the unliveable, throw yourself off a cliff.'

I found her to be an incredible woman. During her last tour of the world she was asked to demonstrate certain yoga positions that she became famous for, but she refused to do that and instead chose to speak about love. She told the students that they had to live to melt and relinquish who they thought they were, and that all we are preparing for in this lifetime is love. At some time we will have to drop the body, we cannot hang onto it forever, so why even try. Enjoy it to the full!

She truly demonstrated what it means to live fully awake. When you live like this, you see love in everyone and every person is beautiful. You see the wounds of others, you see their damage, you see how people try to circumnavigate through their pain. You get an insight into others by the way they sit, the way they talk and the things that they say. You are not continuously in a hurry to get somewhere else because you know wherever you are, is the place you need to be. Things get taken care of because you keep handing it over. It is not that you are without awareness. I, for example, have a very tight schedule, but I keep handing the schedule over.

With this way of being comes a huge sense of freedom.

The Future

In answer to what I think the future holds for me, I would tell you a story from the Native Americans. A boy once said to an elder, 'I sometimes get lost in the cedar forest and I don't know where north or west or east or south is. What do I do when I get lost like that?' The answer that the elder gave was this, 'Wherever you are is a place called here, stand still, if you run you will be lost. Let the forest find you, stand still.' So that is what I would say. Wherever I am is a place called here, there is nowhere I have to be. When I look for security, I am never more bored. When I take risks, I am never more alive. I choose life.

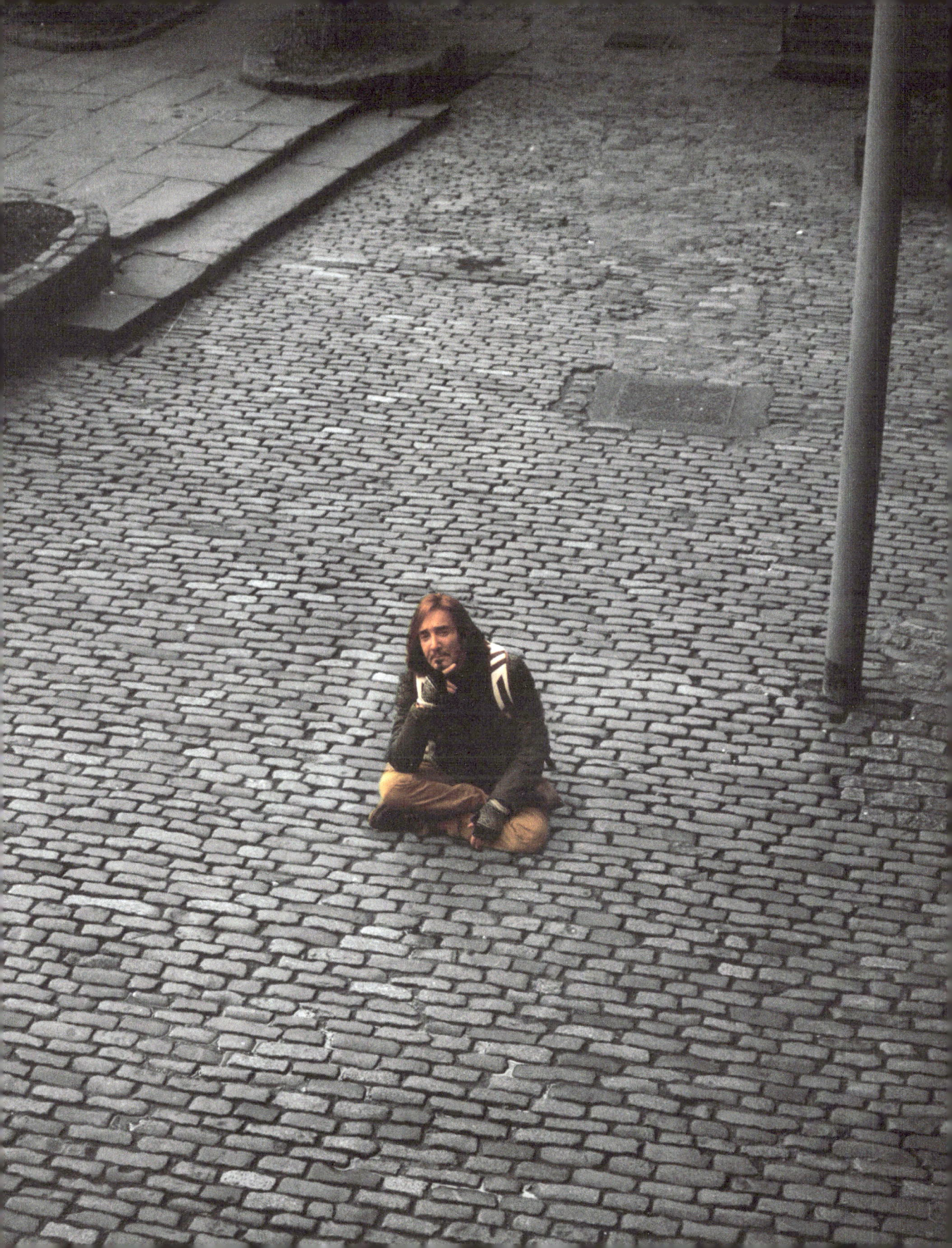

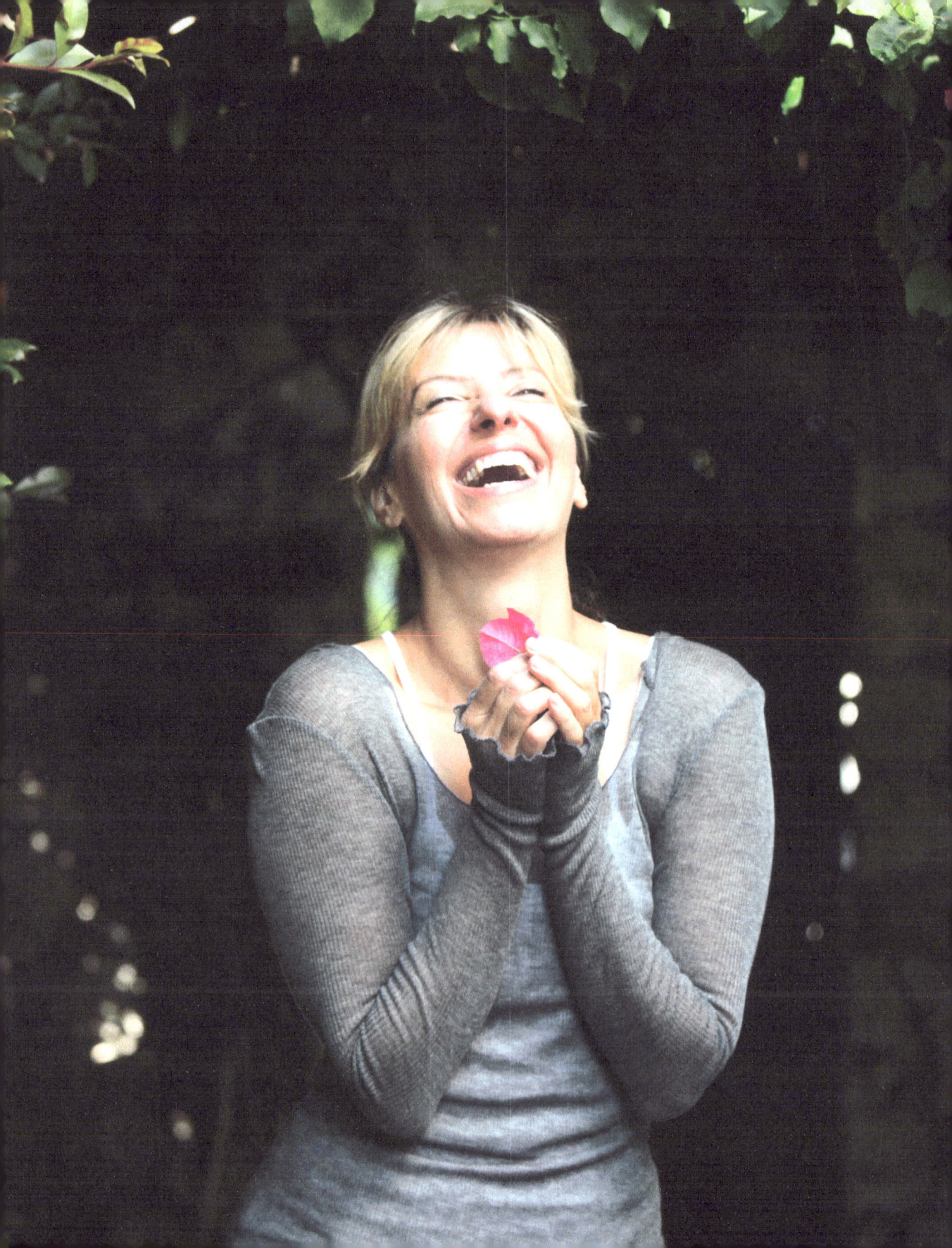

Maya Fiennes
Director of Maya Space, Author and Teacher

Maya Fiennes is a Kundalini Yoga Teacher versed in the art of raising energy in the body in order to create wholeness, connectedness and unity. She has transitioned from a hugely successful concert pianist doing private recitals for audiences, such as the Royal Family and the United Nations assembly, into a Yoga teacher, described by Deepak Chopra as a true example of a pioneer in the field of Yoga.

I used to be a concert pianist and as I got bigger concerts I started getting very nervous about them. Someone suggested I should try yoga because of the breathing, so I started with Hatha yoga and I found that my performance improved as I was more relaxed.

I continued doing yoga because I was curious to know more. I tried both Ashtanga and Iyengar styles of yoga, in order to experience what each technique would give me. But when I came to Kundalini I thought 'This is it!' Things can shift really quickly when you focus on moving your energy. Placing all your attention solely on the physical body is more difficult to effect change and it can take years of practice to get to the point that Kundalini brings you to.

Once I found Kundalini yoga I was committed to it. I trained in London, at a school called Karma Kriya and my teacher was Shiv Charan Singh. He was the first teacher I started Kundalini yoga with and he was amazing. It is through him that I became a teacher myself. He is also a numerologist; he looked at my chart and told me that everything in my numbers said that I had to be a master and a teacher. That was not what I wanted to hear at first, I was a musician. But I started studying, just for my own understanding. Part of the course I was doing required that I teach and I found I really liked it. Teaching yoga was quite a performance and I was already a performer so it made sense to me.

Kundalini Yoga

Kundalini yoga is about freeing our self; so many people are locked into a prison and are not able to express themselves fully. If we are imprisoned, there is no point in asking for something from the universe because we will not be in a position to receive it. We need to know what to ask for and then be opened; this is when we get messages and responses to our questions.

Kundalini yoga is a form of energy work because it concentrates on raising energy up from the base chakra to the crown chakra. Our energy sits at the base chakra in the perineum and it is normally dormant. With a combination of breathing, mantra, meditation, asanas and kriyas, we can achieve a complete body, mind and spirit workout. The practice starts shifting and moving the energy from the base of the spine, to the crown at the top of the head, where it produces an energetic antenna through the crown chakra. This acts as a receiver which enhances our consciousness, allowing us to establish union with the Divine. From here we are able to communicate on a higher and more universal level.

The Chakras

Kundalini yoga brought an understanding of the chakras. These are the seven energy centres in the body and everything that I teach is focused around them. The deeper I go into the chakras the more I realise that the whole body can be harmonised by working on them. The body is really organised and it is through the chakras that you open up all the subjects in life; they incorporate relationships, body organs, health issues and energy levels, everything is there.

Once you begin to clear the chakras you begin to have creativity coming out of your ears. The energy serves to rejuvenate your whole body; this keeps you in the present moment, which means that whatever you see, wherever you go, it is always new. When you make your body strong, you create a good container for the energy and for all the communication and guidance being received. When the creative energy starts moving you, you have no choice but to go with it. However, you need a strong body and mind for this. Everything we do in Kundalini is to prepare ourselves to be a strong receptive container.

Inspiration

I am inspired by the energy! The universe! Life! I meet so many interesting people in my travels and I get really excited about these interactions. If I meet someone who teaches me something amazing I use it straight away. I went to China and learned Chi Kung, which I applied immediately into my classes. I also learned Tai Chi and made use of it straight away, and lately I have been doing the Grinberg Method.

With the Grinberg Method, every adverse emotion you feel – pain, fear and all the subsections of life – you use this modality to intensify it and you really stay present with it. It is only by acknowledging the emotion that you give yourself the space to let go of it. If you keep avoiding it, it will come back and keep bugging you. When this happens, it does not matter who you are with or the situations you find yourself in, you will always be dealing with the same elements and issues. So you need to face it, deal with it, sit with it and even when it feels painful, work with it. Then you can apply the same intensification to the body to disperse the energy out of yourself.

It is an interesting method. There is an exercise that is almost like a dance where you start the thought and you stop, because every thought has a beginning and an end. There are times that we do not know how to end our thought, so with this method we use movement. It is unchoreographed, but you start and stop abruptly. Moving the arms and legs in this manner prompts you on how to start and stop your thoughts. I have been very inspired by this.

Living my Life Purpose

It is almost like somewhere out there I signed a contract in this work and I have to carry on and do it. I feel privileged to be in the position to do this job. I am glad I have my dharma and that I know what I am supposed to be doing! My life purpose is basically about sharing knowledge and bringing this energy of Kundalini yoga out, to excite and energise others. It is an energy that we all have; it is just about believing in ourselves and bringing our power consciously back to ourselves as opposed to giving it away unconsciously to other people. I always tell people that they are the ones who are doing the work; it is about knowing how to use their power.

I remember the days of frustration at the start of this journey, when I was thinking, 'Why am I doing this? How is this going to help me?' But it is amazing, everything I have done in my life has had an exact way of serving. Each step has served the next, nothing has ever been wasted. In a few years, months or weeks, you will look back at the timing and think, 'My God if I had not have done that, this would not have happened!' It is all completely connected!

In one of the lectures that I saw with Deepak Chopra, he said that the way a cocoon becomes a butterfly is a complete mystery. There is no way that you would put the two together. In the same way, a human could become a superhuman. He thinks that if there are enough people thinking the same way we can make that transformation. Looking at how the cocoon creates a butterfly, there is a universal understanding and belief that allows the shift to happen without question.

As human beings we are all made of the negative and positive, yin and yang, male and female, the two extremes always make the whole. We are co-creators and have the potential to become the divine aspect of ourselves. A sign was left in all of us and the journey is about whether we are going to wake it up or not. Not everyone is going to choose the same path, there are different levels and different people. However, as a whole the energy is perfect, there is no duality within it. Kundalini in essence brings us to the wholeness.

The Future

Who knows what the future will bring. I am just going to be opened, to see where it takes me and stay attuned with what is going on within my surroundings. Mainly I think I should be reaching more masses to give them this message so that they can believe in themselves. It is my dream to do yoga with large masses of people. I got to experience this in New York when we had 10,000 people doing yoga all at the same time. It was the most amazing experience; imagine Central Park with 10,000 people altogether singing mantras. Oh my God, that really is powerful! The more people that are gathered creates a cycle and whatever I give comes back. People sometimes ask me if I never get tired, but if you get that energy going it becomes easier with more people. They all become one very quickly. For me this is an absolute joy!

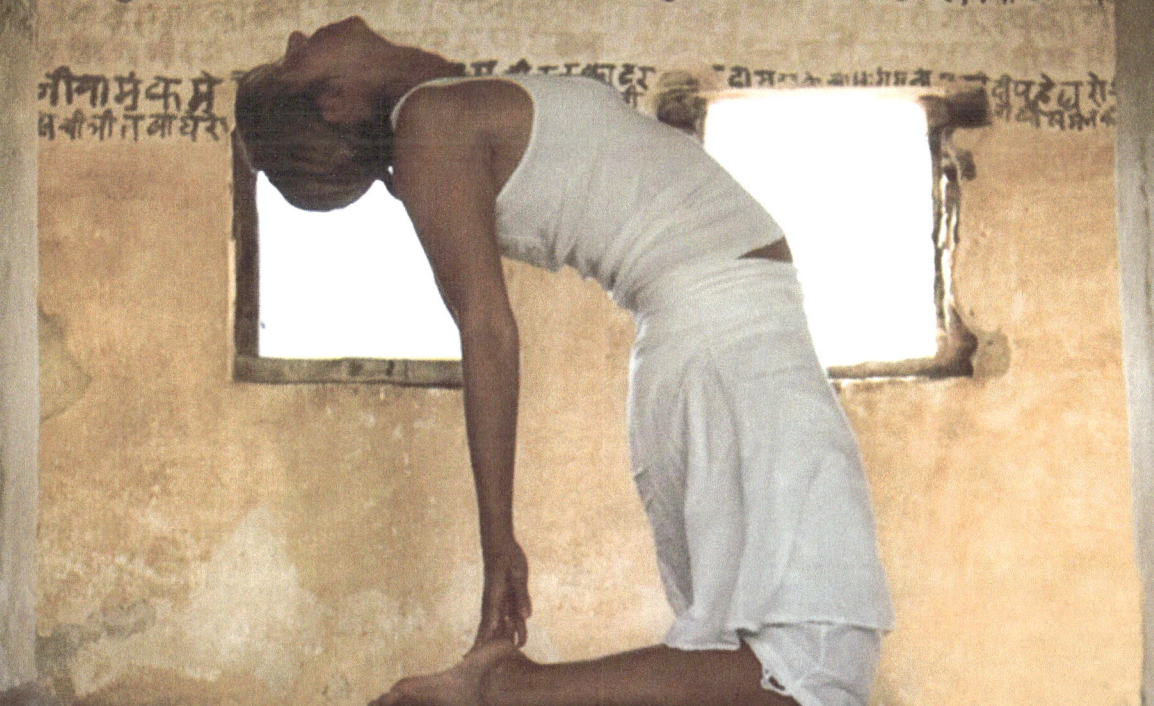

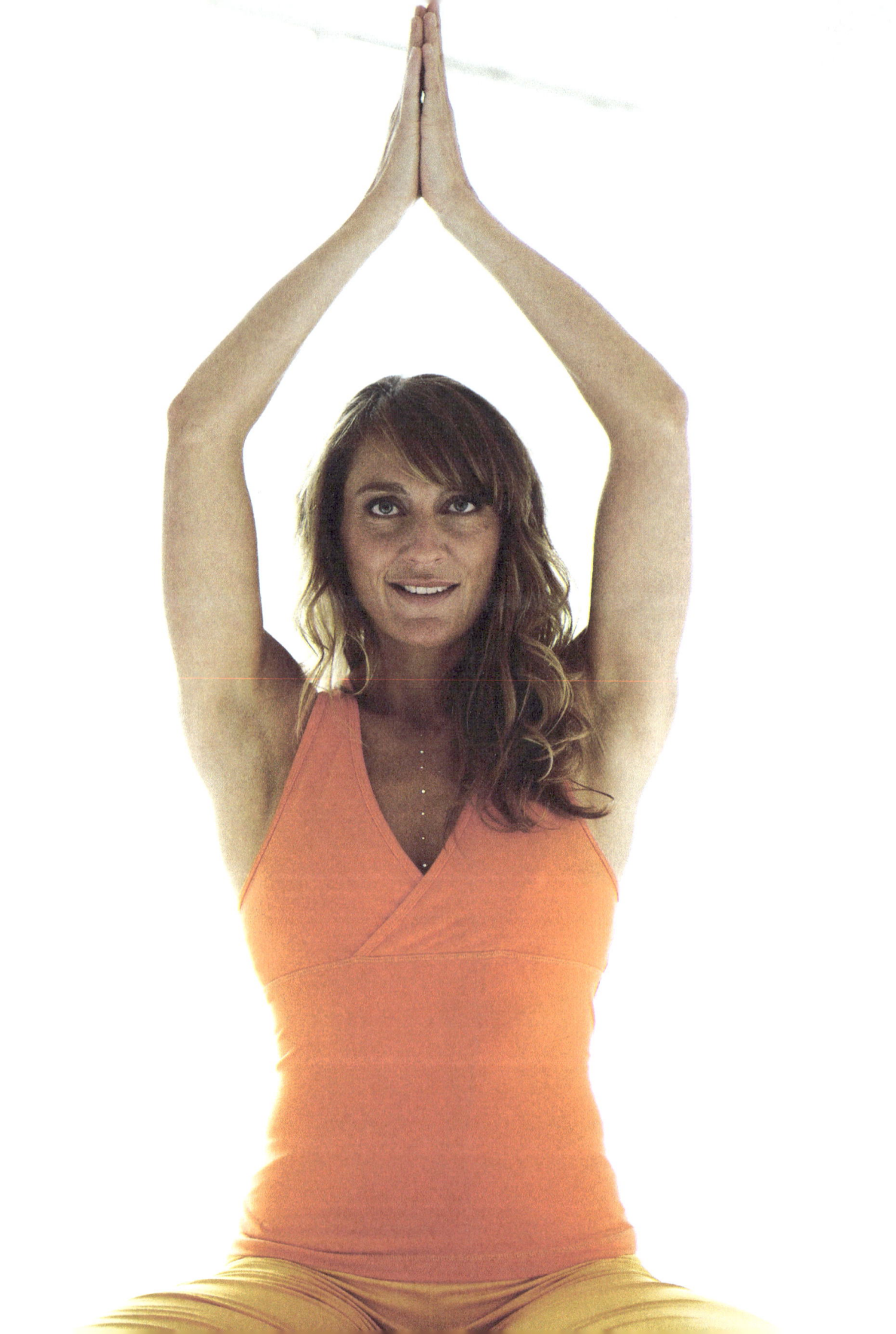

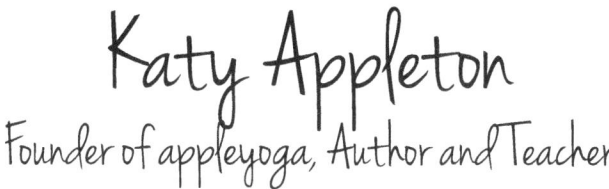

Katy Appleton
Founder of appleyoga, Author and Teacher

Katy Appleton puts her heart into everything she does; this came across very strongly in conversation with her. She left home at the age of eleven to study with the Royal Ballet School. From there she scaled the heights in a career spanning eleven years, dancing with The English National Royal Ballet amongst other companies. She has taken her knowledge in honing the body and invoking different qualities of energy from dancing and combined this with yoga to create a truly unique offering. Her individual style of yoga has gained a huge following and her client list includes royalty and celebrities.

My mum did Iyengar yoga when she was pregnant with me in the 70s and, as a small child, I remember going to yoga classes with her. This is where I first developed a concept of yoga being about physical movement.

Later on in life, as a dancer, I fell upon a yoga session by accident and loved the physical aspects of the practice, but I was put off by the sound work and chanting. I did not have an understanding of what the chanting was about, so it triggered in me a feeling that I had entered into something completely strange and cult like, which made me very wary about engaging with it. I am very much a 'why' person. Tell me the reasoning behind what is being done and I can give myself to it wholeheartedly.

It took me a while to come back to yoga in a class format after that experience. However, there were parts of the session that I loved and continued to use. For example, I completely loved the yoga postures and the breath work. It was such a pleasure to move my body into the asanas, with the realisation that the performance was just for me. Performing as a dancer meant that most of the focus was always on giving energy out to others. The adrenaline high that I got during performances meant that I was constantly up and down emotionally. I used breath work to slow down my nervous system in the evenings so that I could go to sleep.

Interestingly, I have now got a completely different viewpoint of Kirtan chanting. It has become one of my favourite practices in yoga because I have realised, through my own experience with it, that it is a real fast track to the heart. In the beginning, when I was reintroduced to it, the mind would colour the act of chanting in a really taunting way. When something is outside of our comfort zone, there are so many thoughts that can colour the moment, which will then stop us from being opened.

The change in my thinking happened while I was in a yoga class in New York and we were repeating a Kirtan chant over and over again. All of a sudden there was an explosion from within, accompanied by a huge rush of energy. In that moment I understood the gifts Kirtan had to offer and the many blessings it can bring.

Teaching Yoga

I think that understanding the purpose of the practice of yoga appeals to a lot of people because many are not willing to just follow instructions like a parrot. So, for example, I have done a practice on the element of air, which is connected to the heart chakra. The yoga postures were then formed around heart openers and twists, in order to help melt the knots in the heart, which we can carry in our life because of hurts and traumas. I place great emphasis on explaining and demystifying the choice of postures I use and the theme behind them. This allows people to feel empowered and safe within the practice. To me, the practice of yoga has got to be grounded, real and relevant to life.

appleyoga is my life's work. The main reason that I danced was because of my passion for movement and connecting it to the feeling state. In dance, if we are portraying a character, then we have to invoke certain qualities. I use this power of invocation within my yoga practice, where emphasis is placed on consciously invoking different energetic qualities. So, for example, sometimes we need to step into our fire a bit more, or other times we need to ground ourselves and really understand what that feels like. When done consciously, yoga can be an alchemical process.

Also, I really pay attention to the music I play within the classes. Music has been a great part of my life. I am aware of the fact that when people hear music their cells start to move. That said, sometimes silence is just as important, so being able to gauge what is required in the moment is a necessary skill.

The way I choose to awaken people's energies varies. I may, for example, open the class with a quote. I have in the past used Rumi: 'Let the beauty you love, be what you do.' There are so many ways to bless your body. When people hear a quote like that, it changes their movement from robotic to transformational and accentuated because the energy body becomes engaged. The art of being a great guide is to be able to utilise wisdom without it being overwhelming or preachy.

Inspiration

My family inspires me. My mother has been a great inspiration and she has amazing wisdom. I feel incredibly blessed to know her. The same goes for my father and brothers, they inspired me to reach for what I wanted, knowing that nothing was impossible. I think that stood me in great stead in terms of moving into dance. Athletic art careers are tough, there is not a place for everyone inside of them. My family has definitely inspired me to understand that I could move my boundaries and that life is full of possibilities, I really appreciate that blueprint from them.

Also, the magic of dance and music are very deep parts of my life in the sense of inspiration.

Training Teachers

I really love training people to become teachers. It challenges me and moves me in a very beautiful way to step deeper into the practice. I know this is one of the main reasons why I put myself forward to help people to become yoga guides to others. I knew it would shift my boundaries, knowledge and involvement in the practice to a far greater extent than it would have done if I had just stayed on the periphery of the student level. As a teachers' guide, I am telling people what to do so they can inform others. It is a greater responsibility and has a huge knock-on effect.

Yoga is a daily practice, whether you are on your mat or not. That is an ethos which is paramount for me to impart to others. There is the physical aspect of yoga, but there are also all the other elements that potentially make us a better version of ourselves. We need to ask questions like: Am I being kind to myself? What am I learning from this situation? Why am I in this cycle and what do I need to shift in order to make a change? The questioning creates the alchemical process.

Because of my dance background, I try not to make people into slaves to their mats. I have observed how negatively people can react to that. However, if someone is going to hold the seat of being a teacher they are going to have to step towards yoga very differently. Being a teacher is not the same as loving yoga. This point always hits home when trainees qualify and they have that defining moment where they realise people are going to be looking to them to understand what needs to be done within the practice. At that moment a shift happens, many of them really step forward within themselves and they make a commitment to do their practice on a daily basis, rather than as a methodical exercise. As a teacher, if someone has not refined themselves as an instrument of yoga, there is no way that it would be possible for them to go into the heart of the practice. It is definitely a progression that is gained over time.

A Heart-Based Life

I feel so blessed with what I have already done in my life, that everything else is really just a dance. I am very driven which is my nature. I love to do new projects and to get my teeth into different things that inspire me. But I have done a lot in my life. I have written two books, filmed 15 DVDs travelled the world, taught some really awesome people, trained people to be teachers, danced, had the blessing of a very wonderful family and just married the dream man of my life, after waiting a very long time to do that. So I feel very blessed that life for me now, through its ups and downs, is a play. I get to ride it wherever it takes me, I am ready.

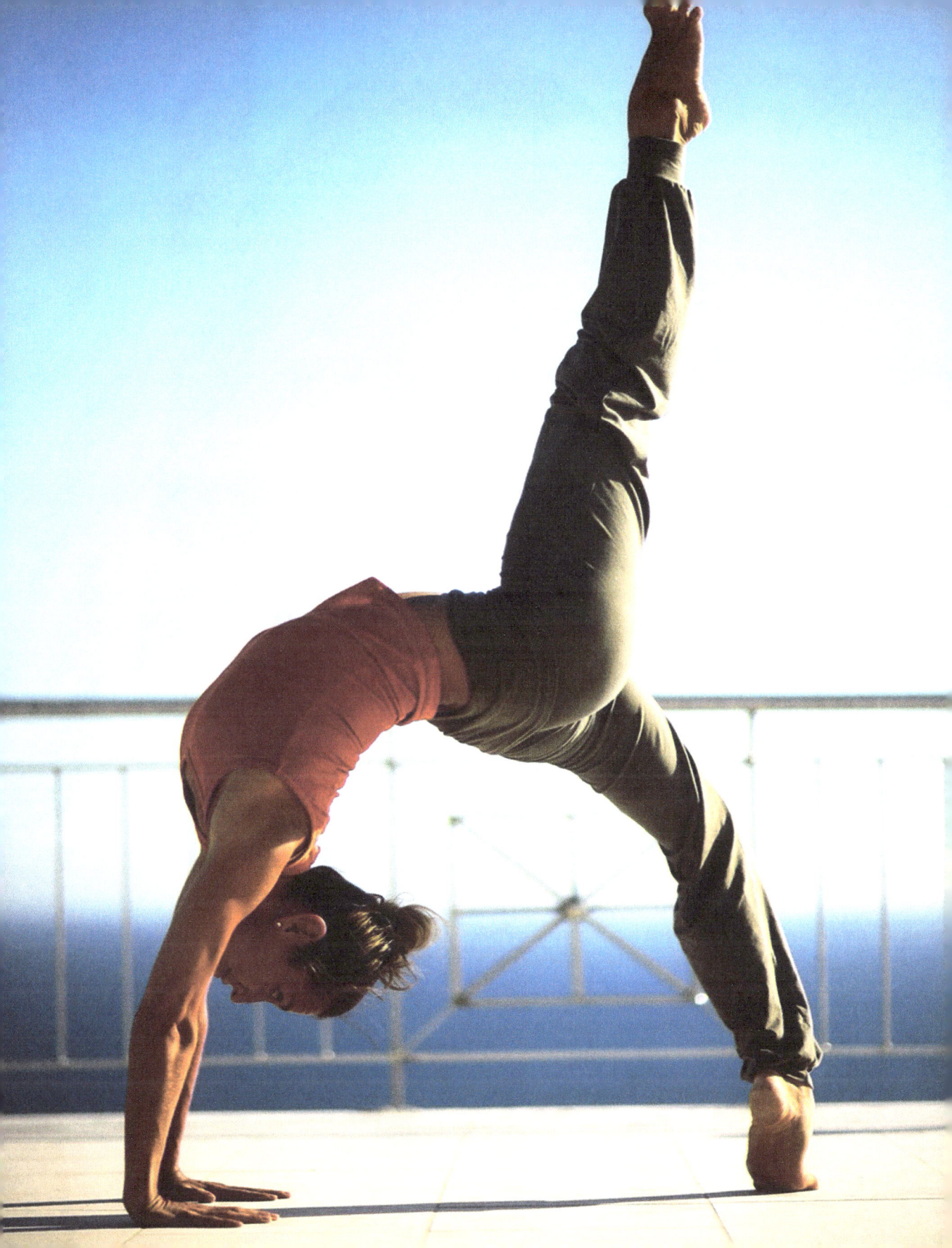

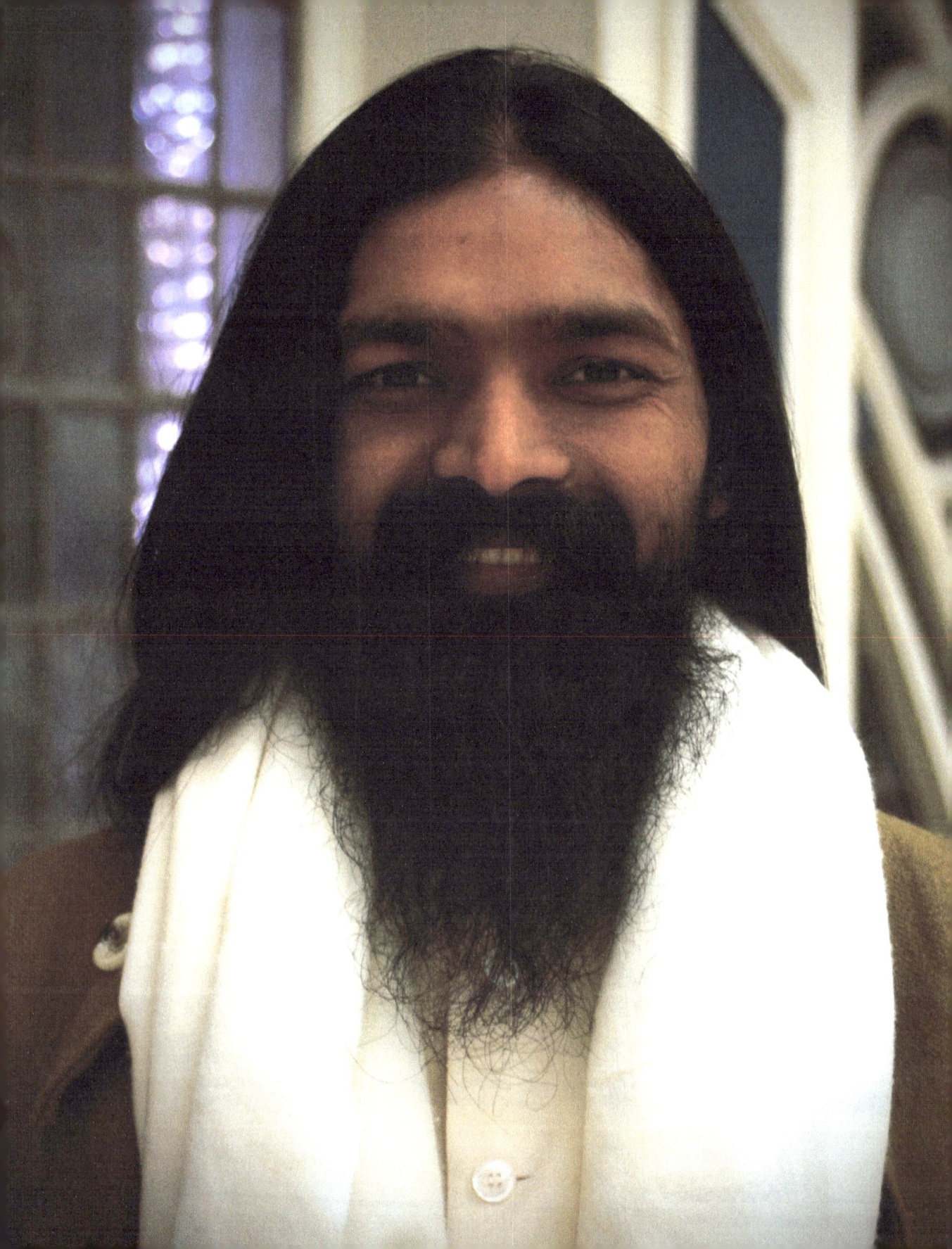

Yogi Ashokananda
Founder of Science of Relaxation Active
Meditation, Himalayan Hatha Yoga, Prana Kriya Yoga

For Yogi Ashokananda, yoga is a way of life and a journey that he has embarked on, in order to explore and discover the fullness of who he is. Yogi is a product of a number of teachers who themselves were grounded and rooted in the embodiment of the practice of yoga. I got a sense of someone who truly understands how sacred, mystical and transformative, meditation and yoga can be and is on a journey to share this knowledge, understanding and experience with us.

Yoga has always been a part of my life. My first teacher was my grandfather, who used to go to the Himalayas every year for the summer months. He would spend time there meditating, practicing yoga and meeting like-minded people. When he came home to the village where we lived, he would do his daily practice and as a child I watched him in fascination. He was aware of my interest and one day put a blanket next to his and invited me to join him.

His way of teaching was different. He never told me how the practice was going to make me feel, he would just set a yoga task and ask me a question related to that task. I had to practise and keep returning to him when I thought I had found the answer to his question. If he was satisfied he would set another task. So my voyage into yoga was made through experience. For my grandfather, the spirituality behind yoga and meditation was considered a sacred and private journey into finding the inner self. He made it understood that I was developing a personal skill to support myself through life.

My Study

I went to university where I studied both Accounting and Computer Science. I was really captivated by the similarities between computer programming and the way the human mind can be programmed. Eventually, though, I lost interest and instead committed myself fully to deepening my understanding and experience of yoga and meditation practices.

My grandfather was my most prominent teacher, because the way I see life and my approach to life has come from him. But I did have a second very influential teacher who I met while I was in university. He was not famous, he just lived a humble life and had a personal practice. When I first asked him to teach me he refused. I continued asking him for three years, but he ignored all my attempts to impress him.

Over time my persistence made him change his mind. He invited me to take a walk with him one day and said that if I came to see him every day he would teach me. I was so excited, I went the next day and he ignored me; I stayed there for two hours before I told him I had to go. This pattern continued. I would get there, he would say nothing and after a few hours he would tell me to come back the following day for my next lesson.

It was intensely frustrating. However, one day he asked me how I felt coming to see him every day. I told him I was angry and disappointed but it did not matter, I would still keep coming. He laughed and said he would see me the next day and then went back to ignoring me. After some time he asked me what I learnt from him and what I thought he was teaching me. I told him I observed myself, my reactions, my judgement, my anger, my frustration, but most of all I learned to be patient. He told me that meditation consisted of patience. In waiting for something to happen you have to be available and have to be present. He said that I had mastered meditation so the next step was developing the body.

I began to realise that he created a space for me to completely melt my ego, because when I showed him my physical practice, he told me that it was all nonsense. He said I was trying to impress him and asked me to show him my practice without making it into a performance. He said I had to let go of my need to perform for the approval of others because competing had no place with spirituality.

Being a Teacher

I came to the UK for the first time in 2005 but did not enjoy it. When I got back to India I told my teacher that I was going to move to the Himalayas and live a simple life. He told me that if I lived in a place where I had nothing, I would never test my ability to be detached, because I would not have anything to be detached from. He said that I had to come back to the West and learn from it. This confused me because spiritual teachers go to the West to teach, not to be taught. His response was that everyone makes a mistake thinking that way. He said that his teachings had come to an end; there was nothing else he could show me. My coming to the West to learn would be a way to repay him for everything he taught me. This was the only reason I came back here for a second time.

From the West I learnt about how the illusion and attachments can be so strong it can really catch people. I realise what my teacher meant, if you have never tested what it means to be attached, it is impossible to understand what detachment means. My teacher told me to go to the place that was most distracting and meditate there. So I went to Oxford Circus and other equally busy and chaotic places every day for three months.

I would lean back against a wall and just watch, for one or two hours every day. Then one day I found that I was able to experience a stillness that was similar to what I experienced in the mountains of the Himalayas. When I told my teacher about this, he said that this meant I could now meditate anywhere. He told me I was not meditating properly previously, because I felt I needed to be in a quiet place or surrounded by certain things. This was creating an attachment to objects when really I needed to be free.

Yoga and Meditation

My teacher had a huge influence on me and the way that I teach. We created Science of Relaxation active meditation together. It is quite an old system that blends mantras, sutras, tantra and yogic techniques. He was a master of many areas of spirituality because he spent his whole life in practice. Unfortunately, he passed away in 2009. During the first class I taught after he died, I felt quite sad. It was a shock for me not having him near but, in helping me to develop, he left behind some very beautiful teachings.

The Science of Relaxation is about experiencing the energy within your own body. People say you can relax through meditation and being quiet. But my teacher told me that you could not call this relaxation, because it was so temporary. Ideas, thoughts and desires create feelings of lack, this traps your energy and you begin to live in a fractured way. The Science of Relaxation bridges the division between the higher and the very human self, healing any split between spiritual self and material personality.

Science of Relaxation uses simple techniques combined with arm movements to move the breath, energy and awareness into and through the most vital areas of the body, where unprocessed emotions and events from our past experiences are stored. In Sanskrit, these are known as Samskaras and are described as impressions left on your soul and body from your experiences, which then forms your personality. If they are left in the body they can dampen your energy making you feel lethargic, depressed, stressed and anxious and can develop into long-term chronic disease. With relaxation comes release from these adverse effects.

It is very possible to experience 100% relaxation twenty-four hours a day. But it is done through practices, patience and meditation every day or as regularly as you can. Through the practice you find prana or energy that will clear the mind and purify the thoughts. This form of meditation is quite dynamic because you use movement and breath work. It is the only thing that I have found to be really effective in completely releasing stagnant or negative emotions.

As a teacher my practice is about how I can take whoever comes to me, into a place where they can find and keep their centre. I have my own style of yoga, it was originated from the mountains so I call it Himalayan Hatha Yoga and I have also developed ancient kriya yoga practices into what I call Pranakriya Yoga, to suit modern life. I take elements of these sacred systems of spirituality and yoga and run courses, workshops, retreats and teacher trainings of varying durations, so that people can learn in their own time, according to their capabilities.

The Future

I am creating community and sustainable projects in Tiruvannamalai, South India, for people to meditate and gain experience in their practice. There is not a big commercial objective, the place is secluded and in beautiful rural surroundings with great energy and views towards the sacred pilgrimage site of Mount Arunachala. I also run other charity projects in the form of a school and medical aid to help the local community there. The way I see myself in society, as a teacher and Yogi, is that I am here to help as many people as possible to find their centre and live from a place that is 100% authentic to them.

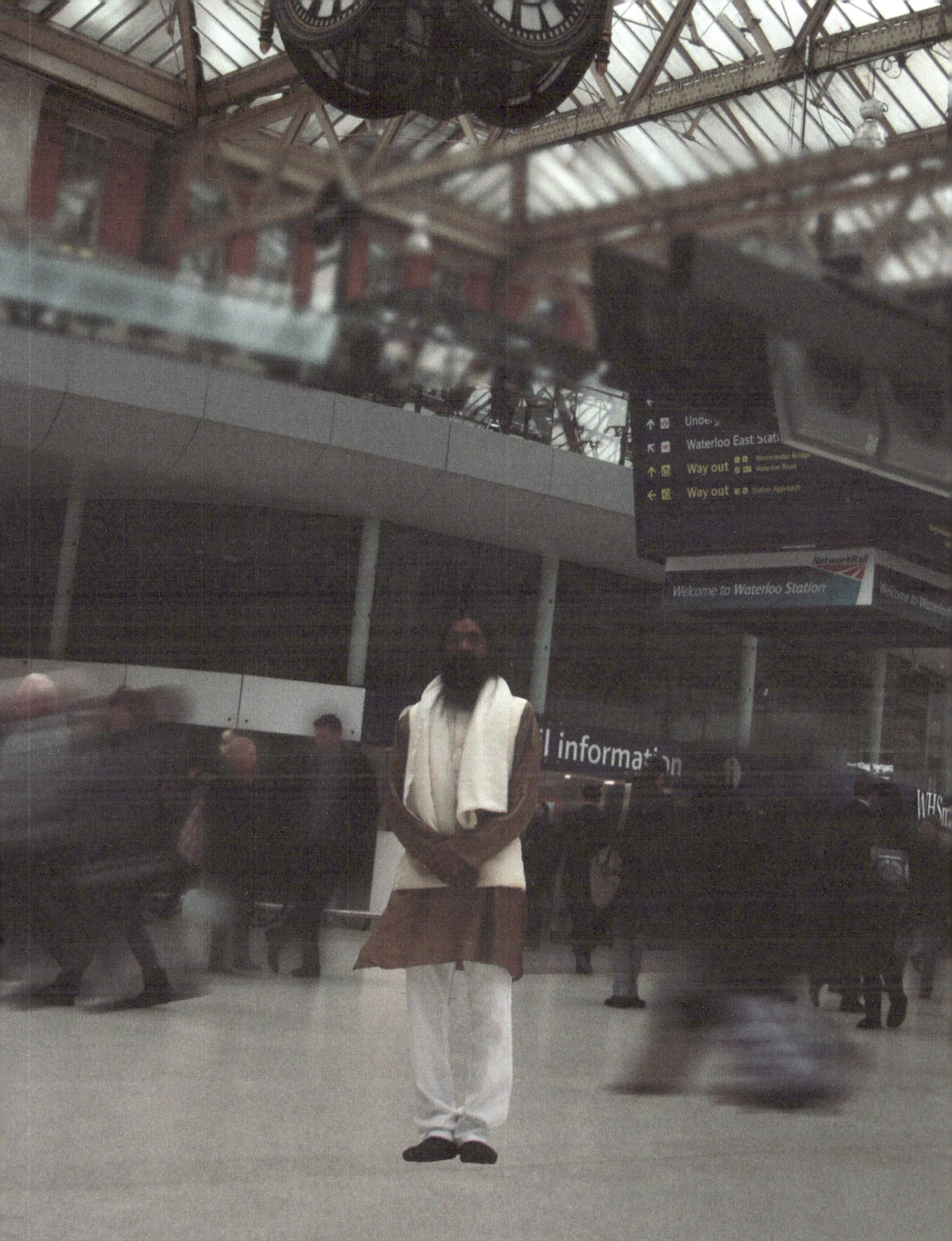

"The more that people tap into the higher aspects of their own energy, the more their creativity starts to flow. This is because the better the filter the better the coffee; the more disempowering beliefs that a person clears the greater the clarity of the mind will be."

- Anna Kitney

Energy Work

There are a number of therapies that deal with managing the subtle or energetic body. The four people who have been chosen to represent this section give a broad view of this area. The Barefoot Doctor has long been an advocate of Tai Chi, energy management, balance and enhancement. Shola Arewa is focused on working with energy in an integrative way by using psychology, chakra balancing, nutrition and exercise. Anna Kitney has been making huge waves in pioneering Theta Healing within the UK and speaks of changing beliefs in order to change energy, and Tina Shaw gives us her personal take on Reiki and its importance in bringing balance.

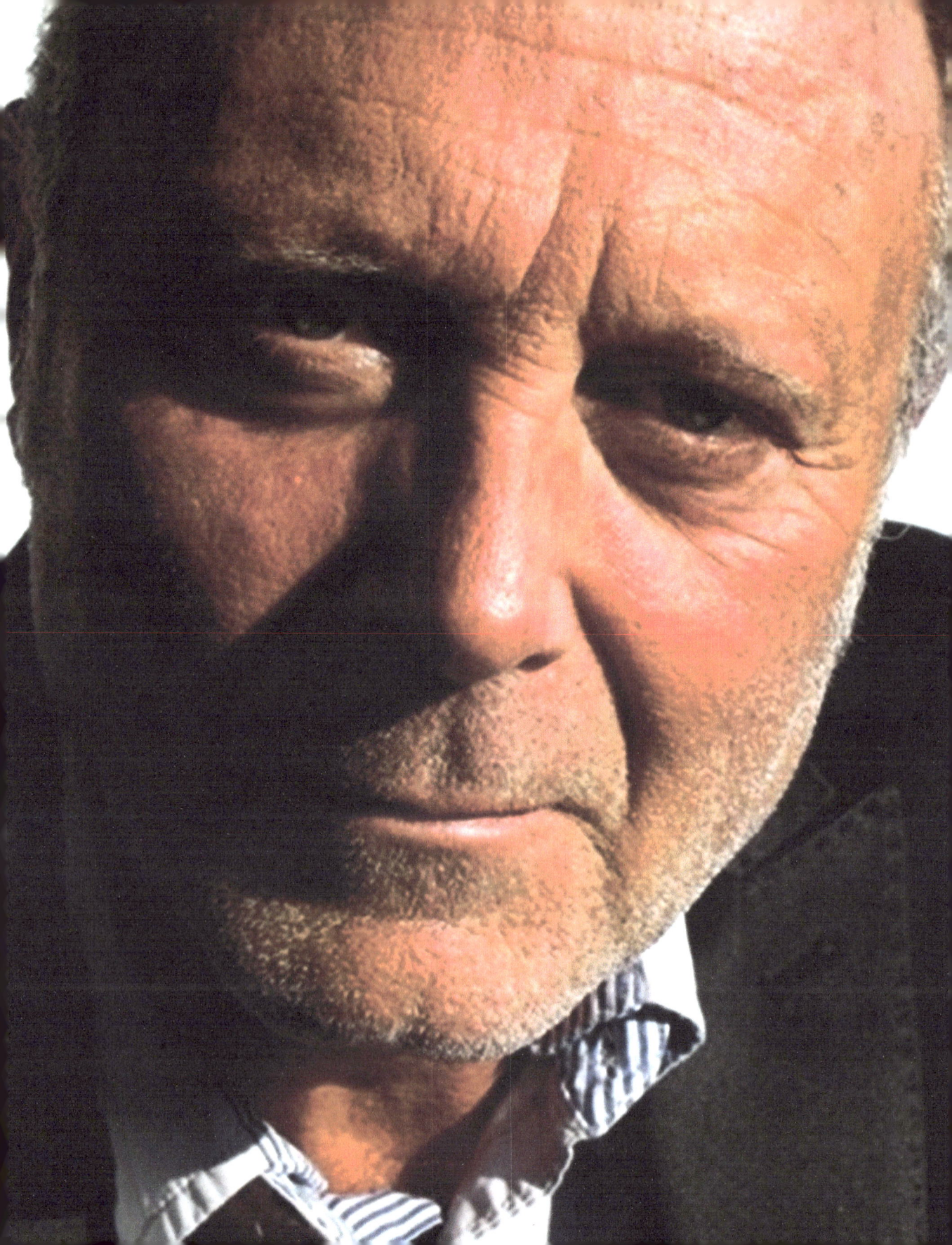

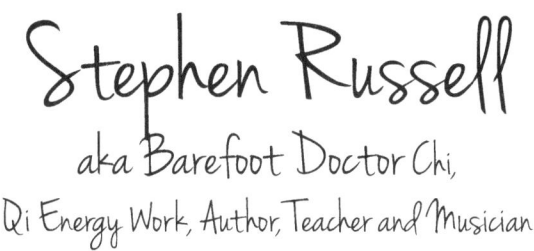

Stephen Russell

aka Barefoot Doctor Chi,
Qi Energy Work, Author, Teacher and Musician

Barefoot Doctor is renowned as a world-class consciousness teacher and the author of 16 books. He's a Taoist Martial Arts master, a master of energy medicine and meditation, and a producer of electronic dance and healing music. As a sound-healing master, his speciality is in helping people to raise their frequency and their game.

When I was eleven, I used to love to fight and was always getting into trouble with the teachers at school. My Dad happened to know someone who was studying Aikido. The teacher was an old Japanese guy who came to London as a healer and based himself in Harley Street. We had a meeting with him, he checked me out and decided to take me on; it was a real honour.

The healing part of the training meant nothing to me. All I wanted to do was to learn how to fight; but the discipline of being with someone who was obviously a master was fantastic. I never came across anyone like him before. There was a time when he told me to punch him in the stomach. I half punched and he asked me to hit him harder. I had three go's before I really went for it. It was like punching an air balloon. There was nothing there, but it was solid at the same time. On the third punch, he flicked his belly and pushed me backwards. I ended up on the wall at the other side of the room. It was amazing! I had real respect for him.

The other guys in the class wanted to learn about healing and meditating, so I was obliged at the end of every lesson to learn to channel energy. I began practising on family and friends and I found it took people's pains away and calmed them down. As a young teenage hippie that was one of the tricks I could do. I liked the place it gave me in society; it was a pleasure to have something to offer. I was learning really great stuff, from Aikido and from meditating about how to be calm. Also, by then I was reading Freud, Jung and Buddhist Text. I was really fascinated by it all.

The Chi or Qi that was moving through the practice of martial arts was indisputable. I switched from Aikido to Tai Chi and I got into Taoism through Tai Chi in my late teens. Around that time I met the psychiatrist R.D. Laing and I studied psychotherapy with him for 3 years. What was driving me was this fascination about how consciousness works, how energy works and how the mechanics of reality all work.

Acupuncture

After studying with R.D. Laing I went to live with the Native Americans in New Mexico for four years. I was teaching Tai Chi for my living and an osteopath friend came over from England and advised me to learn acupuncture as this is where I would really learn about energy, how it flows in the body, how it is produced and how it works.

I ended up being the apprentice to the President of the New Mexico acupuncture board. He was a Chinese hippy and because he was in the hippy culture, as I was at the time, we had a kinship. Otherwise, the Chinese do not generally teach other people that easily. We became friends and I was his apprentice. It was an incredible opportunity.

The healing intention

The mode informing any healing work is one of kindness and the intention is to reinstate the wholeness, that has always been there, under the distortions and the split ups. It is not that people aren't whole, but there is an illusion going on under the surface that we are split up or dissociated, and we live in that illusion. When we come back to being who we really are, there is a wholeness that heals everything.

The job and intention of the healer is to reach that part of the person where they are healed already and then the healing will take place on its own. It doesn't matter what modality you are using, as long as you are good at using it. If you can talk to that whole, healed, healthy part of the person and get that part of the person to realise who's there, the rest of the stuff takes care of itself.

That isn't to say they are going to get better, which sounds like a paradox. In the physical sense they may be too far gone, they may be dying anyway, but the process of dying will become one of grace, rather than pain and suffering.

That is really the other side of it, your motivation is to alleviate suffering and the intention is to create wholeness again.

My Work

Part of my work is to connect people back to source, mostly through sound. Within the Taoist system that I am working with, sound healing is a very intrinsic part of it. There are six Taoist healing sounds, one for each organ and one for the energy field. So I teach people the sounds and I do the sound for them, to heal them with the sound that I am making. As a musician I spend a lot of time creating beats and tunes where I am very careful of the frequency, to vibrate the different areas of the body. I also use my voice, developed over 30 years, as a way of taking people into a trance, so they get in touch with that deepest part of themselves.

Additionally, I felt the need to simplify the essence of the martial arts practice for myself. Not the actual moves, but the internal game of it, the mindset and the way you hold yourself internally. Then the aim was to teach it to everyone, even those who don't do martial arts. If people could find that space, it would transform them in their lives and give them their power base internally. I set about simplifying quite a complex thing, down to seven steps. If you take these seven steps you completely reposition yourself. I created School for Warriors, which is an online training scheme. Every day you watch a video and do an exercise; people have been getting it, it really gives them their power.

The Ego

With the work that I do, the focus is off me and onto others, in the way that I am of service to others. This makes my life work much better for me. My natural inclination is to become egocentric, where it is all about me, how well I'm doing and how I'm going to make it work better. Which is all fine, you really need that as well. You have to have the narcissistic side running, you wouldn't do anything otherwise. We really need it. The narcissistic side drives the vain part of you that needs a hook, otherwise it won't get involved with something. We can't deny that, we all have it. But if your focus is being of service to people or healing people then it does not work as the driving force. Not for me anyway, I can't talk for others. The whole thing only rolls if I let go of me and allow myself to be part of the service. It is not about being saintly or good, it is just about having something you can do.

Daily Practice

I do martial arts, Chi Gong and meditate every day, for an hour to an hour and a half. I get up really early to do it, but it is worth it. I have a condensed version if I am in a rush and only have 20 minutes. It works, but it is not the same. Once I have done the full thing I don't care what happens to me during the day. I don't mind how hard I have to work, what I have to do, how unpleasant the environment. As long as I have done that I am ahead of the game. I feel I can give myself in service because I don't need to feed myself anymore, I have already done it.

The Future

This year I have not been anywhere longer than a week at a time. I have been on the move between Oxford, London, Wales, France, Ibiza, Germany, Italy, and America and back around. I have not stopped, it has been one thing after the other. I love it. I absolutely love being on the move, tuning into new people and new places, overcoming my own prejudices and preferences about what I think I like and don't like, and the vibes I like and don't. I am getting to be at home anywhere on the planet. Living in this way, you have to cut through the disguise that everyone is wearing. It is not always possible, but when it is, and most of the times it is, it is beautiful.

There are 7 billion people on the planet. I would love to talk to every single one and make them smile for five minutes, it would be great.

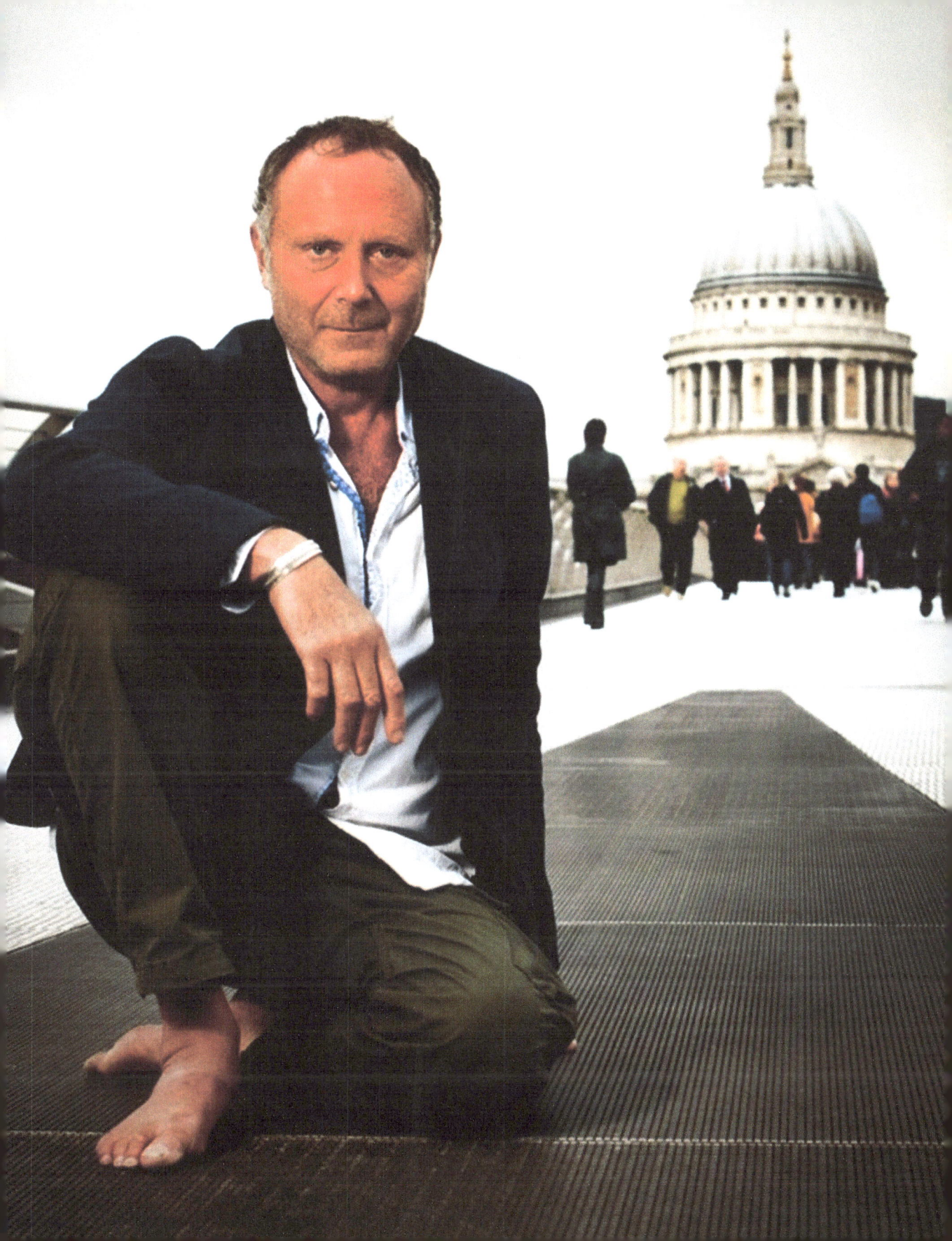

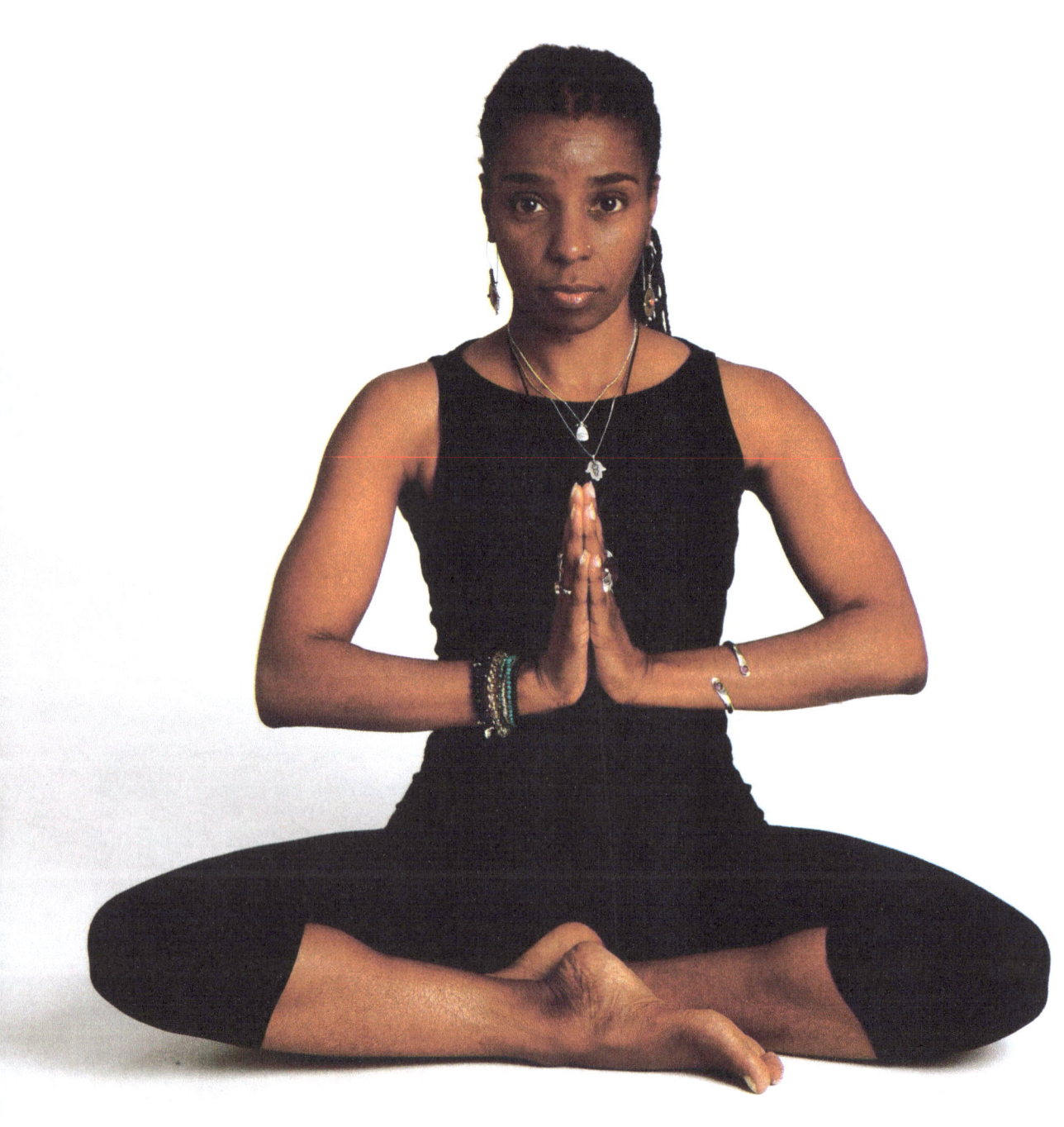

Shola Arewa
Founder of Energy 4 Life, Author and Trainer

Shola Arewa is someone who walks her talk. She started her career scaling the heights of the fashion industry, but this success sparked in her the need for a deeper meaning and understanding of life. Her travels to Asia, particularly India, held the key to unlocking her energy, spirituality and wisdom. It has also been the main contributing factor in the development of her system, Energy 4 Life. Launched in 2008, it continues to create ever expanding ripples outward.

My career started within the fashion industry. It has been a very interesting transition because the physical body is the most peripheral part of ourselves as human beings. So my real journey was from the outer body to the inner core. My fashion business was very successful and I ran it for a number of years, but there was an urge to experience more from my life. So I decided to go travelling and ended up being away for two and a half years. In that time I visited eleven countries in Asia and spent a year and a half in India. It was the time I spent in India that completely transformed my life.

I knew I wanted yoga to be a part of my life, but at the time was not sure of the form this would take. I did not plan to go to India in the beginning, but after I had been away for a while I felt drawn to it. This was mainly because I knew there was a lot that I could learn from yoga philosophy and the practical techniques. I went up to Rishikesh, which is located in the mountains, and started going to the Yoga Niketan Ashram every morning for an hour-long meditation. During the session we were instructed to remain completely still; we could not move, itch or cough. If we did, someone came to haul us out. Not only was it very powerful, but it cultivated a real discipline.

I was eager to experience more through meditation, so in the morning I would climb over the huge gate at the back of the Ashram instead of walking to the front. I would go in, sit down and meditate. They found out I was doing this one day and threw me out. Fortunately, before I left London I bought a yoga book for 50p in Portobello Market and at the back of it there was a programme that I could follow as an alternative, so I began doing this every morning. Somebody saw me practising and asked me if I knew that the Ashram from that book was right next door to Yoga Niketan.

As it transpired, I was obviously meant to be next door. So I ended up in the Ashram of the teacher whose book I was following.

Returning to England

When I came back to England I had changed so much. Before I left I was living the fast life of champagne and parties. On my return everything was different. I wanted to understand what had happened to me, which is why I started studying psychotherapy, in order to make sense of it all.

But it was the energy work that really brought the understanding. I had done yoga, I had worked to develop my spiritual side, studied, practised and taught bodywork. I was a psychotherapist and I had studied expressive arts therapy, so I wanted to find a way to bring it all together. Focusing on the chakras allowed me to take everything I had learnt a step forward and into the core centre. It gave me a clearer, deeper and more expansive understanding of humans. This led to my first book Opening to Spirit. I have spoken at the Mind, Body and Spirit Festival every year for the past 18 years on energy work. I brought my work to the prison service, starting off with yoga for the inmates and then stress management for the staff.

Energy 4 Life

Energy 4 Life was created in 2008. It is something that could not have happened earlier because we did not have enough of the research, information, knowledge and ability to work with energy, in the same way that we have now. In the past I had produced various training programmes, mainly for adult education, but eventually I felt the need to create a programme for myself. This was based on the elements of my work that were fast acting, powerful and potent. I focused on the main issues that clients had and the most effective ways of working with them.

In developing Energy 4 Life, I realised that there were four healing modalities to address. These were: Energy Exercise because one of the major issues that people face is the sedentary lifestyle; Energy Psychology, which focuses on what goes on in the mind and how we can release the things that are holding us back; Energy Food, which places attention on the importance of nutrition, a huge factor in formulating our health; and Energy Balance, which incorporates bodywork, mindfulness, meditation and relaxation.

Yet, while Energy 4 Life is created from these elements, it is informed by a coaching relationship, rather than counselling. Coaching creates a relationship that it is much more empowering and person-centred. It supports the person to get from where they are, to where they want to be, which makes it more progressive in its approach. It does not focus on the past, nor does it hone in on problems and issues. Instead, it looks at what the person wants to achieve and the ways to do that.

Creating Energy 4 Life

I am always interested in looking for common threads in my work and keen to see what really underlies any particular modality. A treatment may be very effective, but my question is why does it work? What parts of it make it work? I then focus on devising a system where you can access the effects in the most direct way. This means that the tools you learn are powerful and get straight to the point, making the greatest impact on the system.

There is a psychological aspect in terms of how we work with the client. We offer support in really identifying what is going on with their own energy, they are then able to focus into the area to be released and let it go. This is the process that we take people through.

Developing as a Teacher and Trainer

Becoming a teacher and trainer was a natural progression for me. I became a yoga teacher in 1985. Within the complementary medicine aspect of my work, I devised programmes, had them accredited with the appropriate bodies, trained the trainers, and then delivered them in Adult Education. As a result, I received the CAM (Complementary and Alternative Medicine) award in 2008 for 'outstanding contribution to the industry', which is an achievement I am proud of. So teaching and training is something I have always done in my work, but I hadn't created an independent training programme yet and I felt that it was time for me to do so.

My Passion for Energy 4 Life

Energy 4 Life is definitely a reflection of my life's work. I specialise in all things pertaining to our well-being as humans. That is what I have done throughout my career as a health practitioner and trainer. So Energy 4 Life really brings it all together by supporting someone in their physical health, psychological well-being, success and fulfilment. One of the great things about working with health is that once we get it right, we are able to fully express much more of who we are.

I was always taught as a child that you could do anything if you put your mind to it.

Because of how strong this belief was, I would fight for that truth. My success in the world of fashion made my belief a reality. I had created a business in Kensington and was making more money than I knew what to do with and I truly knew that no matter where I wanted to take my business, I could make it a success. In knowing that, I could let it go, as I had nothing else to prove. I redefined what success meant to me and I am clear about that now. It is very simple. Success for me is to live with purpose, passion and in peace. I know and seek to embody this truth in every cell of my being.

The Future

I have developed something that is still a new concept in the UK. Energy 4 Life is at the forefront and leading the way in the area of Wellness Coaching and I know we will continue to grow. My work will continue to impact the lives of the coaches that train with me and the lives of the people they offer their service to. Part of my vision when I started out was to put health back into the hands of the people. Through the people I have trained, Energy 4 Life is now in schools, hospitals and the workplace, as well as being in people's homes. I see it growing and expanding, which I am very excited about.

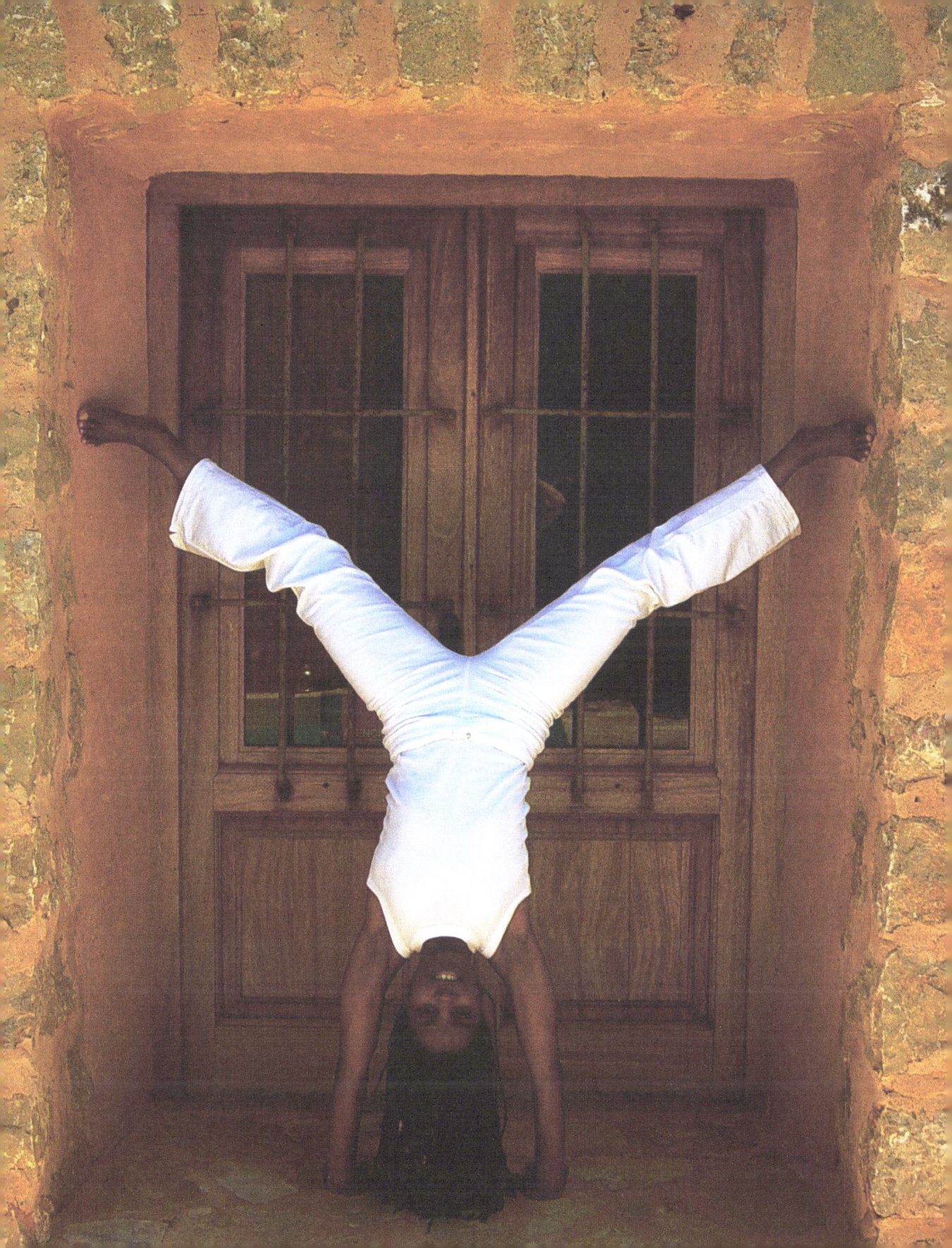

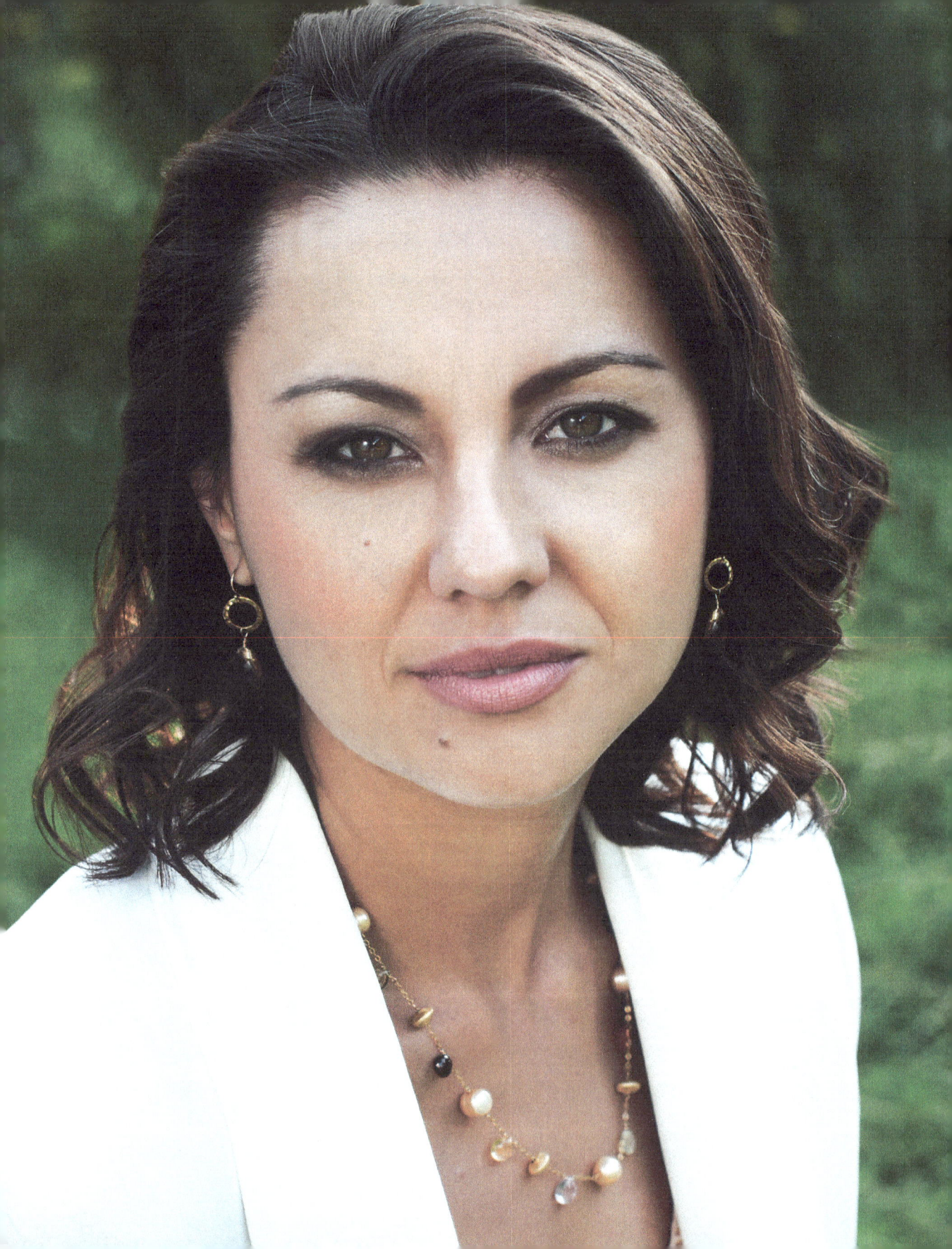

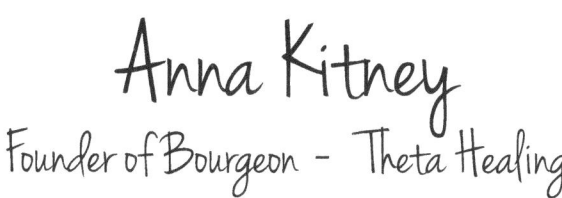

Anna Kitney
Founder of Bourgeon – Theta Healing

Anna Kitney is a true gem in the world of energy healing. She wears many hats including being a Theta Healing Teacher, an Interior Designer, an Intuitive Feng Shui Practitioner and a Jewellery Maker. Each hat is worn with an elegance and divinity that places a particular stamp of excellence on her work. Her ambition is to build a global community of high quality healers and therapists under the umbrella of her company, Bourgeon.

was introduced to Theta Healing through my mum who had first done Reiki and then Theta Healing afterwards. I had lower back pain and had tried a number of things; the pain would get better for a short period after a treatment and then return. As a last resort, I thought I would try energy healing. I was in London and phoned my mum up in Australia to ask for her help. Mum told me she would work on me energetically while I was asleep that night and when I woke up the following morning, the pain was gone!

In our next conversation, she said that the lower back pain was connected to financial support. I was thirty at the time and thinking about having children, but I had fears about being taken care of financially. Stopping work meant my income also stopped and I would become solely dependent on my husband. My mother told me that all of this had been linked to the back pain, without me voicing any of it. I was really impressed that she was able to get so much information intuitively from Theta Healing.

Then, when I got pregnant and my son was born, I decided to do the Theta Healing courses as a way to develop my own intuition, so I could communicate with him. By going deeper into it, I got more than I bargained for. In the past I had attended many personal development seminars and workshops, so I knew a lot about life coaching and goal setting, but with Theta Healing it shifted me from a boxcar to a Lamborghini.

On a personal level, I would always create success and then sabotage it due to my limiting beliefs that I held in my subconscious of not being worthy or deserving, and having to prove myself or having to be poor to be close to my creative source. I was completely unaware of these belief systems because they had been handed down to me by my ancestors without my knowledge. With Theta Healing I tapped into these limiting beliefs and I was able to clear them quickly and easily. That is why I love it.

Theta Healing

I see Theta Healing as a way to tap into your inner truth and your inner knowing. The answers aren't on the outside; we always know our own answers. Theta Healing is a method for personal and self-development. It is a way to access the subconscious mind and change limiting beliefs into empowering ones instantly. It allows you the opportunity to learn your life's lessons quickly.

It is probably out of some people's comfort zone, especially when we start talking about future readings or connections to spirit guides. All of these esoteric aspects of Theta are, however, very valuable when working with the mind, as they give people a way to see their problem in a different light.

As part of my private practice I combine both Theta Healing with Feng Shui. Theta Healing works on the inner world and Feng Shui works on the outer world. Chi, Qi or Prana, whatever you want to call it, is the energy within us and the energy around us. In a dirty, dark, damp place our energy just feels low. Also there are times where the earth energy has witnessed large amounts of trauma as a result of wars being fought; this is where Feng Shui and Theta Healing can work quite nicely together. Healing can be sent to the earth, to release trauma. The earth also needs healing, but we always seem to take. However, when we give to the earth, she gives more.

I work with what the home wants because it carries the energies of the previous occupants. If there were arguments, divorce, abuse in the household, death or a murder, all that energy will be held in the walls. Healing within living spaces is useful because the home is a reflection of who we are on the inside.

We radiate energy out into the home by the kind of family we are. A house contains the vibration of the previous owners and when someone moves in, they take on that vibration. If something is not working in a person's life and the healing work has been done, it could be that the energy in the home is stagnant. Everything is energy so, for example, if you are holding on to clutter, it will start weighing you down. When someone does not feel safe they will feel the need to hoard, whether it is objects or weight. Creating a change in how they feel in the home can be the catalyst for healing to occur.

Creativity

One of my main creative outlets is jewellery making. I got into crystals through Theta Healing and wondered how we could wear healing crystals all the time. Much of the healing jewellery I found was very esoteric and not really to my taste. I am a bit of a fashionista, so I wanted a way where mainstream people could receive healing, regardless of whether they were into Theta Healing or not. It introduces people to how crystals can make them feel and draws them into building a relationship with their personal environment. Even though my jewellery is mid to high-end, I aim to keep it affordable. I therefore work with semi-precious as opposed to fine jewels, and it is a great source of expression for me.

The more that people tap into the higher aspects of their own energy, the more their creativity starts to flow. This is because the better the filter, the better the coffee. The more disempowering beliefs that a person clears, the greater the clarity of the mind will be. Ultimately, everyone who channels the Divine is a filter. Although they are receiving the highest truth, the information has to come through their belief system, and what comes out is the purity of what they are able to translate.

The Healing Process

As a healer, there are generally two main types of healing process. The first type is when the person coming for healing understands how the illness serves them. It may be that they suddenly are getting increased attention or they get to punish certain people for what they feel was done to them. When they can let go of the reason that the illness serves them, they can then have whatever they want without the illness. That is a big leap for some people. The second type of healing process is for the person who is attracted to receiving healing. This is where it is important for the healer not to become too attached to results. The healer needs to have the belief that the person coming to them for healing is fine and perfect just the way they are. The healing process is just about them becoming more aware of their own perfection.

If you view a person as broken and needing to be fixed, their energy will seem dense and the healing will be hard work. It is about asking the energy to show you what needs to be changed and then letting go and being guided. The healing happens more easily, much faster and you don't use your own energy. There are many healers who are exhausted because they do not believe that the creator's energy is enough.

The more you do healing work, the easier your connection to source will become. I remember in the early days I struggled with knowing if I was really connected to my own divinity or not. It takes practice to get a good knowledge of what the creator feels like, as well as their voice and the creator's particular tone.

The Future

I have a grand vision in mind and it is definitely global. I want to expand to offer other modalities. Not everyone is ready for Theta as it can be quite fast. If people fear change, even though they want their problem to be gone, it might be a bit too quick for them. There are some people who are not ready for the whole spiritual experience, so they can come to Bourgeon and enter at whatever point they are ready for.

Bourgeon is about building a community of healers and people who offer different healing modalities. There will be courses, workshops and practitioners available globally. People are drawn to people they like. They pick people they like the look of, or the modality that they think would suit them. I see it being somewhere between The Chopra Centre and Hay House. There will be retreats, books, programmes and meditations.

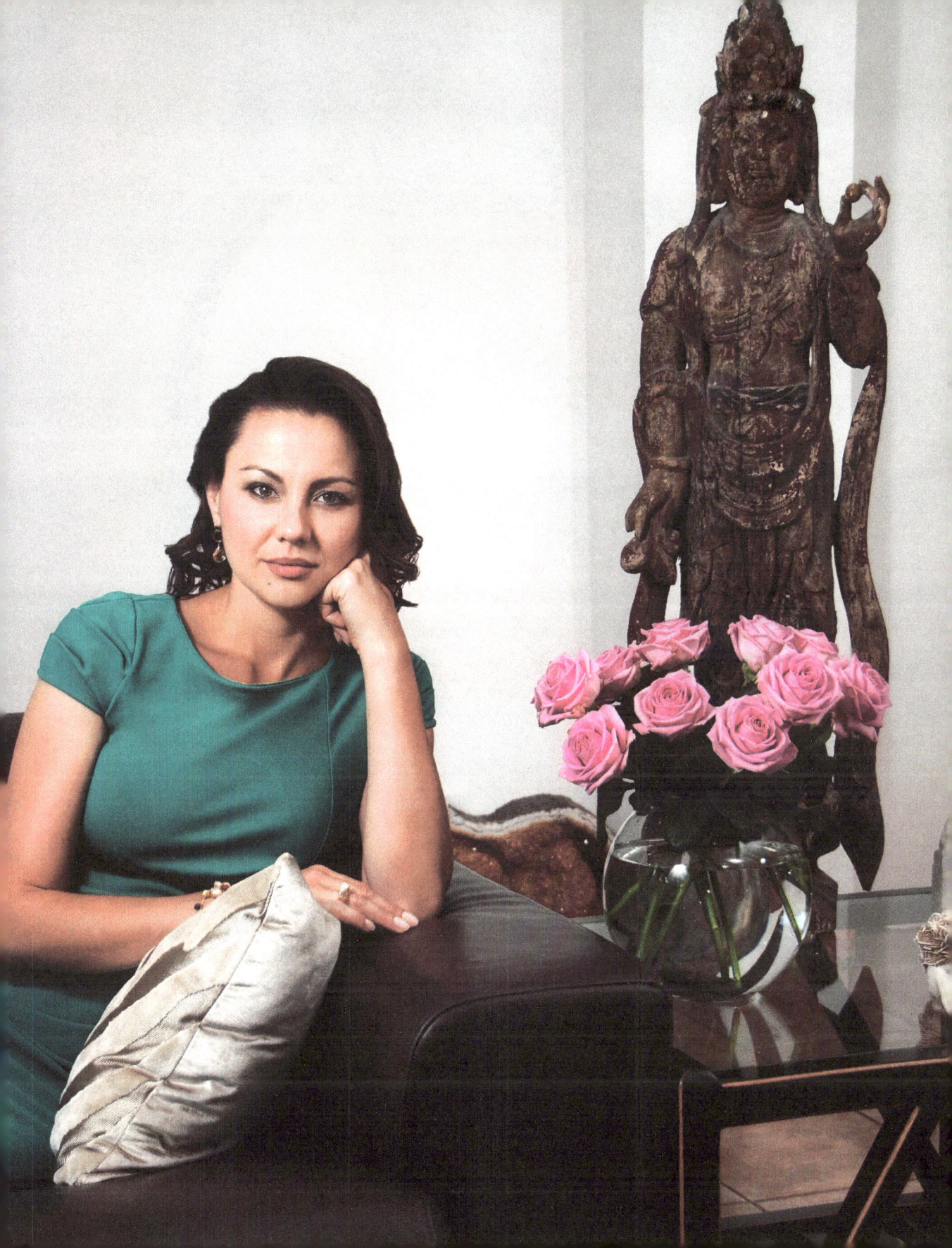

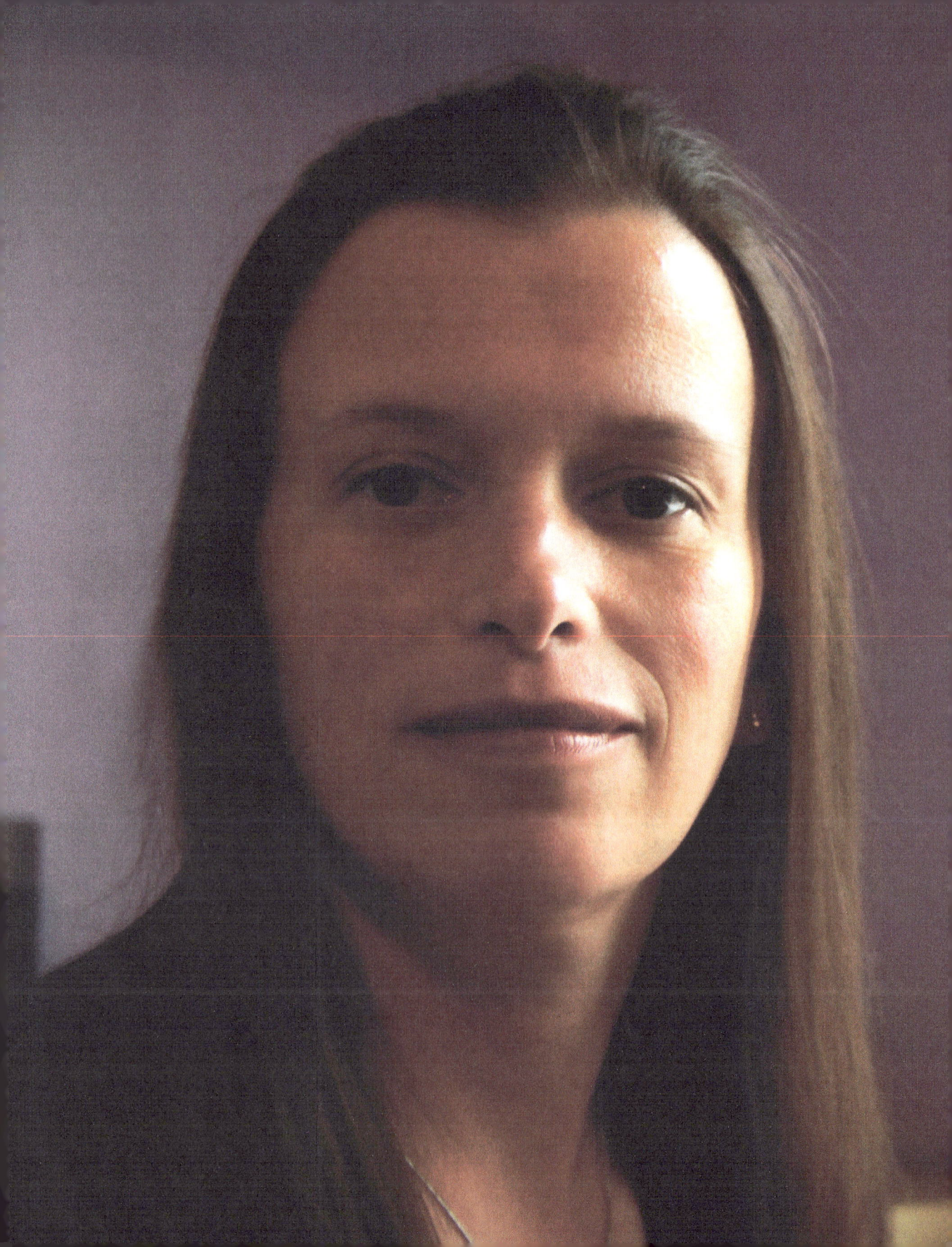

Tina Shaw

Founder of Absolute Reiki, Reiki Master, Teacher, Cognitive Behavioural Hypnotherapist

Tina Shaw began her working life in acting, but soon discovered that she needed more substance from her career. Once she came across the transformative, mystical and elegantly simple modality of Reiki, there was no turning back. It was plain to see how much the system has changed her own life and the difference it was making in the lives of others. Tina who is also trained as a cognitive behavioural hypnotherapist, has become a master teacher of Reiki and has placed a strong focus on the self-developmental aspects of working with this powerful energy art.

I started my career in acting. As a child, films and theatre were a source of inspiration to me. Growing up I became interested in their ability to move and inform people on an emotional level. Fame and celebrity did not excite me, my focus was more on the creative aspect of acting and the ways this could reach other people. Over the last 20 to 30 years the industry has generally gone from being creative and inspiring to being very concerned about celebrity. I became dissatisfied by this and the way I was working as an actress, and wanted to do something that I felt invigorated me.

My first introduction to Reiki was on a night out when a friend gave me some Reiki to get rid of a headache. I was fascinated at the time but then forgot about it. While I was still in acting, I started to evaluate other options and avenues. Reiki came to mind and, as I began my research, it really captivated me. I had always been interested in energy and the way that it transfers between people. I also noticed energetically that feelings could come from me and go into other people and vice-versa, and wondered about that. Once I started my journey into Reiki I realised that I couldn't be both a committed actor and a committed therapist or trainer. I had to make a choice and leave behind the world of acting, so that I could focus on teaching Reiki and my therapy work.

I was also drawn to the Japanese element and Eastern philosophy within Reiki because I had strong roots in Buddhism. I wasn't religious about it, but I liked the philosophy and I applied a lot of its principles to my daily life. I got myself onto a course with Reiki Evolution and immediately knew that I was on the right path when I saw how it was impacting my own life and the transformations it created in others.

Reiki

Reiki is a neutral energy that we can access and use as a tool for healing and personal development. It is an energy that promotes extensive peace and well-being and works beautifully in combination with meditation. My primary focus is personal development because the more centred you are, the more you are able to help others. The beautiful thing about a Reiki treatment is that everything you give to the other person you also give to yourself.

There is such a simplicity to Reiki as a modality. All you need to do is tune into the energy and allow it to move through you. In the act of the practitioner letting go and letting the intelligence of the energy work, transformation can occur and great things can happen.

At every level of Reiki there is a focus on our personal development and transformation. The energy helps us to increase our self-awareness and mindfulness as we follow the practices we are given. Each level also helps to enhance our work with others and opens us to the more subtle aspects of the energy. Using Reiki we can focus our work in specific ways to heal physically, emotionally, mentally and spiritually.

Reiki gives us a tool in which to experience the concept of oneness and connectedness, which allows us to use energy in a way that transcends time and space. I work with symbols and sacred sounds called the Kotodama that help students to access these energies and states quickly. Over time they develop such a strong connection with these states that they may no longer need to use these tools to trigger them. Symbols have power because they have been used so many times by so many people, which has served to reinforce the intention behind them. However, they are not the only way to work with the subtle energies within Reiki and intention is one of the most powerful tools.

Usui, the Founder of Reiki

Reiki was founded by Mikao Usui who was a Japanese Buddhist. No one knows the absolute truth about how he created the system, but it is clear that he developed a level of mastery in his understanding of spirituality and energy. His approach and way of teaching was flexible and he worked with many people from varying backgrounds. He fine-tuned his work to fit with the individual, incorporating energy healing, meditation, sacred sound and the use of symbols to help focus his work.

He developed the system primarily to gain an understanding of himself. Reiki was then expanded to be used as a self-development and healing modality, to help others get a better understanding of who they really are. The foundation of the system rests on five principles. These are: Just for today, do not anger, do not worry, be humble, be honest in your dealing with others, and be kind to yourself and others. 'Just for today' is at the heart of these principles, demonstrating that we should be present to people in the here and now.

Self-Development

The most profound aspect of working with Reiki is that it helps people to get a better understanding of themselves by bringing with it a feeling of being calm, centred and aware. Once people feel centred, they begin to understand what they really want to get out of life and Reiki supports them in the process of actually making it happen. It also heightens and expands people's intuition. In my opinion, intuition is a very natural thing. It's not a special gift that only certain people have. Each of us can tune into it. The subconscious mind is capable of understanding much more information, compared to the conscious mind. Intuition is just a way of tapping into the subconscious elements of who we are. This contains the millions of bits of information we absorb in every moment and every day.

Working with Reiki often means living by a whole different set of values. In the western world we get trapped by the idea that we're only worthy if we have certain material possessions. When we are able to look past the solid and physical world, we are left with who we really are and what we can bring to the world past the labels we have tagged ourselves with. Reiki helps shift people's viewpoint in that respect.

Another fundamental aspect of Reiki is self-acceptance. The more people are able to come to terms with the strength of the energy within themselves, the greater is their ability to love themselves. Once someone is able to treat themselves with love and kindness, everything else moves in the right direction.

The Future

There always needs to be a level of flexibility in terms of the future, as you never know what is going to happen. However, in terms of Reiki, I am placing my focus on developing courses. I love doing the treatments and that is an element of my work that will always be there. But I really do believe that people are better off if they learn to work with the energy for themselves and integrate it into their daily lives. Reiki was always meant to be inclusive. It is not a modality designed only for people who want to operate on a professional level.

One of the things I absolutely love about Reiki is its simplicity. Because it is just uncovering an integral part of who a person actually is, anyone can gain an understanding of it through the experience of it. I am focusing what I do now towards making sure that those people who just want to do it for their own personal development still have the opportunity to do so without getting involved in the dogma that can sometimes surround it.

Another area I have been focusing on is intuition. As mentioned before, I believe that this is a natural part of being human, rather than something that is only gifted to those who are special. I am really expanding this element of my work to help people to advance this side of themselves. I am very passionate about Reiki and nothing makes my heart sing more than seeing others empowered by the transformation that this subtle, but powerful, system enables within us.

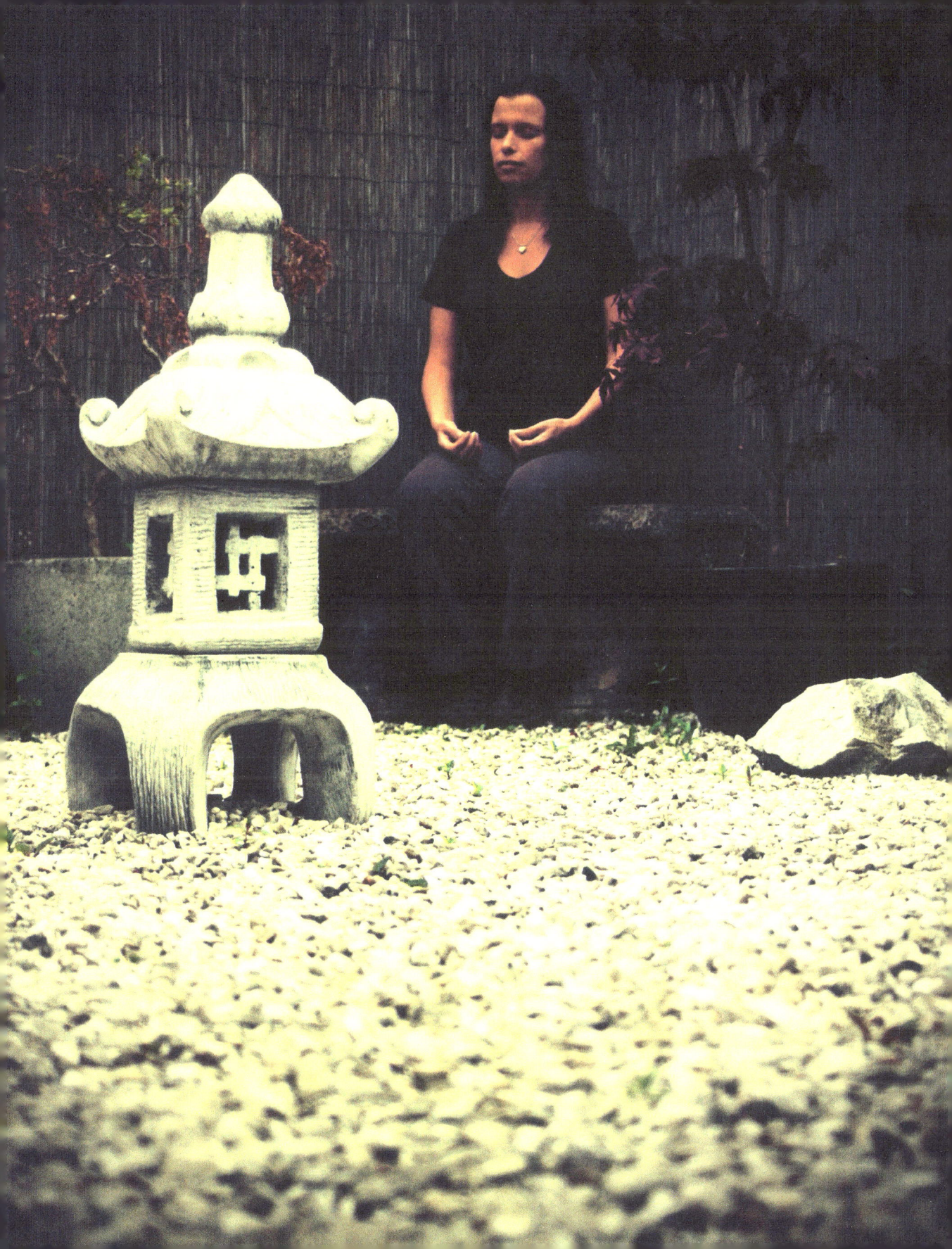

"All music is perfect, I very much believe in the orchestra of life, we are all instruments and everyone has their perfect part to play. If you are not attuned to your instrument and how it's meant to be, you will find yourself in a section of the orchestra where you do not belong and that feels really discordant."

- Nikki Slade

Sound Therapy

Sound therapy uses intonation, sound frequency and vocal expression in order to promote health and create balance. Through the four individuals in this section we get an understanding of how drums can build a feeling of community; how vocal expression can hold the key to freeing our ability to operate authentically and fully; how musical frequency can be used to effect change in the body; and how chanting specific tones can change our resonance. We all have an innate understanding of how much sounds can affect us. We respond in varying and contrasting ways, for example, to heavy loud beats, soft soothing melodies and the sounds of nature all around us. Sound therapy brings a greater awareness to the gifts that our auditory experience can bring us.

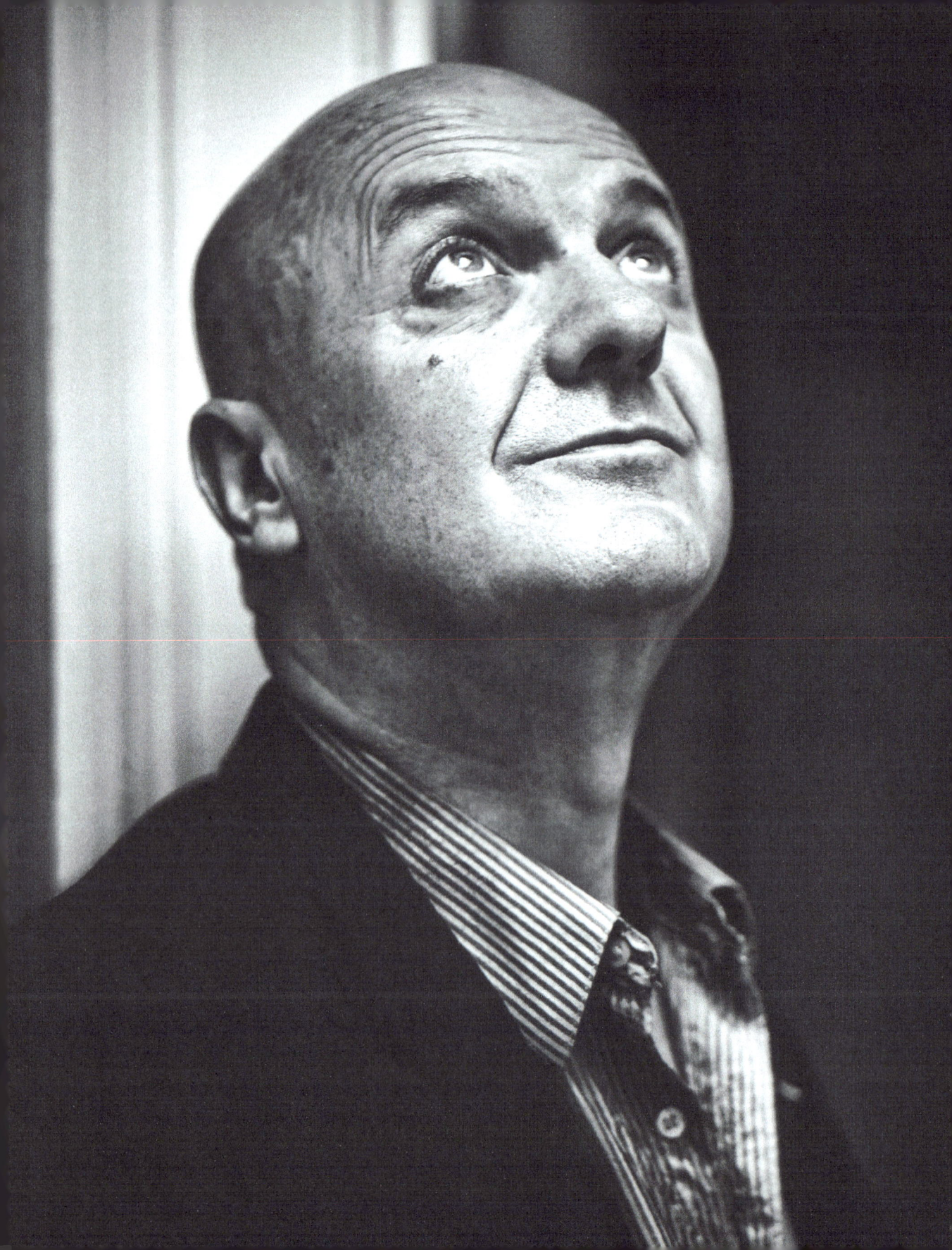

Tim Wheater

Musician, Sound Therapist, Performer and Teacher

Tim Wheater has been an amazing conduit for the intelligence, wisdom and healing that music has to offer humanity. He has co-presented the deeper concepts of sound in arenas with some of the greatest transformational influencers of our time, including the Dalai Lama and Deepak Chopra. He has a huge exuberance when communicating his thoughts on music, and his passion for it, which he conveys with joyful warmth. It was an insightful experience to take a look at the healing elements of sound through his eyes.

Music was a salvation for me in my early teens, once I had discovered it and realised I had an aptitude for it. I started developing ideas on how I wanted to work with music and the parts of it I wanted to explore. I was fifteen when I got started on my musical path and by seventeen I was going to art school and doing a lot by way of musical practice. My passion and enthusiasm ensured that I got a scholarship to study in London.

After graduating, I started working in the pop music business, but I had an inner calling and internal draw to start writing music that was more akin to what I do now. This wellspring of ideas led me to write slower music and, by chance, a few people I knew circulated it. As a result, it got used as therapy in America within psychiatry. I found this interesting and it was very inspiring for me. I then started to think about performing, which at the beginning felt like an odd situation for me. I did my first ever Mind, Body and Spirit Festival in London and within 30 seconds of starting my performance, a very eminent healer called Matthew Manning approached the organiser and asked to work with me. There have been a lot of therapists who have locked on to the music since and found it to be quite useful in their work.

So, from the outset, I did not intentionally set out to create therapeutic music, I was just answering my inner impulse. It was the therapists themselves who recognised its benefits and it began to evolve and expand into that world. It was only after I personally interacted with music on a healing level that I started to get an insight into how powerful it could be in creating positive internal and physical changes in the body.

Experiential Healing With Music

I had an experience a few years down the line where I was poisoned. At the time I looked for my own solace and healing through sound and it worked. This really took the scales off my eyes and enlightened me about music's profound effects. It changed the dynamic of my energy and brought me to a place of balance, and also affected the cellular structure within my body. There are large noticeable physical changes when you open yourself to receive music in this way. As a result of the poisoning, I had developed a condition that paralysed my limbs and I noticed that music caused definitive positive shifts to my paralysis, which gave me an insight into the potency of music sound.

Creating Healing Music

I have created a repertoire of music that has been used successfully by a lot of therapists and has now become a body of work. I am always fascinated to do more and more research on the power of music and I am very enthusiastic about its effects. My awareness of what sound can do continues to become deeper as I work with it. I see music as a sacred divine transmission. We receive it and it affects the water content of the body, heart, soul, mind and emotions. It is very extraordinary when you examine it. It is beyond just art and the Arts.

I feel very lucky and blessed indeed. However, music is mixed up among all the other parts of life going on and, as we all know, life can sometimes create a distraction. I find that when I work I never take the phone or the computer with me so I can immerse myself in the whole journey and exploration of sound. But once I come out of that state and return to normal, there are other things going on.

Using the Instrument of The Voice to Heal

I felt that I had my own method and unique way of singing and toning, which came to me spontaneously and instinctively, and I found that I could share this with others. So aside from developing my own voice, I was interested in encouraging others to develop theirs as well. This is what created the expansion of my work into workshops. The voice is a convenient instrument to access because we carry it with us at all times. I try to make it easy for people to discover their voices. I often will tell an audience that in two minutes I will get them to sing like the most magnificent choir in the world. I start off by getting them to consciously link with their breath and then I bring the voice work in. It is usually quite profound.

I am always very keen to reach as many people as possible, through the awareness and experience of sound and voice. I find this work is especially pertinent in these extraordinary and changing days, when there are enormous shifts going on in the world. Statically they say that we are experiencing the biggest global shift for the last one hundred years. It is both social and economic, so it is obviously huge.

A lot of people ask me where my inspiration comes from. I always think that the world and people offer a tremendous kaleidoscope of energies to observe, witness and to be in harmony or compassion with. We are all in the process of observing a massive evolution of society and human kind. I think there is a lot more to come and there is a necessity for us as a humanity, to find our core centre of peace and harmony. What we are really seeking is unity.

The Future

I am very optimistic about my personal life development. I am very creative and that is why I encourage other people to find their own creativity, because I think it is a beautiful outlet. I obviously love music and I am completely and unashamedly getting more commercial with it at the moment. My aim is to convey to a much broader audience the understanding of the effects of the harmonic content of music on our feeling body. In my experience the younger generation is a lot more switched on. I sometimes work with people who are half my age, so my style is very broad and quite popular.

I am also developing my core work of sound healing much more. I have worked with sound in a big expansive way and I am now honing it down to smaller more malleable ways. For example, I am working a lot with tuning forks, producing very specific frequencies. These align themselves to the mathematical codes in our body and nature, which can aid us in our quest to centre and balance ourselves.

I think music and all the arts is a language that allows people to have a glimpse of their own divinity and sacredness. Even for people who normally would not have access to this way of being, sound can just give them that.

My Inspiration

My inspiration comes from so many places. I think the Dalai Lama is a very beautiful man, he has a unique way of bringing peace to the world. Nature I find to be very stunning, in its display of the creativity we witness and are a part of every day. The human race is also very interesting. It can move us in a compassionate and empathetic sense, when we realise that we all have very similar feelings, emotions and needs. I feel a lot of empathy for the human condition. With that empathy comes an emotional aspect, which can inspire me to deliver more poignancy in my work.

It is a very exciting time to be alive. We are at a time where we are able to express ourselves in ways that are both expansive and enlightening. There is a hunger and thirst within humanity, but also a confusion. We are all slightly bewildered by the challenging events; however, this is a time for many of us to examine our purpose in life and recognise our duty to step up to service and expand our awareness of ourselves and our world. It is a real wake-up period, in which we all need to come together in unity, in order to offer guidance and help to others. It is my hope that I can be an inspiration to those who will be responsible for being catalysts for transformation.

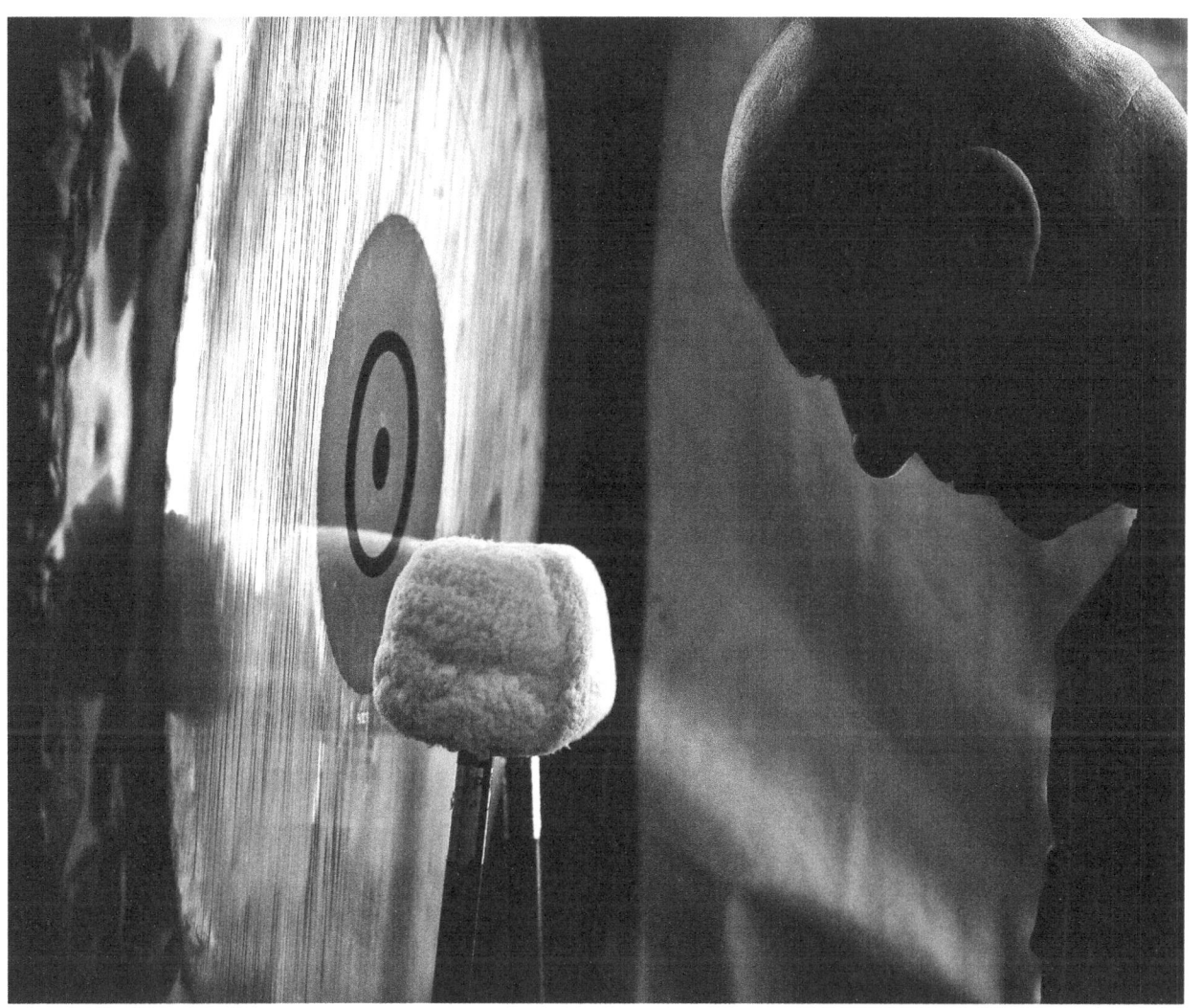

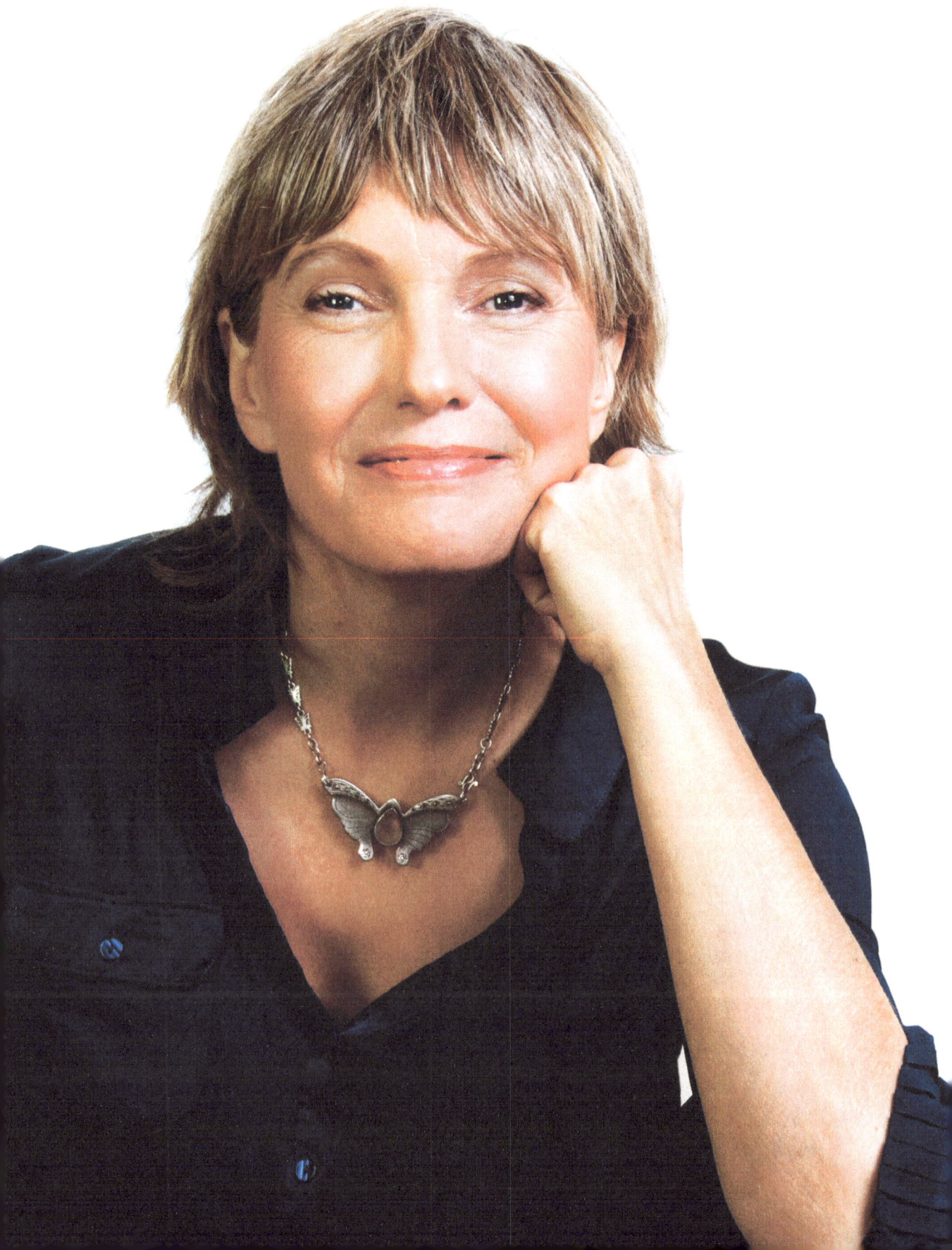

Nikki Slade

Founder of Free The Inner Voice and Chemistry At Work, Teacher, Author, and Facilitator

Nikki Slade is a pioneering facilitator in the field of natural voice. Her work has been recognised in wide arenas ranging from prisons to corporations. She is a renowned Kirtan leader and has released a number of chanting CDs worldwide. Nikki has made a colourful journey from being an actress and singer, playing venues such as the Royal Albert Hall and the Royal National Theatre, to today being a leader in the field of unlocking our potential through the power of primordial chanting, voice and free self expression.

As a child I always loved singing. This is the gift I was born with, but at the time I didn't know what to do with it. My uncle was the late theatre composer Julian Slade who wrote a musical called Salad Days in the 1950s. I loved going to see his plays. Something opened in me when I saw people singing and dancing on the stage, it looked really free. It was the nearest thing I found at that time to the kind of feeling that was inside me.

My friend's mother overheard me singing one day; she was connected to the theatre and brought my talent to the attention of my parents. From that moment on I was actively encouraged. Yet being a traditional performer in front of an audience did not come naturally at first. There was a fear of standing up, being visible and being counted. It was alright doing it in my own little world, but to actually be in front of people engaging with them was an issue.

Later I realised that my life's work was to answer the question: 'How do you be yourself, expressing the full being that is you to the world, and be completely confident whilst doing it?'

The Transition from Theatre to Vocal Work

Traditional theatre fulfilled me to a certain extent and I did quite well. In 1987 I was cast in a Dickensian musical The Mystery of Edwin Drood and I was the understudy to Lulu. There was a Buddhist in that production and Lulu was practicing meditation, yoga and chanting. I was really curious; her energy was so vibrant and I was attracted to it, so I made enquiries.

It was from that point on that I began to explore the natural voice. As I delved, I got less interested in becoming someone else and more interested in becoming myself. Having been to a lot of ashrams in the past, where chanting was included, I wanted to create my own thing. I braved my first workshop in 1990, in a healing centre opposite Brixton Prison. This had resonances for me because there we were freeing our inner voice, yet faced with this prison. Many years later I took the work into Wandsworth Men's Prison.

Working with Creative Sound

People come to me for all sorts of reasons: to overcome issues of confidence, to tap into their creativity, to be in a bath of sound with others, or just to have fun. The work developed into a therapeutic side, without me being labelled a therapist. If anything I am a creative sound artist. The labels, as you know, don't really mean anything, it is the personal experience that is important.

In terms of experience people report that they have breakthroughs in their relationships with their colleagues, partners and friends. They also open themselves to things like public speaking and giving presentations. Through the voice we work on the fabric underneath the words, which is where my expertise lies, we work with the vibration that permeates everything that we do and say.

I am passionate about creating a space where people can attune to the melody that is really them. They can then begin to see how they would like to play in the world, what they want to express and who they want to attract. This is where it becomes really delightful.

A Journey from Inner Expansion to Outer Expression

There was a time when I searched for myself in all the 'wrong places', although ultimately nothing is ever really 'wrong'. I used the path of addiction between the ages of 14 to 27 and crashed quite badly with that. My awakening came between ages 27 to 31, which is that classical Saturn return phase. I had both an emergence and an emergency, with everything coming up that had not been dealt with. In fact, I spent four weeks of my life in 1989 on a psychiatric wing; they did not know where else to put me, I was going through different states of consciousness. However, ultimately I had a lot of understandings at that time.

As a result of my experience, for the last 20 years I have been the resident voice facilitator of the Priory Hospital on the addiction treatment wing. I go there every

Wednesday and share this work with recovering addicts. I am who I am because of all of that. I have no shame or defensiveness in saying where I have come from, because there is a totality about it today that is very rich.

What I tell people at the Priory every week is that my journey past addiction has just been one day at a time for 22 years. We are all asking questions like, 'What is the meaning of life? Where is bliss?' It is just that we sought the answer in all the wrong places. But how can it really be wrong if it has brought you onto your spiritual path?

All music is perfect, I very much believe in the orchestra of life. We are all instruments and everyone has their perfect part to play. If you are not attuned to your instrument and how it's meant to be, you will find yourself in a section of the orchestra where you do not belong and that feels really discordant.

The work I offer to people is for them to hear where they have to be and through the power of attraction they bring in the other ensemble players. We attract where we are, our feeling is the point of attraction.

My Love for My Work

I love to see people go out there and embrace what they've got. So in short I am here to empower people quickly, so they can use what they've got and go out there and make a difference. There are times when I feel something close to what Michelangelo may have felt. Amazing potential walks into the room with each person and the voice that they have. As I listen my ear becomes a chisel that taps away to find the treasure.

One area that has been amazing for me is the developments I have made in the corporate world. My work within corporate businesses has been a huge part of my life for the last 10 years. It is exciting because I get to play a part in helping people to make a shift towards more heart-based business. Anything I can do in that arena I am really inspired by. Once you have had an experience with sound, it is very hard to stay in your head. If someone has really looked into the eye of their colleague, they can't go back to monosyllabic passing each other at the water cooler.

With M&C Saatchi for example, I was working with one of their creative directors privately and he was inspired enough to give me the opportunity to work with his team. He took a big leap of faith putting me in front of 20 account holders and they all absolutely loved it.

Alchemically when people are in their own true note and they are in accord inside, they get on better, they feel happier and brighter, their energy is fuller and their productivity is greater. The work is completely experiential and unique to each individual. This is why I love it.

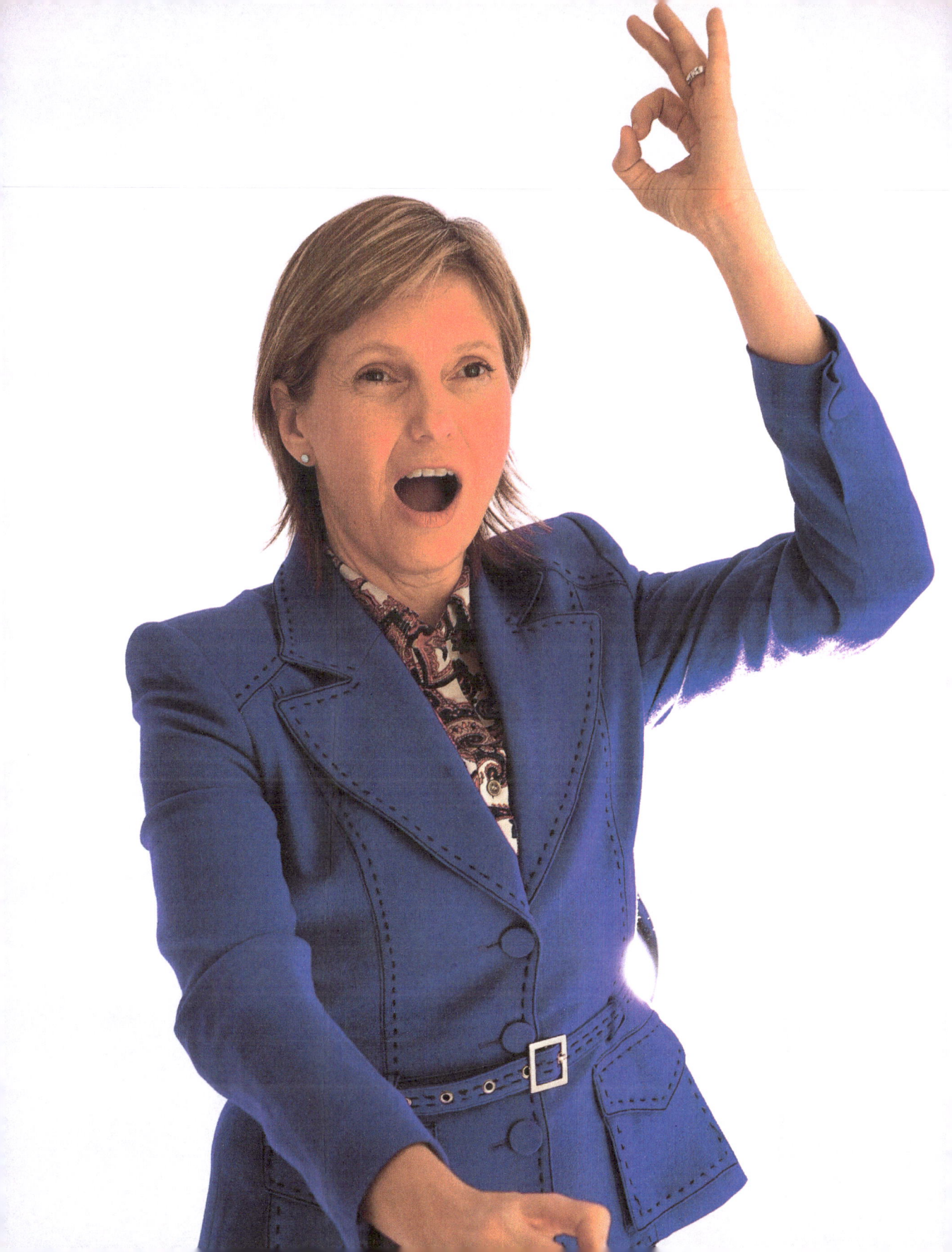

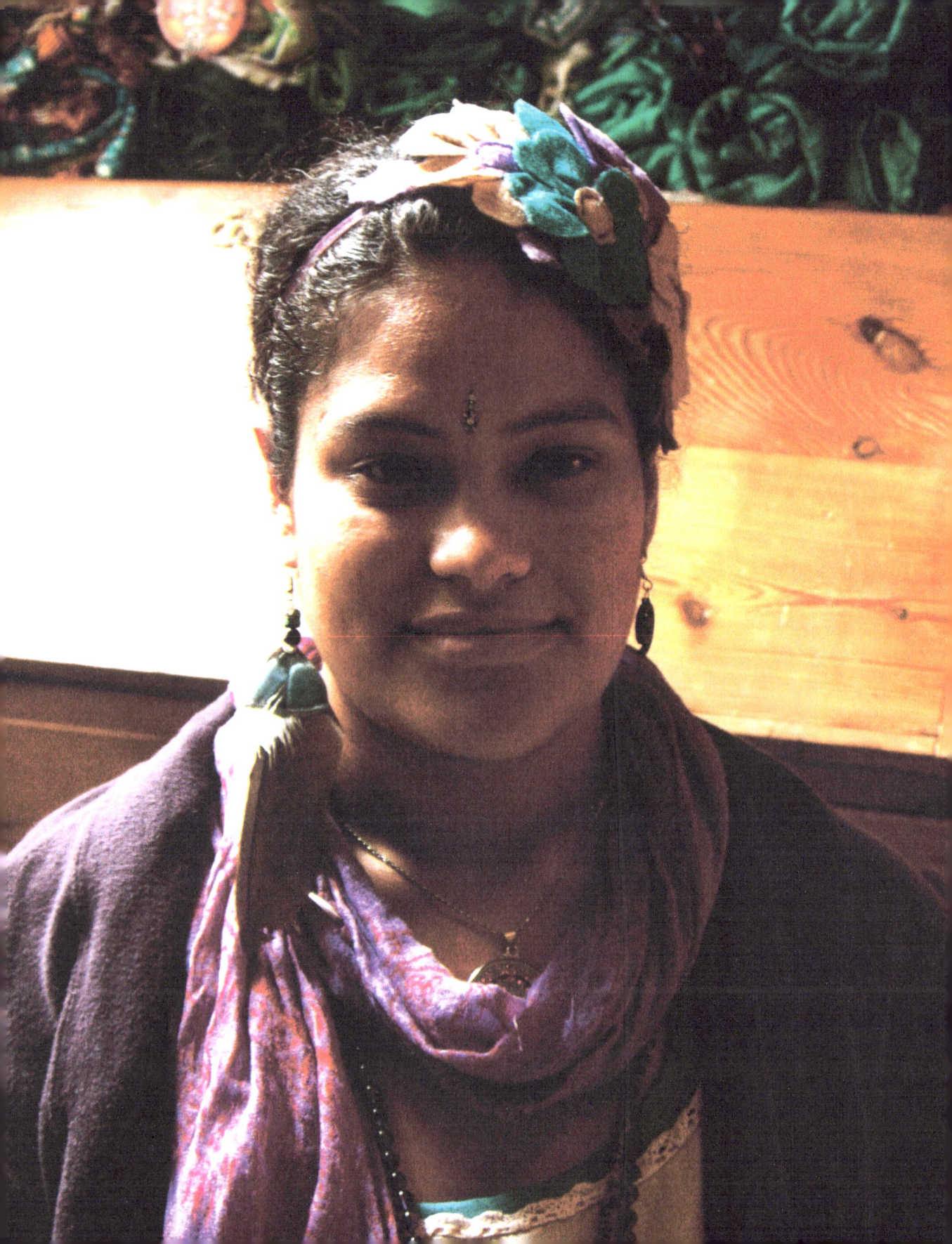

Naomi Francis
Kirtan Facilitator and Shakti Dance Yoga Teacher

Naomi Francis, AKA HariPyari, acquired her pseudonym while travelling in India. She is a colourful and creatively expressive character with a feather in her ear and a beautiful array of hues and textures in her wear. But you get the sense that behind the youthful playfulness lies an immensely deep thinker. Although she is opened to exploration and learning, there is a respect for Kirtan, which has seen her immersing herself and honing her understanding. Yet it is clear that even with an intellectual and academic knowledge of her subject, what matters most to HariPyari is that she connects to her practice through her heart and through her love. It was a joy to get her take on the powerful art of Kirtan.

People always ask me how I came to Kirtan, but I do not have a clear recollection of when this happened. I was into yoga from childhood, because my mother used to do it. However, when I was around ten years old she developed more of an interest in Tai Chi, while I still maintained my love of yoga. This was when I got initiated into developing a yoga practice for myself independently; the whole process happened quite organically.

I went to boarding school and at the gym there were yoga classes, which I attended. Once I left school I began working at the Special Yoga Centre and my practice blossomed from there since I was able to go to as many classes as I could. I worked on reception and every Wednesday there was a Kirtan session in the room just opposite. It was the last class that I had to sign people into, so I used to sneak in a quarter of the way through. I loved the experience of Kirtan and this was where my practice began to expand.

Kirtan

Kirtan is the joyful chanting of mantras which express devotion and love. The mantras are sung in Sanskrit, which is the language of Hinduism, and is a powerful way to activate the energetic body. Each of the mantras contain a sound formula and through the act of singing we ourselves become the instruments for the sound.

It impacts people on a very personal and individualistic level and its meaning is linked to the feelings and emotions it inspires.

The Sanskrit letters all directly relate to the seven chakras or energy centres within the body. The chakras are usually symbolised by various numbers of lotus petals, so for example the base chakra has four lotus petals, while the throat chakra has sixteen. Each petal represents a letter in Sanskrit and there are the same number of lotus petals as there are Sanskrit letters. Each Sanskrit word that makes up a mantra is a combination of those letters, which once blended together produce very specific sounds. These sounds activate the energy contained within the chakra. So by chanting the sounds you tap into the energy of the chakras that they correspond to. Through Kirtan, we are given the opportunity to play and tune our energetic system.

Working with Mantra

There are a lot of layers to working with mantra. If we come from the understanding that we are using the mantra to turn ourselves into a musical instrument, then pronunciation is really very important. The way I was taught by my teacher was to place a high level of focus on pronouncing the mantra well, but also making it clear when teaching others that it does not matter as much how you pronounce the mantra as long as you are doing it from the heart with a pureness of spirit and devotion.

When it comes to Kirtan, it is the love with which you do your practice that is really important. There are so many elements to the process, it would be quite easy to reduce it to a purely academic viewpoint. But the reality is that when we are practising Kirtan, chanting it from a space of love is really the ultimate key. During the session we don't even get into the fact that we are playing notes through the sounds we make. It is more about opening ourselves to the energy of the heart. When we connect to our heart, we are making a connection to the guru and the light within ourselves. To open our voice from this space of love is the most important thing that this practice teaches us.

My Experience of Kirtan

Through Kirtan, I have had the most amazing meditative experiences as it has opened up a sacred space within me. Once I discovered its potential I fell in love with it and went to every form of Kirtan practice imaginable. With some of these sessions there was such an embodiment of the practice, they generated powerful feelings of bliss and a deep sense of love. But it is not a kind of love that requires anything in return, instead it is an experience of oneness and unity with all things.

As a facilitator of Kirtan, I lead the session and hold the space so that the environment is in tune with the practice. But each person who attends is an important part of the process, so there can be no ego involved. I love the idea of tapping into the guru within. For some people the focus is placed on unearthing an external guru, but for me it is on finding the internal guru, and this is what the Kirtan is about. Tapping into the light within and letting ourselves shine and flow this light freely.

Kirtan in the Real World

We all have the propensity to make judgements on ourselves and others. Everything that you think you take on, so every judgement that you make has to come through you first. Impurities are in the mind predominantly, before they manifest physically. I have personal stresses in my day-to-day life. I have had people I love, leave me through death and there have been challenges to be dealt with. At times, all of these things express very obviously and very painfully in life. But the more I do this work, the better I am able to deal with the difficulties that may arise.

Your perception of things is what you project into the world. You see things in a certain way because of your thoughts and your experiences, but if you look at them with a different mindset they look completely different. In the practice that I do, it is about looking through the heart rather than the mind. When you do this, you are then able to see with eyes of love and beauty. When I was younger I had so many judgements about people, but more and more I have realised that although we are at different stages of our path we all have the divine light within us. This makes every person glorious if we are willing to see that, it is such a joy when we are.

Being a Teacher

I love to learn and I think that this is a key element about being a teacher, you need to be the ultimate student. You are constantly learning about others while you teach, which creates a circle. Teaching has allowed me to go deeper into my practice. As you go deeper into something you unravel more layers of it. With Kirtan the depth of the practice has made it more and more profound for me energetically. When we are new to something we are normally a bit tentative, dipping our toe into the water. Whereas the more we do it, the more we can swim with ease, which allows for the practice to do its work without resistance getting in the way.

Large cities like London often contain big concentrated areas where people are spiritually unconscious and unaware. Having a practice of Kirtan is even more profound in a place like this. There is a quote by the Dalai Lama that says: 'You can't achieve world peace without first achieving peace within yourself'. When we take the time to work on ourselves, we have a positive effect on the world around us. The more people we come into contact with the more sparks that we give off. By finding the peace within ourselves we inspire others to do the same. We have so many types of energy exchanges within our lives and once we develop an awareness of this, we begin to realise how important it is to be steeped in our own practice. When we are at one with ourselves we have a definite idea of the energy that belongs to us and the energy we choose to take on.

As a teacher I have always observed people at the start of a session, where they may have come in tired or with the weighty energy of their day. At the end of the session, when they leave, they always look beautiful and radiant. This is what makes what I do so great. It returns people to their guru essence.

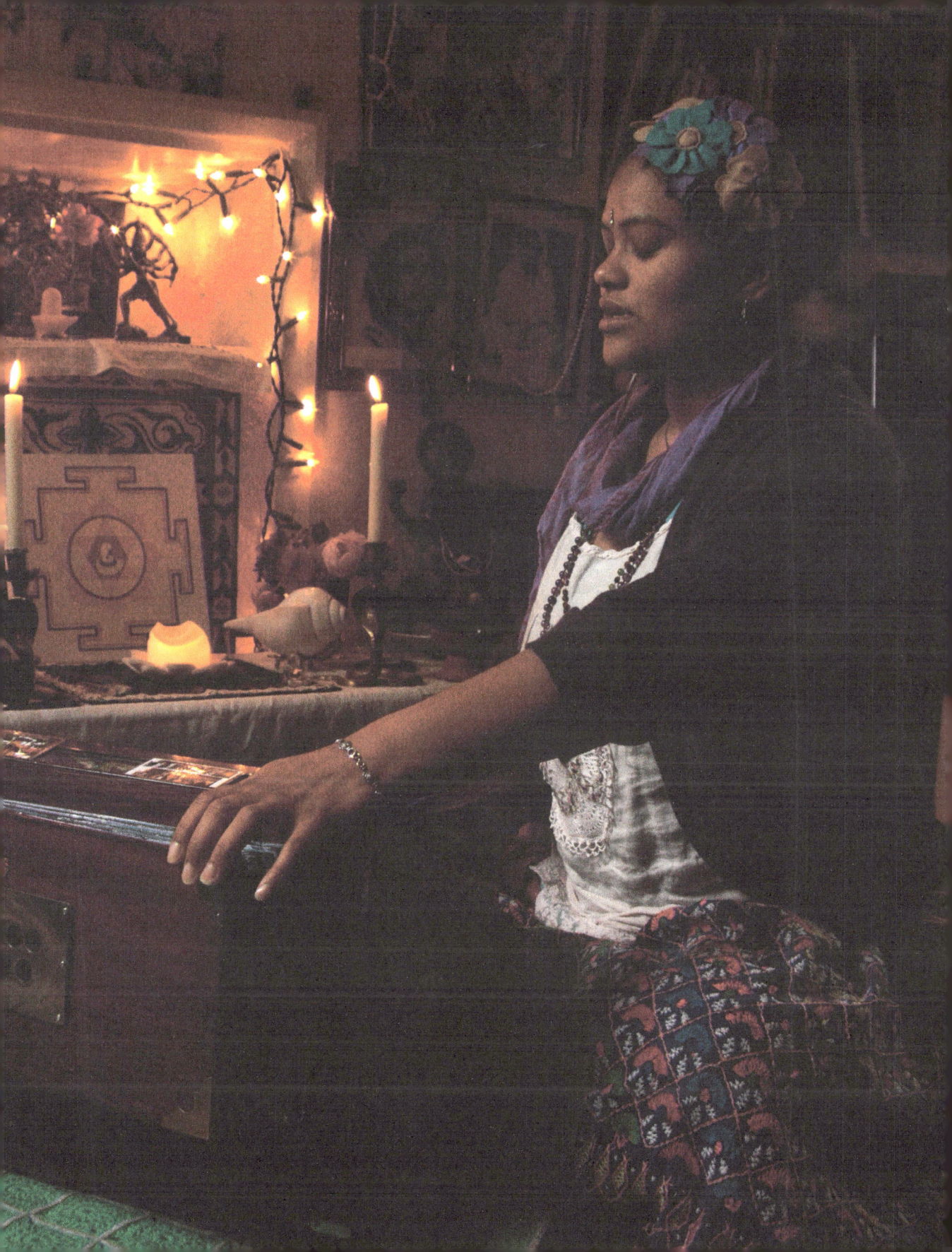

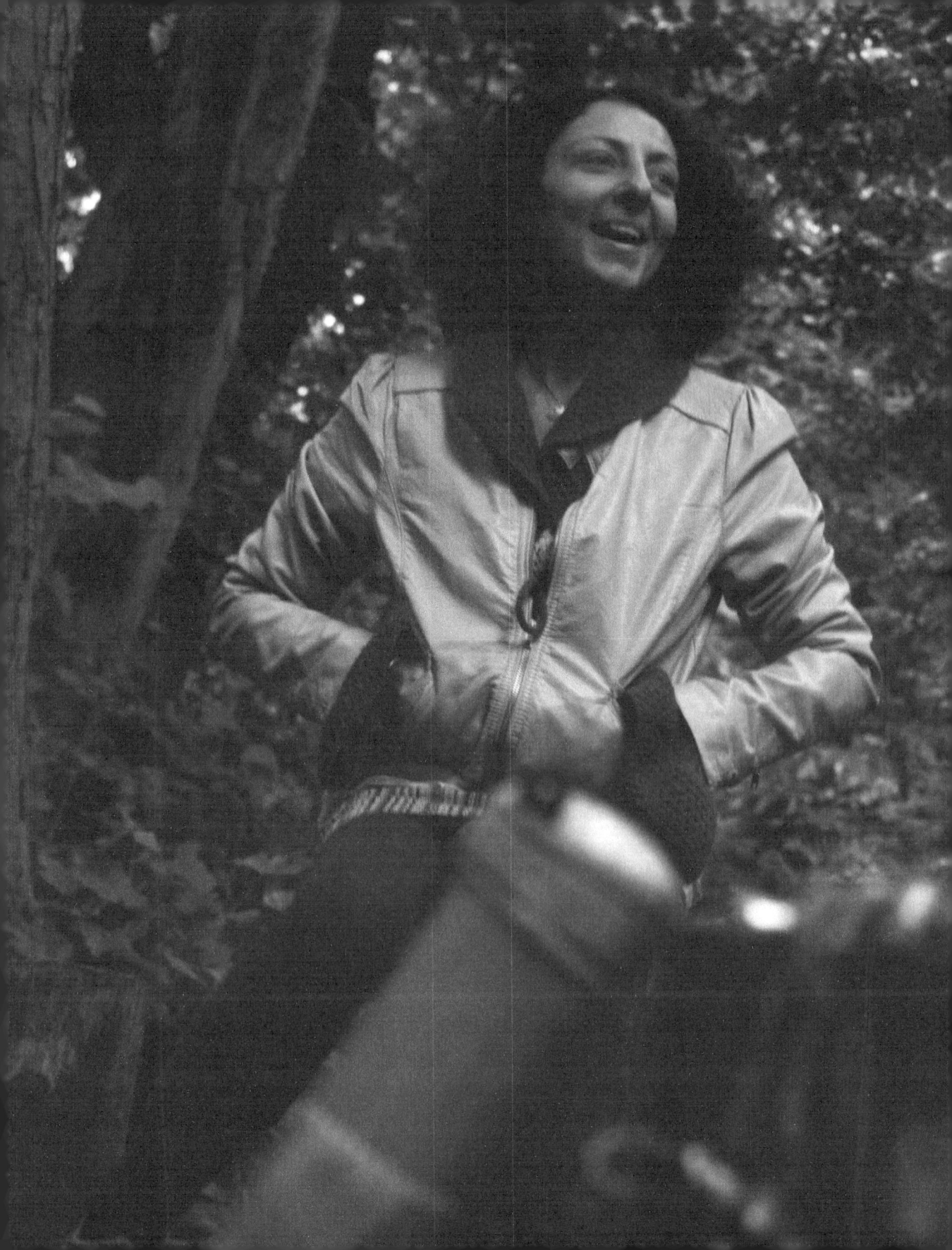

Laura Valenti
Director of Harmonic Inspiration

For Laura Valenti, the timeline between being an Italian Lawyer and a Sound Therapist residing in London has been filled in with colourful flair and a mountain of discoveries and realisations. Through her, one is given a view of how infinitely changing life can be and the beauty that can be created through surrendering to one's heart and one's path. It was a treat to speak to her about Sound Therapy and her love of the drums.

In Italy I studied law, specialising in Sociology of Migrations. I was interested in the aspect of law that dealt with human rights and, specifically, in the protection of women. This covered areas, such as human trafficking, smuggling and domestic violence. As a child, I always had a strong sense of justice. I remember watching certain incidences on the news and crying if there was suffering involved. I guess there was also a lot of interest coming from my family as well. My dad studied law and my family is very academic, so it was interwoven into my background. I did not feel that I really dared to open my imagination at that point in life.

While I was studying law, I started to read about and investigate the theatre. At that time there was one book that influenced me greatly, called Meetings With Remarkable Men by Gurdjief. He was quite an interesting character who spent a lot of time travelling in Asia. He spoke a number of languages and brought lots of information about Asian culture to the West. His books spoke about exercises that he would do with his students, many of which came from the theatre. So my interest in the theatre was sparked by a craving to know about life. At the time I was still in my 20's and in a place where I was searching. I found in Gurdjief someone who had travelled all over the world. He was a pioneer who used his practices from the theatre to help people to be present, to expand their consciousness, and to be more mindful, open and curious. It was all the things that I wanted to be.

Opening People up to their Expression

The road of expression has a very powerful path to it. Especially as it relies very strongly on the individual being willing to be animated by their expression. It does not have to be very complex to be profound though. For example, from time to time I work with a charity that looks after adults with learning difficulties. One week I led a class and brought in drums as our instrument and we did some very simple movements and voice work. Then something incredible happened. For thirty seconds they managed to be in complete silence. I have never seen that in a whole year of being there. It seemed like the sound allowed them to empty themselves of something, which created a space to support the expression of silence.

Sound Therapy in Social Healing

I have worked with the drug and alcohol rehabilitation of battered women, some of who are involved in domestic violence and trafficking. But this I have done with sound, where as previously I did it with law.

I think it is possible to use sound to experience pleasure and a sense of feeling good within the body. If there has been abuse that has left a person emotionally very vulnerable, their sense of self-esteem is normally low, which in turn inhibits their ability to have pleasurable sensations through the body, or feel good about the body. If sound creates a positive physical vibration and the person is conscious of this – even if it is only for 30 seconds – a new map can be created. This opens up the possibility for the person to feel good again. It becomes something to build on.

I am not interested in giving solutions to people, I prefer to work in a space where there are questions that will allow a person to find what works best for them. Some of the feedback I get immediately after a session expresses that people feel free and equal within the circle. They do not feel judged and the space around them offers a playground to them.

The inner map that we all have is so rich, deep and changeable. The more alive we are internally, the more information comes to us. Sometimes this comes with a strength that is difficult to ignore. Awareness brings an understanding of what the sensations within the body are telling you. For example, it may be that you need to hold yourself a bit more gently or to take more care of certain areas in your daily life.

My Journey to Sound Therapy

I was practicing law in Italy, but it became evident after a while that I could not do that within a contained office for the rest of my life. Then an opportunity of a grant from the European Community to go to Budapest arose. So I joined an NGO in Hungary that was working with women. From there I travelled to Denmark to visit a theatre company and was told about LISPA (London International School of Performing Arts), which spurred me to come to London to study. LISPA is an amazing place because it expands our awareness of our journey as human beings. It focuses on opening the body, being fully in the body and working with neutral masks.

Working with masks is very shamanic and archetypal. One of the biggest lessons I learnt is that the mask we wear changes with our journey. The question is, how do we stay opened when everything is off balance? How do we allow ourselves to be off balance, embrace all that is and then move forward? I learned that there is a necessity to be in the present moment, to be opened even when it hurts. These are such wonderful teachings.

My Journey Through Cancer

At the end of the first year at LISPA, I could not continue because I discovered that I had cancer. This led to the start of a whole new journey. I began studying and researching al-ternative and complementary health. I completely changed my diet, danced a lot through my chemo, cycled through snow in London, went to the Lake District and walked twelve hours in a storm. I kept challenging myself in ways that I found fun. I took cancer as a part of my life's adventure. I was in a lot of pain, but I tried to have fun through my experience. I enjoyed having no hair, I wore broad hats and big earrings. At times I loved being provocative and showing up to places completely bald. Many people thought I was a monk because, through it all, I still looked healthy.

I made a commitment to myself and my health. I had a very long break from my family be-cause there were many things that needed to be healed and I needed a strong break. I de-toxed, went for enemas and colonic irrigation, and just kept things simple food wise. Through it all, I had a lot of support around me. This experience really brought out the question of how we are with each other and how we can support each other with kindness in a healthy way, so that it does not become dysfunctional. To be healed from cancer, I had to create health in so many different areas of my life.

My Work

I would like to learn more about living in communities in a sustainable way, how to create them and how to work with them. I will also be developing my work within adult learning difficulties because I really love this area. I have fun and so do they, and I am paid for it. Some people with learning difficulties live in a bubble, others have more awareness and are conscious about being a victim of stigmas. They crave things like having a job, a family and going on holiday. Playing the drums makes them feel like they are playing music. The beauty of the drums is that there is no need for lessons and they can keep a very simple beat. With this work, I give something and then the person receives it and they give something back. In this way it is constantly multiplying and I find that very nourishing. Every time I do it, I feel better within myself, so I do it with pleasure.

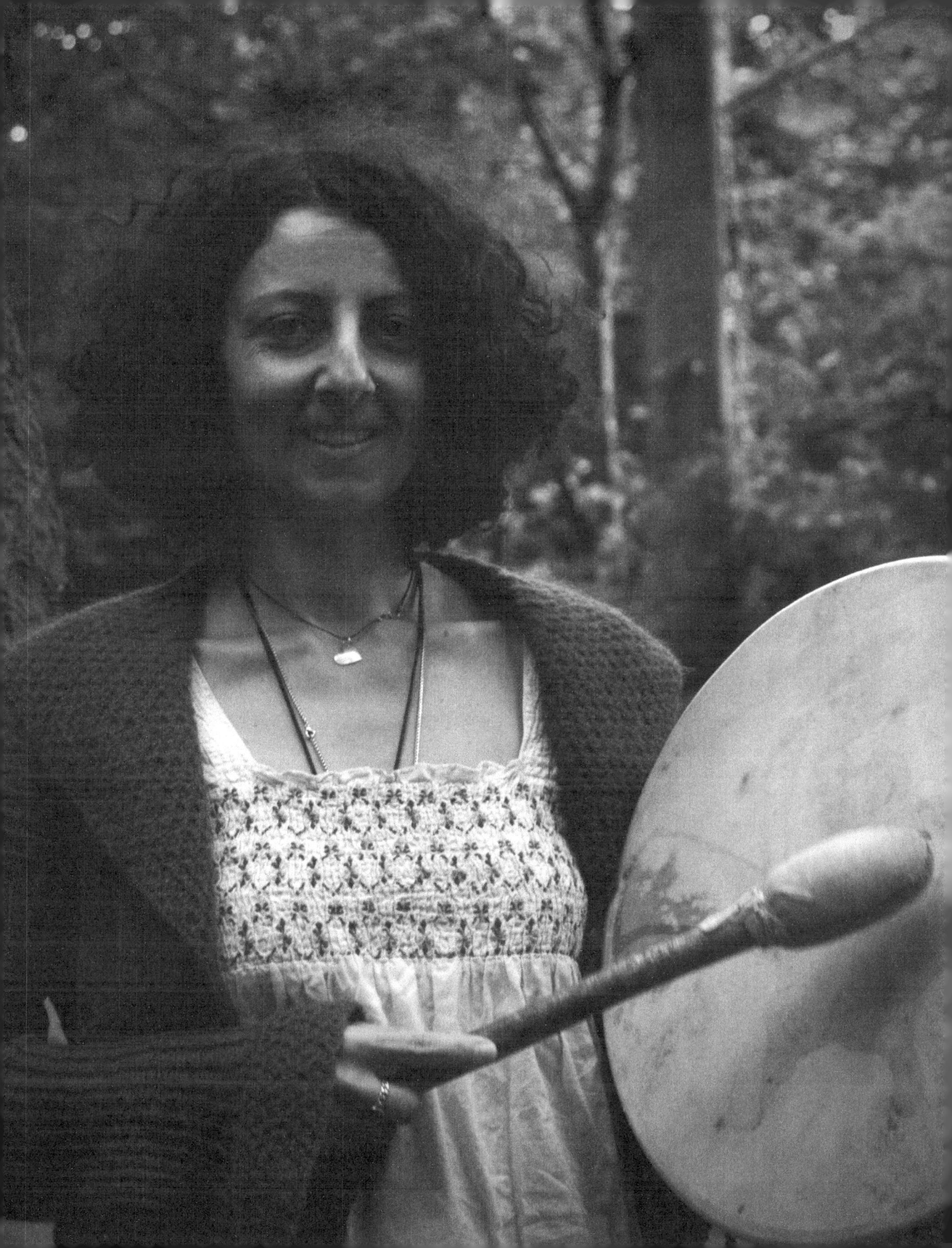

"During my session with a client I try to bring ultimate relaxation, not just on the surface but deep down to the kidney level, which is the deepest organ in the body energetically. This kind of relaxation makes a huge difference, they can respond to chal-lenging situations in their life far more easily."

- Sinsook Park

Acupuncture

Acupuncture is a component of Traditional Chinese Medicine. It focuses on harmonising the balance of energy within the body by working on a series of channels or meridian lines that run in various directions along the body's surface. Along each of these meridian lines are a number of points directly connected to our organs, blood circulation, emotional system and specific physical areas. The Acupuncturist develops a sensitivity for checking the blood flow through the pulse and also checking these meridian points for either excessive or sluggish flow. By working with specific points, it is possible to reduce stress, increase circulation and alleviate ailments in the areas they represent.

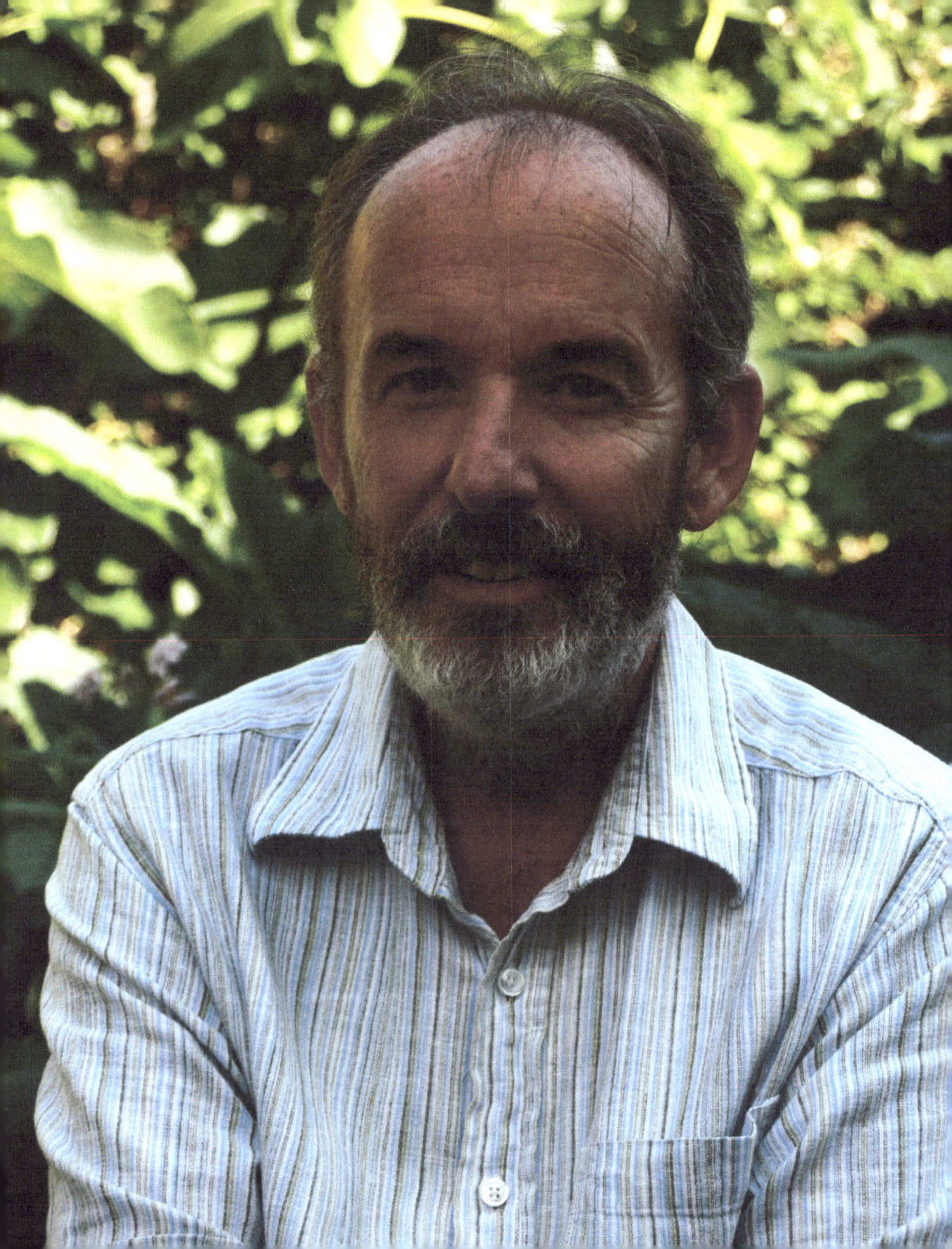

Merlin Young

Founder of Moxafrica, Acupuncturist and Author

Merlin Young is one of the mavericks of his field. As co-founder of the project Moxafrica, he has had to communicate succinctly with the medical and scientific world in order to bring their awareness to his cause. Yet on the other end of the spectrum he is well versed with the intangible, subtle and yet deeply powerful world of Chi or the energetic life force that permeates everything. The two languages are very different yet he has gained a fluency in both. In our conversation he highlights how a simple mugwort weed may be key to enhancing the lives of millions.

Before I came to acupuncture I was working within construction and got sick with autoimmune disease. I tried a number of different health modalities in an attempt to get better, but nothing seemed to work. When I decided to have acupuncture I was totally sceptical and my expectations were low. However, I found the treatment to be very profound. It did not miraculously cure me, yet its positive effects could not be denied. After my session I experienced the world with a clarity not felt for fifteen years. There was no doubt that my acupuncturist was a very gifted healer.

Acupuncture had created such a shift in my own life that I began thinking about becoming an acupuncturist myself. I was excited by the opportunity of facilitating the same experience within others. The next time I saw my acupuncturist I asked for her advice and she said she always felt I would make a great acupuncturist. She became an enormous advocate and support system for me, I would not have completed the training without her help.

When I was much younger I dreamt of studying the Chinese language and acupuncture gave me an opportunity to do this in a lot of ways. But it was a very different world to the career I had in construction and it took me some time to redefine myself as an acupuncturist. Sometimes it seems that things happen exactly when they are meant to. By the time I came to acupuncture, I was at a stage of my life where I had a few knocks and I understood what it was like to suffer from a chronic problem; this gave me a much better perspective on being a practitioner than I would have had previously.

Acupuncture

Traditional acupuncture is based on theories that go back around two thousand years. In essence, the theory of acupuncture is about regulating Chi or the energetic life force within the body. The acupuncture I do is with silver needles and often I do not insert through the skin. This means that there are no cellular or nerve responses to the physical intrusion, allowing me to work solely with the Chi. In the old Chinese acupuncture texts they talk about the nine needles, only one of which could be described as an acupuncture needle. At the time that the books were written, it would have been extremely difficult to make thin wire, so acupuncture needles as we know them today, would have been very expensive and probably only the resort of the elite. Most of the acupuncture that was done traditionally would have made use of the other eight needles, some of which could only be used on the skin surface. The field of acupuncture has largely ignored this.

The first time I came across this technique within acupuncture was in Holland in 2001. There were four teachers that came over from Japan, three of them were blind and the fourth was visually impaired. One of them was the most gifted acupuncturist I had ever seen. I remember him saying that when you are looking for an acupuncture point, imagine that you have a piece of tissue between your finger and the skin and you do not want to move the tissue. He said that you must allow the Chi to invite you in. Most people have preconceived ideas of what acupuncture is, so this method of performing a treatment would be viewed as being very different. There are times during a session where you get a sense that you are meeting the Chi well above the skin and therefore this is where the acupuncture takes place. If as an acupuncturist your focus is on regulating the Chi, then understanding and developing this technique is invaluable.

Acupuncture and Science

One of the things that makes my expression as an acupuncturist a bit different, is that I am committed to the project Moxafrica. The project requires that we investigate moxibustion and its ability to create an immune response in TB patients, which demands that I now operate in two completely different ways. If you can imagine a continuous line, at one end you have traditional acupuncture and the other end you have biomedicine. If you live at the biomedicine end, you will only do evidence-based acupuncture. This will limit your treatment to maybe five main areas - back issues, knee issues, migraines, nausea and dental pain - and we have good research in these areas. For real science fundamentalists, those are their only areas in which acupuncture should be used. On the other end of the scale are the people who deal with Chi and are more creatively flexible treating a variety of complaints, which is how acupuncture was used in the past. Most acupuncturists live somewhere in the middle of that line. I, on the other hand, operate at one end of the field with one hat on, regulating Chi and being creative in my treatment methods, but I am also in the medical-based field on the other end, getting sound research and talking only in the scientific language of immune systems. It is definitely a curious place to find myself.

Being in a position of working in two quite separate arenas has brought the understanding that as complementary therapists we should never be complacent. We need to have the confidence to be critical of ourselves, because that is the only way we become better at what we do. If you were to put a group of scientists together to discuss a topic not everyone is going to agree. There may in fact be major fallouts, but it is through the questioning and probing that growth is achieved. As complementary therapists this is something that we need to emulate in order to expand the field.

Tuberculosis (TB)

The project Moxafrica works to get sound research on the effects of Moxa treatments on TB, particularly drug resistant TB. TB is caused by an airborne bacteria and is generally infectious. In most healthy people, their immune system will be strong enough so that their body's natural defences will contain the bacteria and stop it becoming an active disease. However, if the immune system is compromised in any way then the bacteria will grow, leading to active infection and the symptoms of this will develop sometimes years later. 95% of people who die of TB today, live well below the poverty line.

When you start exploring it, you realise that there is more TB in Africa than there is in anywhere else in the world: 640 million people in the Sub-Sahara are latently infected with TB and in at least 10% this will develop into an active disease, added to which you have the HIV component. The two diseases together are the most appalling, destructive combination. Almost 80% of Africans who have HIV die of TB so it is ultimately the killer disease.

Moxafrica

A friend and colleague, Jenny Craig, was the one who introduced me to the idea of acupuncture in Africa. We were doing an advanced two-year training course in acupuncture, which we attended three times a year for long weekends. Jenny grew up in Zambia and Malawi and after the very first weekend of the training we were sitting outside a pub having a drink. She asked me to get involved with putting a project together using acupuncture in Africa. All I could see was the issue with needles in a situation like that and the fact that training and ongoing support would be a real challenge, and assumed it could not be done.

On the very last weekend of the course the subject came up again. I had a light bulb flashing moment and thought, 'Moxa!' This is one of the components within the acupuncture tool kit. It would be a simple treatment to implement, safely applied to the skin by burning a cone made from the mugwort weed and there are no needles involved. I remembered that Moxa was successfully used in the 1930s to treat TB in Japan and this could be replicated in Africa. We only realised the scale of the issue when we began our research. It took us 20 months to get the project running and we have deliberately gone down the route of focusing on research. We are aiming to provide sustainable treatment for millions of people, but we cannot do that without first proving that it works.

We should be publishing our findings by the end of 2014. The day-to-day research itself has been entrusted to a professor, a doctor, a TB sister, a TB nurse and a data manager, in Kampala, Uganda, and I could not ask for a better team. I go over every four months to ensure that everything is on track and going to plan. So much now hangs on this investigation, millions of lives can potentially be changed for the better, which is a humbling thought. In the greater scheme of things I think that TB is trying to teach us about our wider humanity. It is trying to teach us to look after each other, the poor just as much as the rich. Simple Moxa treatment and the humble mugwort weed could possibly go a long way to aid this process.

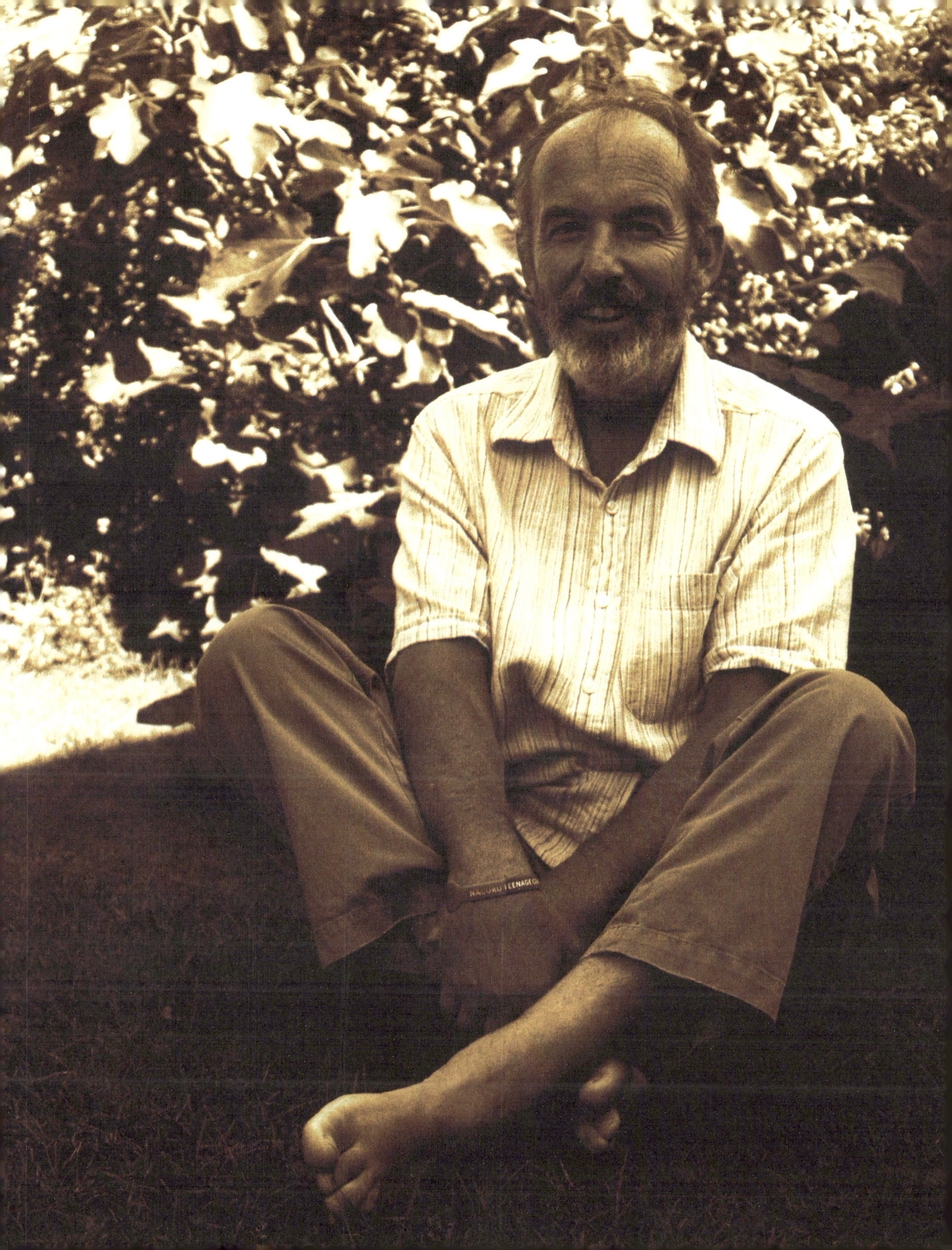

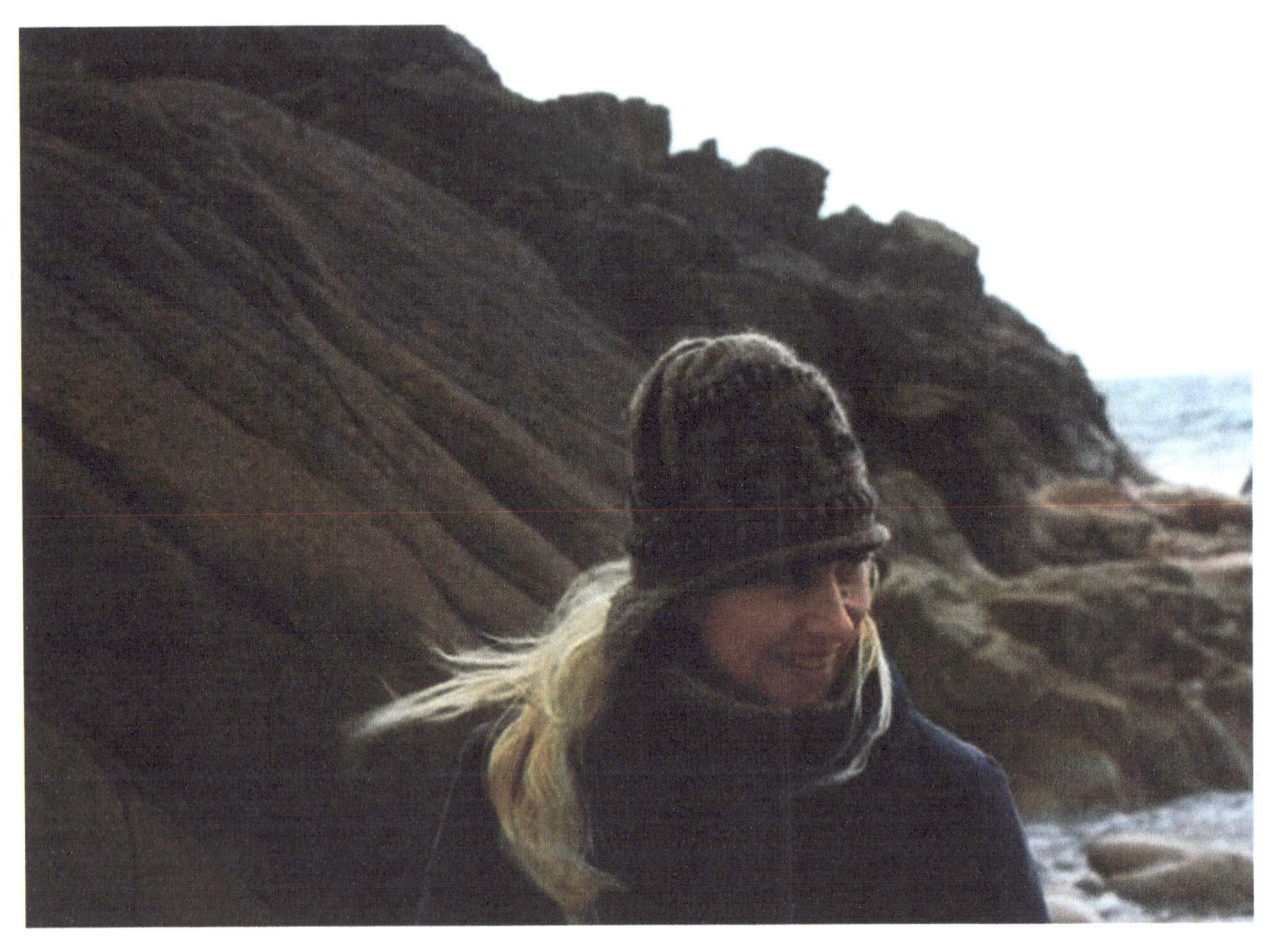

Sarah Prichard

Founder of Healing Path, Practitioner, Author and Teacher

Sarah Prichard has made the journey from acting and the arts to Chinese Medicine and acupuncture. Throughout our conversation I got the sense that her path has been very much about following her heart-based instincts and finding ways to use her creative expression to its fullest potential. In order to satisfy her inner artist completely, she writes and sings professionally as well as being both a teacher and practitioner of all aspects of Chinese Medicine. Expressive outlets both professionally and creatively feed, inform and add colour to who Sarah is, and the contributions that she makes through her work.

I trained for three years at The Royal Academy of Dramatic Arts and the course included modules in meditation, Tai Chi and Chi Gong. As I began to integrate these modalities into my life, I became very interested in how the performing arts and the healing arts interrelate. During my early years in performance, I lost my voice on a number of occasions. Eventually a friend of mine, who was also an actress, said I should go to see the 'pin lady'. This was my first encounter with acupuncture and the very first question asked by the acupuncturist was, 'What is it that you are not saying?' This question, combined with the treatment, was a profound trigger for me and a huge catalyst for change.

My fascination grew from there and I got fully immersed in the philosophy of traditional, classical Chinese medicine, which is based in Taoism. I found a book by the author Giovanni Maciocia, called The Foundations of Chinese Medicine, which was the primary learning manual that they were using in the acupuncture colleges at the time. I had no idea that this was the case when I bought it. I just thought it looked substantial and interesting and I felt that it would give me a well-rounded understanding of what acupuncture was about. Once I began reading about acupuncture, there was a familiarity about it and it just made complete sense. The language of Chinese medicine, particularly the classics, is very poetic. It is science and art at its best.

During this period, I was still working in performance but at the same time pursuing my interest in Chinese medicine. While the love of theatre, plays and acting was very strong in me, I did not really have the personality that enjoyed the aspects of networking, self-promotion and public relations that being an actress entails. So it became clear that I had to find a different form of work.

Becoming an Acupuncturist

I knew acupuncture was going to be my path forward. So the next decision I had to make was on which avenue was going to be the best choice to pursue it with studies. I had already studied for three years at drama school and I was not sure how I was going to pay for another big course. Then I came across the London School of Yoga and Shiatsu Studies, which had loads of Chinese Medicine courses at the time. I enrolled to do Tuina Chinese Massage. One of my main teachers was Robert Cran, a herbalist, acupuncturist, Tuina practitioner, Shiatsu practitioner and an exceptional guide for others. He was a Glaswegian whose knowledge of the theory of Chinese Medicine was brilliant; he worked us quite hard, physically and mentally, throughout our course.

After qualifying in Tuina, I went to Nanjing in China and studied at the University of Chinese Medicine. I was there for six weeks, working in their hospital. Then I spent another twelve months doing clinical studies in what used to be The London College of Traditional Acupuncture and Oriental Medicine. I also studied in Beijing to give me a different perspective because, while the Nanjing-style of treatment is more graceful and flowing, the Beijing-style is tougher, harder, faster and stronger.

Defining Acupuncture

Acupuncture works with energy channels within the body and the spirit or essence of each acupuncture point. Every point has a name and each name was specifically chosen to denote a particular meaning. For example, the names given to energy points include spirit door, bubbling spring and a hundred meetings. They describe what the point is meant to do and how energy operates when the point is stimulated. We use the nature of the point to work alongside the individual's constitution in order to harmonise the energy within the body.

When people think of acupuncture they think of the classical channels on the body's map, which are primary meridians. But there is a huge network of additional channels, which can be used to take pathology from the body's interior to its exterior to be released. The body is clever; it always moves negative energies outwards and away from the internal organs.

When applying acupuncture I work with different patients in varying ways. Once I feel the person's pulse, this will direct me on what the treatment is to be. So the work then becomes more instinctive and creative.

The Power of the Therapist's Touch

In the moment that the therapist touches the patient, it creates the potential for change. Anything can come back to alignment with the resonance of one person to another, through touch. During my studies in Beijing I met Wang Ju Li, a brilliant acupuncturist, who has been practising for over 40 years and is now in his 70s. Even with his level of experience he still feels for every acupuncture point. He says you must feel for every point because they are different on every patient, even on the same patient they may change from one week to the next, as the fascia changes.

I went through a phase where I was approaching my work by studying a patient's case file. I would look at it from every possible angle and compile a series of points that would be perfect for their session the following week. They would then come along, I would be completely prepared, only to find that there was nothing wrong any more. The issue they had the week before no longer existed. Again, this really drilled home how important it is to work and be in the moment with each person I see.

The Treatment

The therapeutic relationship is established with the quality of the very first connections that are made within the session. These include the presence of the therapist in listening, questioning, feeling the pulse and looking at the tongue. All of these elements build the foundation for the actual hands- on treatment, whether this be through massage or needles.

Often the first session for a patient takes longer because I need to find out who they are. It is only by listening that I can gauge their physical element and then decide which channels stand out as the ones to balance the system. There are times when I will refer to Chinese astrology to get a fuller picture. This is because Chinese astrology is one of the stems within classical Chinese medicine, meaning that if someone comes in with a fire element in their sign for example, their constitution will most probably be informed by this. I will usually keep the person's astrology in mind during my work, especially if a certain element is being expressed quite strongly by them.

The Contribution of Creative Outlets to my Work

The contribution that acting has made to my work as an acupuncturist is immense. Acting is very much about being in the present moment. When you are involved in communicating with an audience, you have to be in the moment. Also there is the whole aspect of the breath; a lot of emphasis is placed on breathing in acting and vocal training. Breath, of course, is a tool that can be used to bring us to the present moment.

As a teacher of acupuncture, I am always making my students aware of the first touch, whether it is with their hands or with the acupuncture needle. I get them to become aware of questions like, 'Am I in my body?' 'What sensations do I have?' 'Am I present?' 'What is my breathing like?' Bringing your presence to the person you work with changes the way you approach your treatment with them. For some people who come for treatment, just having their pulse felt can lead to therapeutic changes. The pulse contains the blood, which in turn carries the emotions and the movement of energy. This is what the acupuncturist is tuning into and it should be given due respect.

Additionally, I love expressing myself vocally and I sing using my own lyrics. I have also recently begun doing beat box poetry with a jazz guitar as accompaniment. In the end, all my creative outlets tie in together and inform each other. The acupuncture grounds me, while music and poetry feeds my creativity. The grounding element I get from acupuncture helps me to channel my creativity. My work as an acupuncturist is fed by my creativity because it teaches me how to be opened enough to flow with the moment. They harmonise each other, which brings harmony to me.

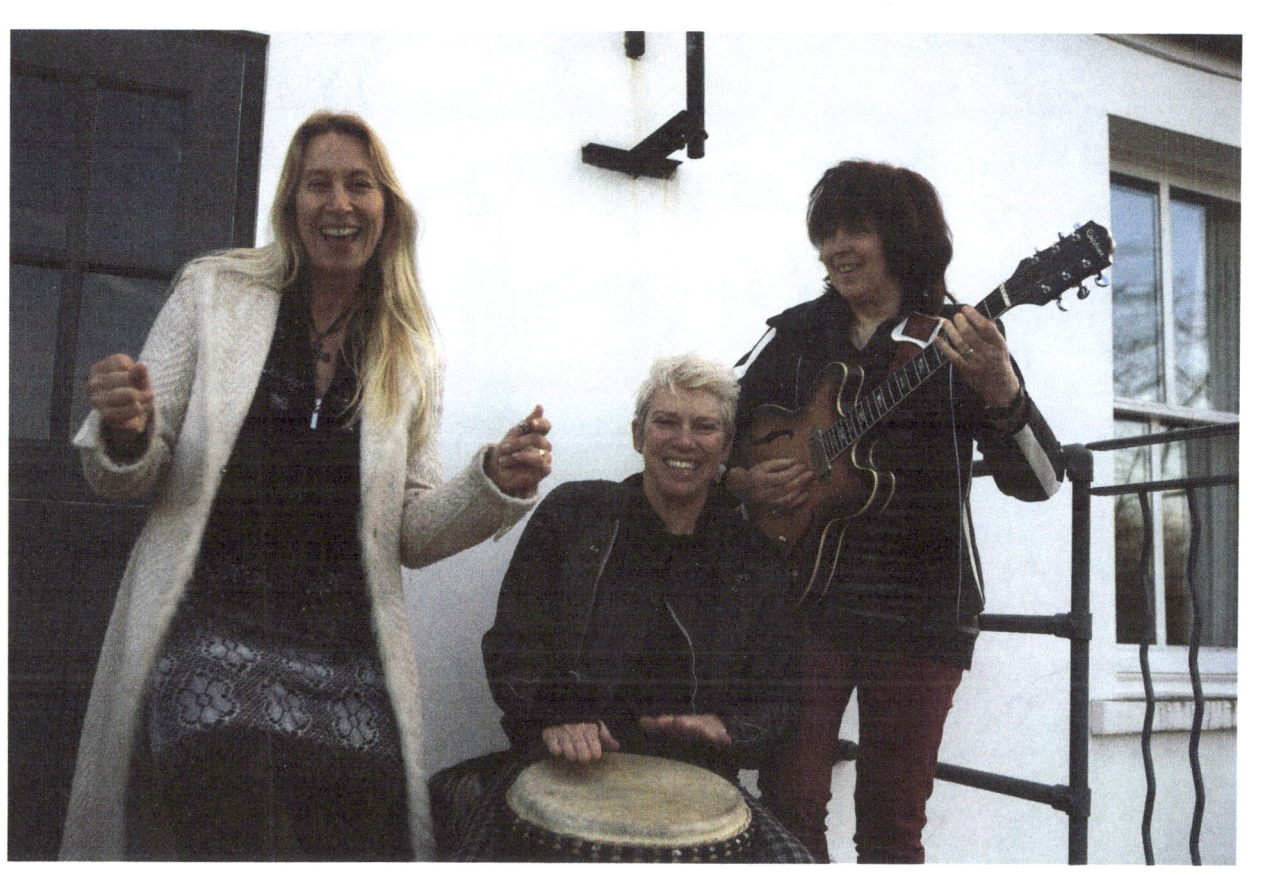

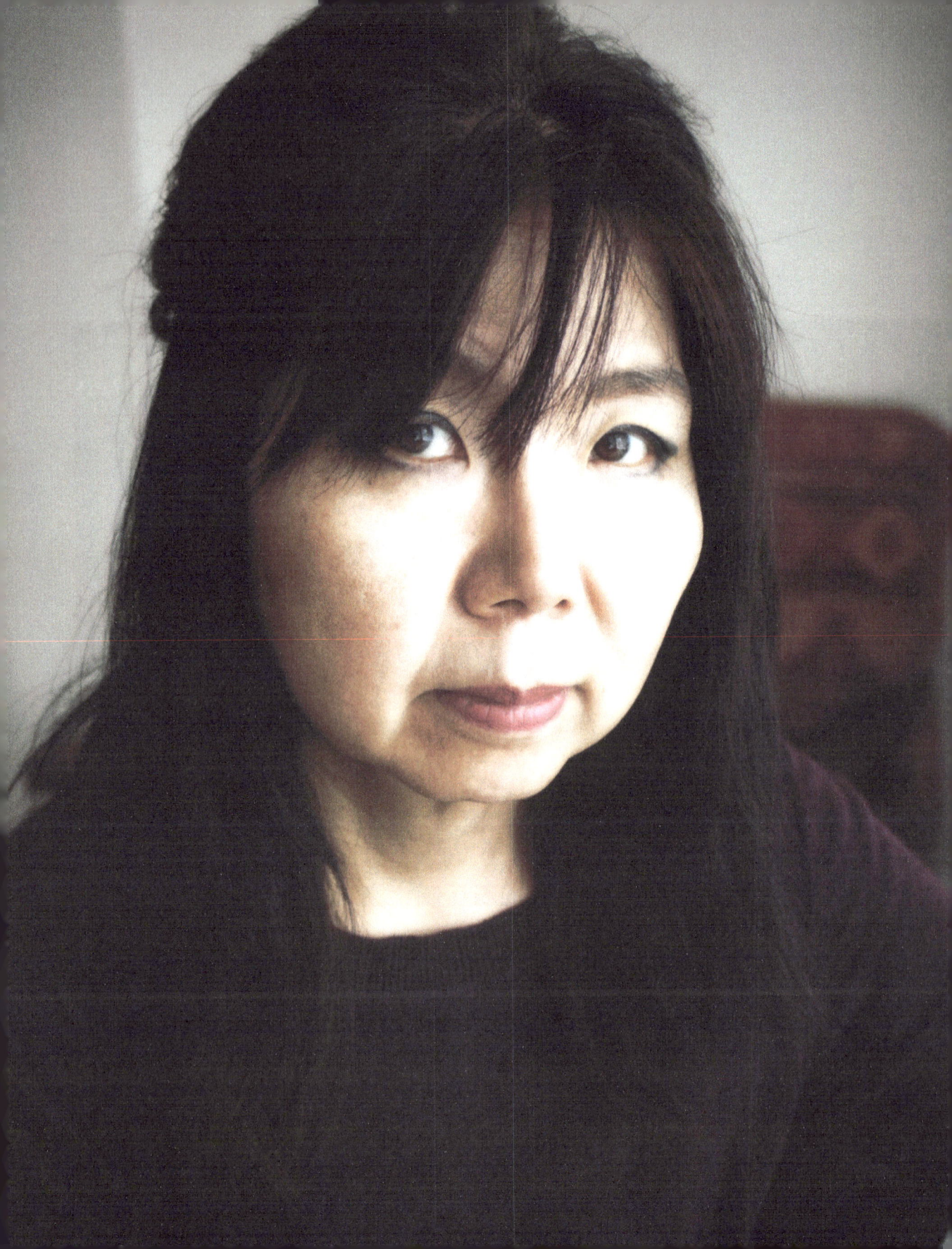

Sinsook Park

Acupuncturist

Sinsook Park runs a very successful private practice in acupuncture and Chinese Medicine. She is renowned in the field and people have been known to travel cross country for an appointment with her. She combines western medical knowledge, gained from working as an A&E nurse in a very busy teaching hospital in Korea, with the Eastern Chinese Medicine expertise that is so engrained in her cultural background. The result is someone who has a deep understanding of what it means for us to be out of balance physically and energetically, in medical terms, and how we can be returned to our true essence of balance and harmony, in the most natural way possible.

My career began in Western Medicine, as a nurse in the A&E Department at a large teaching hospital in the heart of Korea's capital, Seoul. I would see on average 70 patients a day and, as a nurse, I was often the first person that patients would communicate with. It was important for me to be able to first recognise the health problem a person was presenting and then prepare the right equipment for the doctors to treat them. This was invaluable in developing my skill to identify an individual's physical disorders. In Korea, Chinese Medicine is still regarded as one of the main forms of treatment for the majority of the population. It is often used alongside Western Medicine and we have developed a way for the two to work together in harmony.

After I moved with my family to the UK, my son became ill. It seemed natural to take him to a Chinese Doctor, but I was really disappointed by the experience. She charged a lot, both for the treatment and the herbs and was very distant and detached. There was almost no verbal communication. This experience was partly responsible for spurring me to become an acupuncturist myself. The other motivating factor was that my command of English wasn't great when I arrived in the UK. I knew I had to retrain in order to work, and doing acupuncture and Chinese herbal treatments seemed like the most sensible way forward. I got into the very best acupuncture school at the time, but the language barrier proved to be a challenge and I had to assimilate a huge acupuncture textbook from cover to cover. To this day, I can still recall which page to go to in order to find a specific piece of information.

My Personal Experience With Acupuncture

I had a huge amount of determination to excel and I found acupuncture to be both amazing and fascinating. With my cultural upbringing, a lot of the principles I read about made perfect sense to me. Additionally, I was able to experience first hand how powerful it was as a modality. When I was 12, I got a kidney infection after having the flu. From that point on, I never seemed to feel as well as I did before. It was recommended from time to time that I should visit my doctor in order to have a full system check-up. Every time I visited I was given all sorts of tests to try and find out what the cause of my ill feeling was. Each time the results showed there was nothing wrong and yet I would leave the appointment feeling as awful as I did when I arrived. I also had a sense of helplessness, as no one seemed to understand what I was going through and all the medical tests said I should have been fine, but I wasn't.

My body would get really bloated, my face would be visibly swollen and I felt heavy and lethargic, which meant I had to take at least two naps a day. For a teenager who previously had boundless energy, this was a truly miserable existence and I couldn't understand what had happened to me. However, when I started to study traditional acupuncture, I got to the section on the kidneys and I just couldn't believe it, all my symptoms were there.

My fellow acupuncture students found the theory, philosophy and practice of acupuncture very rewarding, but it was even more so for me because of the difference it made to my personal suffering. My passion grew and I couldn't stop reading about it. My love for the subject was evident and, even though my English was very limited at that time, my academic score was always near the top of the class.

The Effects of Acupuncture

Through my years of work, I have discovered that Chinese Medicine is really about living life in line with nature. Human beings are a part of nature, so we have to keep in tune with the natural rhythms in order to maintain our equilibrium or homeostasis. The daily and seasonal changes give us our recipe for what needs to be done. Furthermore, we need to achieve emotional peace and harmony in order to maintain our body's balance. Western Medicine also recognises that emotional hardship can sometimes manifest itself as physical symptoms and signs.

As a whole, my practice is gradually moving towards working with the individual's emotional and mental side. I do this by listening to and harmonising their responses to the situations in their life. With the creation of balance being my main aim, a large part of my practice involves simply helping my clients to switch off and relax, which can sometimes be difficult in modern life.

Kidney Energy

Nowadays, due to the relentless pace of modern life, people often use energy too excessively and unsustainably. Having an abundance of energy means that the person is operating at an optimum level rather than an extreme. The way I perceive excessive energy is that the person's head seems ready to explode like a pressure cooker. Paradoxically, they may tend to feel very lethargic, because there is not enough energy in the lower part of the body to offer grounding and stability. If we think of a tree with a big tree trunk, it may seem impressive in size, but it would be impossible to sustain if the root was rotting.

When we apply this analogy to the body, the root can be represented by the kidneys. In acupuncture, when a person dies we could equally say that the kidney energy is completely gone. Kidney energy is not normally used in our day-to-day life. Instead, it bears a similar resemblance to water in a reservoir, which is held as a reserve, rather than freely flowing when we turn on the tap. It is there to support us in the case of an emergency. If the kidney energy is depleted, the person feels unwell, becomes vulnerable and ages quickly.

To sustain kidney energy we need to top up our life force on a daily basis. This means following nature's daily cycle. During daylight hours we need to open our eyes, get up, go out and be active with our bodies. As the sun sets and the day draws to a close, our body has to be gradually quietened. In the evening we should give ourselves the opportunity to return home, rest our energy and decrease our level of activities. With regards to the seasons, in the summer season it feels natural to be more active and in the winter we are more inclined to reduce our activities and become more introspective. Diet also plays an important part and the more natural our food products are the better we feel. When our modern lifestyle follows nature's rhythms, it ensures that the decline in our kidney energy is a lot slower and far more natural, meaning that we age in a graceful manner.

During my session with a client I try to bring ultimate relaxation, not just on the surface but also deep down to the kidney level, which is the deepest organ in the body energetically. This kind of relaxation makes a huge difference and they can respond to challenging situations in their life far more easily. The session allows them space, rest and enables them to recharge their batteries so that can engage with their lives in a balanced way.

The Recipe for Success

I have learned enormous lessons from various people's attitudes and ways that they lead their lives. I have especially learnt the importance of understanding and accepting others for who they are.

To be successful in any business, it is crucial to be passionate about your clients. In my field of work this can be displayed through kindness, compassion and understanding my client's situation on a holistic level. It is only through establishing this emotional and spiritual connection, that my clients are able to absorb my treatments far more effectively.

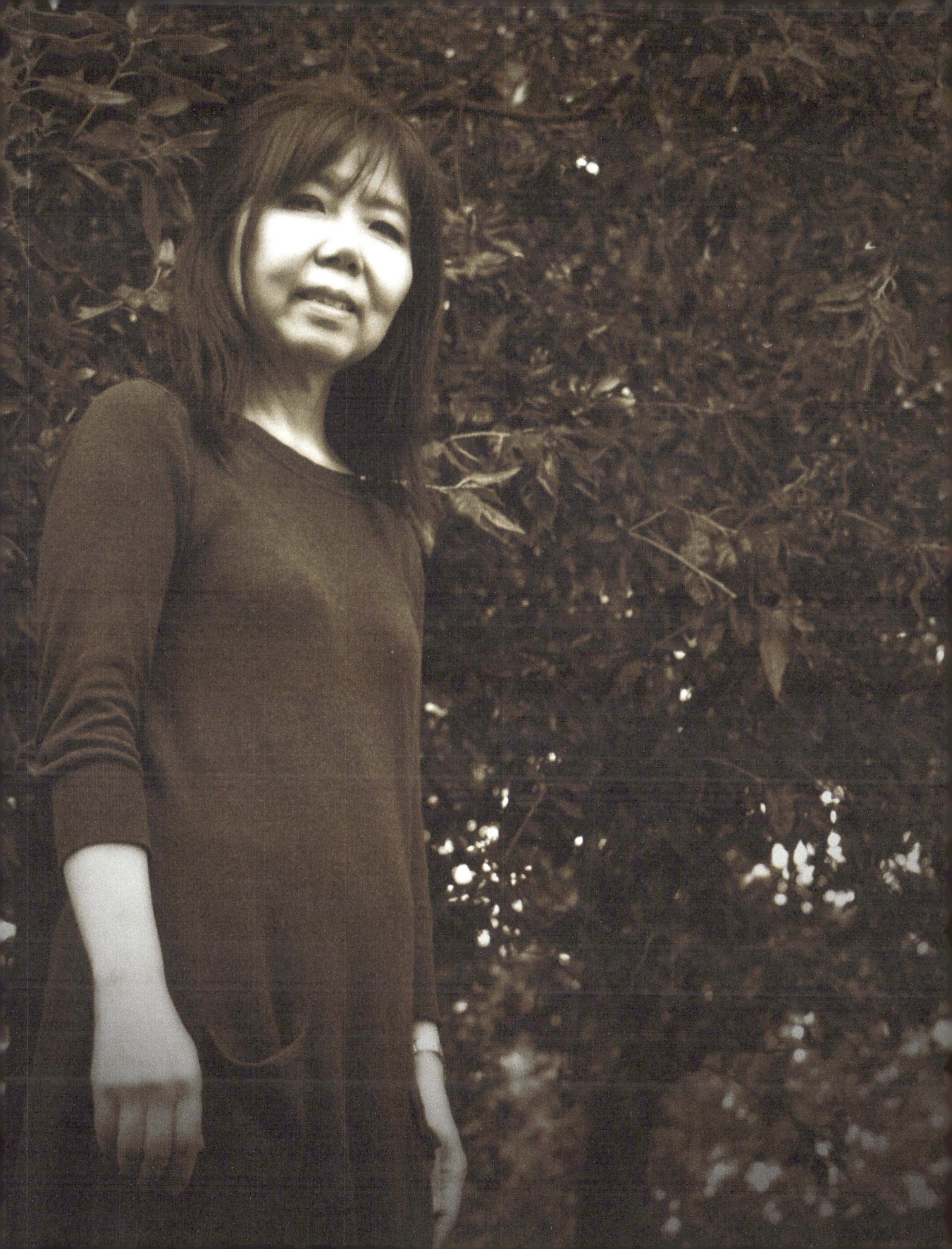

Artists of Health Contributors

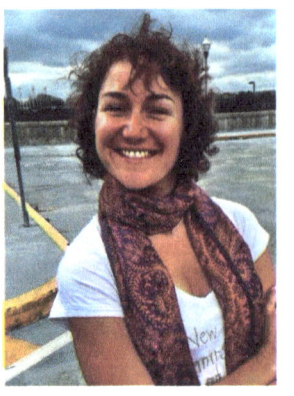

**Artists of Health Photographer
Karyn Schafer Campbell**

Freelance photographer & curator
www.kscphotography.co.uk
info@kscphotography.co.uk

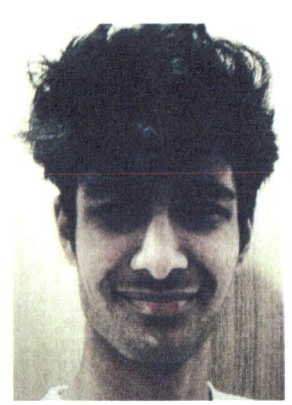

**Artists of Health Book Designer
Ahad Sheikh**

Founder of BluRoc Designs Ltd
www.blu-roc.com
www.pph.me/blu-roc
ahad.sheikh@blu-roc.com

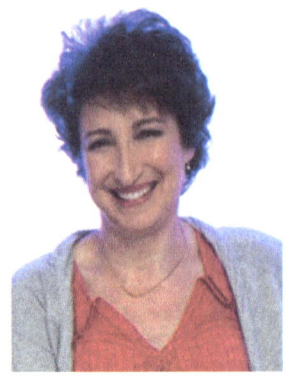

**Artists of Health Proofreader
Etty Payne**

Translator | Proofreader | Copy-editor
etty@elegantwords.co.uk
www.elegantwords.co.uk

Artists' own photographs provided by:

- Beata Aleksandrowicz
- Karen Downes
- Patrick Holford
- Emma Roberts
- Gerry Gajadharsingh
- Anna Barnsley
- Valerie Austin
- Jacqueline Hurst
- Teresa Hale
- Ali Campbell
- Ed Percival
- Nina Madden
- Gladeana McMahon
- Stephen Russell
- Anna Kitney - Photographer Samjhana Moon
- Shola Arewa - Photographer Jonathan Perugia (Meditation) / Anne Marie Newland (Handstand)
- Maya Fiennes
- Katy Appleton
- Nikki Slade
- Tim Wheater - Photographer Natalie Shaw
- Sarah Prichard

Lightning Source UK Ltd.
Milton Keynes UK
UKOW06f0653221114

242022UK00002B/15/P